Viral Hepatitis in Children

Mei-Hwei Chang • Kathleen B. Schwarz
Editors

Viral Hepatitis in Children

Prevention and Management

Springer

Editors
Mei-Hwei Chang
Department of Pediatrics
National Taiwan University College of Medicine
Taipei, Taiwan

Kathleen B. Schwarz
Department of Pediatrics
Johns Hopkins University School of Mediine
Baltimore, MD, USA

ISBN 978-981-13-0049-3 ISBN 978-981-13-0050-9 (eBook)
https://doi.org/10.1007/978-981-13-0050-9

Library of Congress Control Number: 2018961383

This Springer imprint is published by the registered company Springer Nature Singapore Pte Ltd.
The registered company address is: 152 Beach Road, #21-01/04 Gateway East, Singapore 189721, Singapore

Contents

1 The Challenges of Conquering Viral Hepatitis Beginning in Childhood: Introduction of the Rationale and Importance of Controlling Viral Hepatitis Starting from Children

Kathleen B. Schwarz

Abstract

The purpose of this first chapter is to take a more global view of the challenges of conquering viral hepatitis beginning in childhood, to analyze the problems from the viewpoint of the key players: governments, the pharmaceutical industry, third-party payors, physicians/professional societies, and educators. The chapter will conclude with some suggestions for novel approaches to the major challenges of conquering viral hepatitis beginning in childhood.

1.1 Introduction

In consideration of the many challenges of conquering viral hepatitis globally, it is essential to start at the beginning of life. This is especially true for the two hepatitis viruses: hepatitis B virus (HBV) (which is sometimes complicated by co- or supra-infection with hepatitis D virus (HDV)) and hepatitis C virus (HCV). These viruses are usually characterized by chronic infection resulting in stigma and social isolation during childhood and the evolution of chronic liver disease, cirrhosis, need for liver transplantation, and/or hepatocellular carcinoma in adulthood. However on occasion infection with either virus may evolve so aggressively that end-stage liver disease and attendant consequences can occur in young children [1, 2]. In addition the importance of preventing acute hepatitis secondary to the two vaccine preventable RNA viruses (A and E) in children cannot be underestimated, both because of the associated morbidity and mortality and also because of the public health costs. Finally given that the number of cases of hepatitis C virus is increasing in young injection drug users [3], it is clear that there is a mandate for a safe and effective HCV vaccine.

The global disease burden of viral hepatitis is staggering. Unlike most communicable diseases which are actually declining, the rates of infections with hepatitis viruses and related morbidity and mortality are increasing. According to the Global Burden of Disease Study in 2013, between 1990 and 2013, deaths from viral hepatitis in the world increased from 0.89 to 1.45 million. In 2013, viral hepatitis was the seventh leading cause of death globally compared with tenth in 1990 [4]. Figure 1.1 is a graphic representation of the viral hepatitis-related age-standardized mortality rates by the various Global Burden of Disease regions of the world. According to this study, which uses country level and regional causes of death data to determine the various

K. B. Schwarz (✉)
Department of Pediatrics, Johns Hopkins University School of Medicine, Baltimore, MD, USA
e-mail: kschwarz@jhmi.edu

M.-H. Chang, K. B. Schwarz (eds.), *Viral Hepatitis in Children*,
https://doi.org/10.1007/978-981-13-0050-9_1

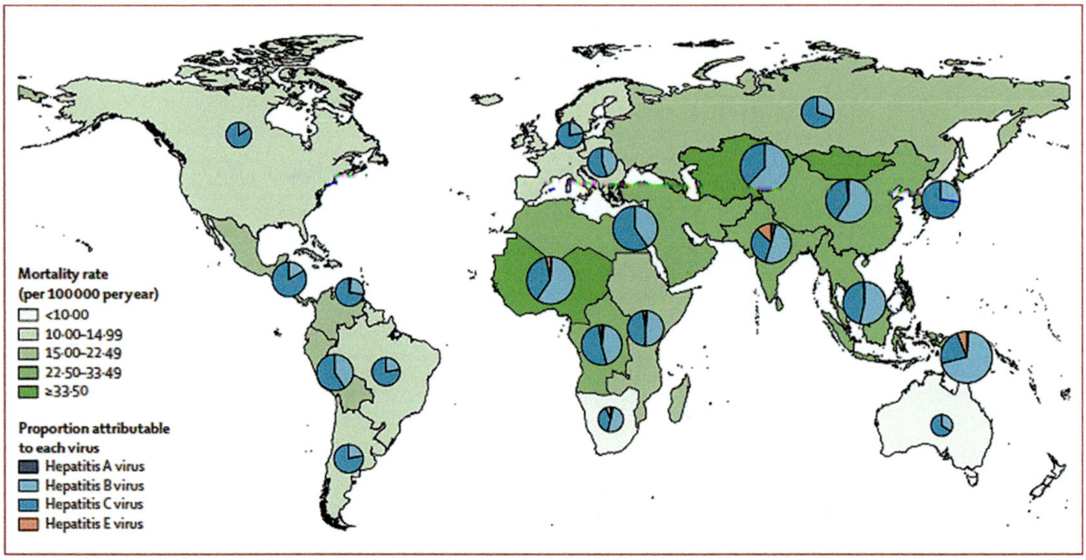

Fig. 1.1 Map of viral hepatitis-related age-standardized mortality rate by Global Burden of Disease region. Overlaid pie charts indicate each virus type's contribution to the total hepatitis-related mortality; the size of the pie charts are proportional to the region's hepatitis-attributable mortality rate. GBD=Global Burden of Disease (Reproduced with permission from Ref. [4])
Springer Nature remains neutral with regard to jurisdictional claims in published maps and institutional affiliations

underlying causes of liver cancer and cirrhosis deaths, chronic HBV and HCV infections are the leading causes of death from liver cancer and cirrhosis globally [4].

Although there is a safe and effective vaccine for hepatitis A virus (HAV), the World Health Organization estimates that the number of cases of acute HAV occurring worldwide increased from 177 million in 1990 to 212 million in 2005 and deaths from HAV decreased from 30,283 in 1990 to 30,245 in 2005. The age group 2–14 years was one of the groups with the highest increase [5]. Despite having made major progress in developing a safe and effective vaccine for HBV and having administered >1 billion doses worldwide, the number of people infected with the virus is actually increasing, from 223 million in 1990 to 240 million in 2005 [6]. HBV affects an estimated 248 million people globally, and mortality rates are high [7]. For example, there were 786,000 deaths due to HBV in 2010 [8]. There are approximately 170 M people in the world infected with HCV including 11 M children [9]. In the United States alone, associated healthcare costs are very high. For example, in the United States in 2011, total healthcare costs related to HCV infection were $6.5 billion and are expected to increase to $9.1B in 2024. Table 1.1 is a dramatic demonstration of the effect of age of infection on cost burden, with the lifetime costs of a child infected at 0–4 years of age being by far the highest, for example, over twice that of persons infected at age 40–44 years ($51,610 for males and $67,880 for females) [10]. And finally hepatitis E is an emerging infection for which the healthcare costs have not yet been estimated globally but are likely to be high because this virus is the most common cause of acute viral hepatitis worldwide. Case fatality rates are particularly high in pregnant females [11].

Table 1.1 Lifetime cost by age, HCV infection, and gender (in 2011 Dollars)

Age (in years)	Male	Female
0–4	$116,600	$147,130
5–9	$105,950	$138,360
10–14	$94,810	$128,440
15–19	$83,430	$117,590

Reproduced with permission from Ref. [10]

Thus if infants and children could be protected from infection by these four viruses by safe and effective vaccines and if safe and effective treatments were broadly available for children unfortunate enough to become infected with HBV and/or HCV, the morbidity and mortality as well as the healthcare costs described above could be drastically reduced. In the ensuing 15 chapters of this book, the biological, virological, immunological, and pharmacological issues regarding each of these viral infections of children will be addressed in great detail.

1.2 The Role of Governments Including Global Health Organizations

In elaborating a national strategy for the prevention and control of hepatitis B and C, the Institute of Medicine in the United States has identified the underlying factors that impede current efforts to prevent and control these diseases, including those in the area of governmental responsibilities [12]. These include a lack of knowledge about viral hepatitis among policy makers, particularly if there is insufficient understanding about the extent and seriousness of this public health problem, so inadequate public resources are being allocated to prevention, control, and surveillance programs.

There are inadequate disease surveillance systems for acute and chronic hepatitis virus infections and therefore underreporting; thus the full extent of the problem is unknown. This deficiency was dramatically highlighted as far as it impacts the health of the young by a careful study by Delgado-Borrego et al. [13] who estimated that from 2000 to 2009, only 12% of the children in the state of Florida who were estimated to have HCV infection were identified as having positive anti-HCV tests. Furthermore, only 1.6% of those with positive tests were actually followed by a pediatric gastroenterologist. For the United States as a whole, she estimated that only 4.9% of the expected cases were identified. Figure 1.2 from her study demonstrates that for large areas of the United States, there were no reported cases, suggesting that no surveillance was being done and/or that surveillance was grossly inadequate, given that the prevalence of HCV in children in the United States is 0.2–0.4%, according to NHANES data [14].

Globally governments need to develop much more effective screening policies for identification of individuals with infection with acute infections with hepatitis A virus (so as to improve HAV vaccine policies) and hepatitis E virus. Data regarding the prevalence and global disease bur-

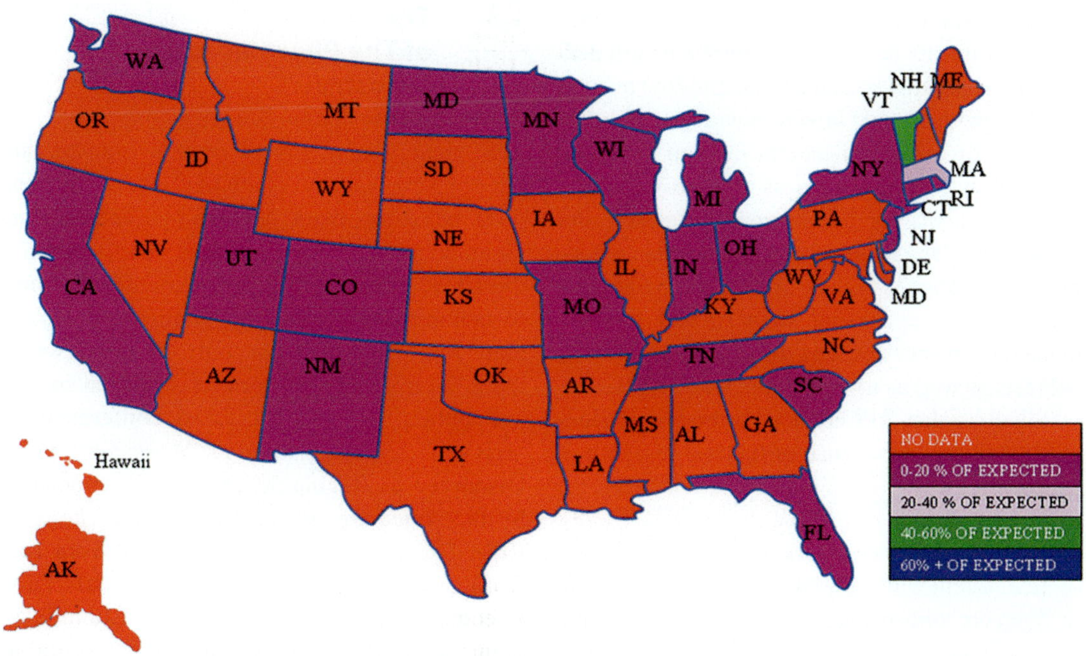

Fig. 1.2 Percentage of expected cases of hepatitis C virus infection in children in the United States actually reported to health authorities. (Reproduced with permission from Ref. [13])

den of HEV are needed in order to better evaluate the cost benefits of making an HEV vaccine available in countries other than China, which is currently the only country in the world with such a vaccine [15]. Governments need to develop more effective screening policies for chronic HBV and HCV infection particularly aimed at reaching high-risk individuals from endemic countries and mandating prenatal screening. However, individuals with the highest risk of chronic infection (incarcerated, homeless, immigrants, nursing home residents, and hospitalized persons) tend to be underrepresented in current prevalence figures leading to an underestimation of the true prevalence of chronic hepatitis B and C virus infection.

Governments and global health organizations need to understand the cost-effectiveness of supporting better vaccine policies for effective administration of the HBV vaccine, including the birth dose [16]. In those countries where a high percentage of infants are born at home [17], governments need to support the administration of nucleoside analogues for highly infectious mothers in the third trimester of pregnancy or even during the entire pregnancy, a practice which has been shown to be safe and to decrease maternal-fetal transmission of HBV [18].

Governments need to direct public health dollars to cover antiviral therapy for children as well as adults with chronic infection with HBV and/or HCV, and regulatory agencies need to be aware of the clear cost-effectiveness of approving antiviral treatments for use in young children and adolescents. The Institute of Medicine has recognized that infected people often have inadequate access to testing, social support, and medical management services, and this pertains to young subjects as well as to vulnerable adults [12].

Finally policy makers need to be knowledgeable about the importance of funding research in several areas:

1. Antiviral treatments which will truly be effective in achieving at least a "functional cure" in subjects with hepatitis B – probably a triple drug therapy – including (a) agents to eliminate covalently closed circular HBV DNA (still a major challenge for molecular virologists) [19], (b) safe effective nucleoside analogues to rapidly decrease the viral load (both entecavir [20] and tenofovir [21] have been shown to be safe and effective in the young), and (c) drugs which are capable of boosting the immune response to HBV (still a research challenge).
2. A means of interrupting maternal-fetal transmission of HCV.
3. A safe and effective vaccine for HCV.
4. A safe and effective vaccine for HEV.

In summary policy makers in governments and global health organizations have the opportunity to make major progress in eliminating the staggering global burden of viral hepatitis by first becoming more knowledgeable about the problem, by promoting the development of effective surveillance programs, by developing and funding more effective vaccine programs for HAV and HBV vaccines, and by supporting antiviral treatments for children and adults with HBV and HCV, as well as directing research dollars to the four top priority areas enumerated above.

1.3 The Role of The Pharmaceutical Industry

It is clear that members of this industry are key players in the challenge of conquering viral hepatitis, from developing, testing, and manufacturing both vaccines and antiviral therapies, bringing them to regulatory approval to making them broadly available and affordable. Major progress can only be made where there is effective collaboration between private and public sectors. The 2016 conference on "HBV Treatment Endpoints Workshop: From Discovery to Regulatory Approval" sponsored by the American Association for the Study of Liver Disease, with thought leaders from academia, pharma, and the Food and Drug Administration, was a wonderful example of how such collaborations can lead to solutions. Approximately 30 new technologies to either diagnose or treat hepatitis B were discussed, holding much promise for the future and improving mutual understanding between all parties involved.

In addition to the obvious imperative of developing safe and truly effective antiviral therapies for HBV, pharma can play a very positive role in funding investigations on the other priorities described above for government research: interruption of maternal-fetal transmission of HCV and developing safe and effective vaccines for HCV and HEV.

Pharma has been very generous in funding educational programs regarding the many challenges of caring for adults with chronic HBV and HCV. There is a growing recognition of the need to sponsor research in antiviral therapies for children with HBV and/or HCV and bring these therapies to regulatory approval. Pharma should also be strongly encouraged to fund educational programs which are specifically focused on pediatric issues related to viral hepatitis.

Finally pharmaceutical industries are strongly encouraged to reduce the cost of vaccines and antiviral drugs so as to make these affordable to all who need them, including our youngest subjects. It is clear that mass treatment of the millions infected with HBV or HCV will require very low-cost drugs. The availability of low-cost antiviral drugs will be aided and abetted by expiration of patents. For example, Hill et al. [22] have reported on the feasibility of making low-cost entecavir available on a mass scale. The annual cost of entecavir for the United States for an adult with HBV in 2015 when the patent expired was $15,111 for the brand drug and $6127 for the generic version. The global lowest price was $427. However the authors calculated that production of the active pharmaceutical ingredient was only $4/year based on quotations of generic suppliers. Adding $20 per year for formulation and packaging and a 50% profit margin, entecavir was estimated to cost a minimum of $36 per year, much lower than current originator and generic prices.

1.4 The Role of Third-Party Payors

Given that there is ample data on the cost-effectiveness of treating chronic HBV in adults, which can decrease liver disease and mortality and decrease the need for very expensive liver transplantation [23], third-party payors should avail themselves of this information because support of these treatments and the resulting health benefits will not only benefit the patients themselves but be cost-saving for the insurors as well. Likewise, there is ample published information about the cost-effectiveness of treating chronic HCV in adults, especially with the new highly safe and effective direct-acting antiviral agents [24], and third-party payors should become very familiar with these analyses. Although there are few published data of the cost-effectiveness of treating children with these chronic infections [25], it is predictable that early treatment of the young is likely to be highly cost-effective given the life span of the child as well as the fact that smaller quantities of drug are necessary for smaller individuals, given weight-based dosing.

1.5 The Role of Physicians and Professional Societies

The Institute of Medicine 2010 study examined underlying factors that impeded current efforts to prevent and control viral hepatitis and concluded that one of the major impediments was a lack of knowledge about viral hepatitis among primary care and social service providers [12]. Physicians and their professional societies need to develop educational programs to increase knowledge about whom to screen for HBV and HCV and how to do it. They need to educate patients who have been identified with these infections as to how to decrease disease transmission to family members and friends and how to best manage pregnant females with HBV or HCV and their offspring. Primary care physicians need to understand the indications for treatment of children with HBV or HCV and when to refer to pediatric hepatologists for management of these treatments, which of course can be a collaboration between the specialist and primary care provider. Finally they need to develop better educational programs to overcome irrational vaccine phobias in their patients and families [26].

An excellent example of the need to educate primary care providers about the importance of screening high-risk individuals was the study by Chu and colleagues [27] who surveyed HBV screening practices and barriers to screening of 217 Asian-American primary care providers (PCPs) who treat Asian adults living in the United States. This was a web-based survey of Asian-American PCPs with at least 25% Asian-American patients in their practice. Although 95% of Asian-American PCPs report ever having screened a patient for HBV, 41% reported that ≤25% of their Asian-American patients had ever been screened. The most important reasons reported for HBV screening in Asian-American patients were elevated liver enzymes, elevated liver function tests plus a family history of chronic hepatitis B or liver disease, and birth outside the United States. The most common reasons for not screening for HBV were a (false) perception that the patient was not at risk, lack of symptoms of chronic hepatitis B or liver disease, HBV vaccination, prior screening, patient refusal, and lack of insurance. The question about HBV vaccination is interesting because families who have a child infected with HBV will frequently have the child vaccinated so as to be able to complete the school form with that affirmation, even though they are aware that HBV vaccination is ineffective in infected individuals.

Figure 1.3 is a dramatic example of the gaps between the number of HBV-infected individuals in the United States, the number aware of their infection, the number referred for treatment, the number potentially eligible for care, the number actually entering care, and the number referred for treatment [28]. Much more aggressive strategies by primary care physicians are needed to screen high-risk patients (those from countries where the HBV endemicity rate is 2% or higher and those who indulge in high-risk practices such

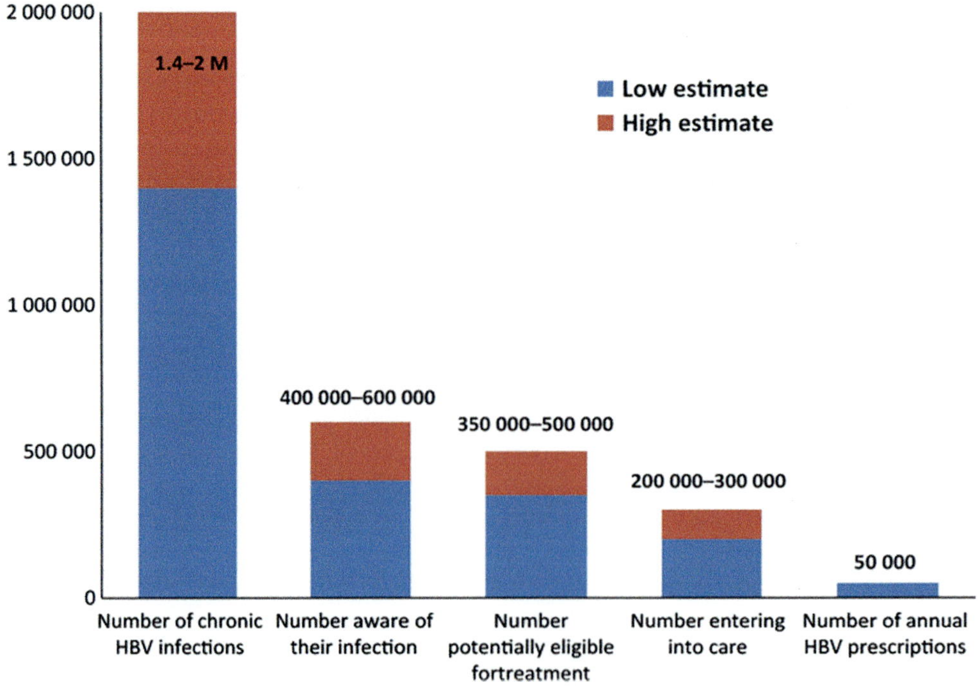

Fig. 1.3 Gaps between the number of individuals in the United States estimated to have hepatitis B virus infection and those aware of their infection and actually receiving treatment. (Reproduced with permission from Ref. [28])

as injection drug use), to educate their patients about the disease, and to refer appropriate individuals for treatment. Putting such strategies into place could drastically reduce these tragic gaps to care and treatment suffered by the majority of HBV-infected individuals.

1.6 The Role of Educators

Beginning with preschool age children, educators in public and private schools, as well as high-risk settings such as homeless shelters have a golden opportunity to educate children and adolescents about ways to protect themselves from acquiring hepatitis B or C. A wonderful example of such tools is the clever coloring book: Olivia and Oliver, Meet Your Miraculous Liver [29], which educates young children about the functions of the liver and how to keep their liver healthy. A prospective randomized controlled trial of a culturally appropriate HBV video vs a smoking prevention video shown to homeless youth and their families demonstrated a significant positive impact of the HBV video, not only on HBV knowledge and acceptance of an HBV vaccine at time of the initial visit but, remarkably, increased return rates for the follow-up HBV vaccine [30].

Educators can also help improve the quality of life among children with viral hepatitis by educating their classmates on the low likelihood of horizontal transmission, thus helping to decrease the irrational stigma and discrimination suffered by so many with chronic viral hepatitis [31]. Finally educators are encouraged to be sensitive about the reduced health-related quality of life and depression suffered by children and youth (particularly adolescent males) with chronic HBV [32].

1.7 Innovative Solutions

A number of innovative strategies have recently been found to be promising. These fall into the categories of improving vaccine distribution and compliance, innovative screening techniques for HBV, new educational modules for pediatricians, improving the safety of food and water contamination with HAV and HBV as well as recommendations to base global responses to control of viral hepatitis by learning from the successful strategies applied to the HIV epidemic.

Some have suggested consideration of one dose of HAV vaccine in resource poor countries [33]. Lawler reported that government recommendations improved HAV vaccine administration rates by 20%, and government mandates increased rates still further by an additional 8% [34]. Bundling of the HBV vaccine with other infant vaccines has recently been shown to have a dramatic positive impact on rates of administration of the HBV vaccine [35], and smartphone technology could be employed to increase vaccine compliance in underserved areas [36].

One of the difficulties in widespread screening is the problem of performing venipuncture in nontraditional settings such as health fairs. Venipuncture is particularly problematic in screening children for HBV and HCV given the need for parental consent and the need to employ phlebotomists. Finger-stick blood samples are much easier to obtain in young children. Dried blood spot technology has been in place for HCV screening for several years and has been successfully employed in screening high-risk homeless children [37]. Recently dried blood spot technology has been developed for HBV as well [38]. Although this useful technique is currently not FDA-approved, it is to be hoped that the FDA will take a positive view of this technique and escalate approval so it can be put into place in the United States as well as globally.

It is important to note the need for enlightened food safety practices to decrease transmission of HAV and HEV. The same advice applies to the need to develop better techniques to eliminate viral pathogens such as HAV [39] and HEV [40] from sewage and repurposed water supply. Kobayashi et al. [41] tested the impact of a down-flow hanging sponge (DHS) reactor for treatment of municipal wastewater and health risks associated with utilization of the effluent for agricultural irrigation. The rates of contamination of the waste water with HAV and HEV were 11% or below, so they were unable to demonstrate high log-fold reduction of these two viruses. Nonetheless, for the most part the technique did drop the viral burden considerably, and therefore the technique or a future improved version does hold promise for reduction of HAV and HEV by agricultural waters.

Table 1.2 outlines some very useful strategies which were successful in mounting a global response to the epidemic of HIV infection. The problems are strikingly similar to the challenges in conquering the global epidemic of viral hepatitis, including the needs for affordable drugs, to simplify international guidelines, to decentralize care strategies and involve patients and local healthcare workers, to develop deliverable goals and then to hold players responsible, and to develop effective financing [42].

Table 1.2 Creating a global hepatitis movement using lessons from HIV response

Issue	Actions
Affordable drugs	Voluntary and compulsory licensing, large pool of prequalified generics, and high-volume procurement
Simplification international guidelines	Simplified care models, drug regimen trials, single fixed-dose regimens, and simple point-of-care diagnostics
Task shifting international guidelines	Operational research, job aids, low technology point-of-care diagnostics, integration, and decentralization, patient and community
	Build treatment literacy up front, engage, resource, and support community health workers for early identification and adherence, monitor treatment access, especially among marginalized groups
Delivery goals	Accountability (execution focus, delivery of therapy) then integration of therapy into care
Financing	Build international and national commitment, provide new, dedicated financing to kick-start antiviral treatment

Reproduced with permission from Ref. [42]

1.8 Summary

It is true that the challenges of conquering viral hepatitis beginning in childhood are daunting, but by working together and staying focused on this laudable goal, the tools do exist to make major progress. Surely the children of the world deserve nothing less!

References

1. Chang MH, You SL, Chen CJ, Liu CJ, Lai MW, Wu TC, Wu SF, Lee CM, Yang SS, Chu HC, Wang TE, Chen BW, Chuang WL, Soon MS, Lin CY, Chiou ST, Kuo HS, Chen DS, Taiwan Hepatoma Study Group (2016) Long-term effects of hepatitis B immunization of infants in preventing liver cancer. Gastroenterology 151(3):472–480
2. González-Peralta RP, Langham MR Jr, Andres JM, Mohan P, Colombani PM, Alford MK, Schwarz KB (2009) Hepatocellular carcinoma in 2 young adolescents with chronic hepatitis C. J Pediatr Gastroenterol Nutr 48(5):630–635
3. Suryaprasad AG, White JZ, Xu F, Eichler BA, Hamilton J, Patel A, Hamdounia SB, Church DR, Barton K, Fisher C, Macomber K, Stanley M, Guilfoyle SM, Sweet K, Liu S, Iqbal K, Tohme R, Sharapov U, Kupronis BA, Ward JW, Holmberg SD (2014) Emerging epidemic of hepatitis C virus infections among young nonurban persons who inject drugs in the United States, 2006-2012. Clin Infect Dis 59(10):1411–1419
4. Stanaway JD, Flaxman AD, Naghavi M, Fitzmaurice C, Vos T, Abubakar I, Abu-Raddad LJ, Assadi R, Bhala N, Cowie B, Forouzanfour MH, Groeger J, Mohd Hanafiah K, Jacobsen KH, James SL, MacLachlan J, Malekzadeh R, Martin NK, Mokdad AA, Mokdad AH, Murray CJ, Plass D, Rana S, Rein DB, Richardus JH, Sanabria J, Saylan M, Shahraz S, So S, Vlassov VV, Weiderpass E, Wiersma ST, Younis M, Yu C, El Sayed Zaki M, Cooke GS (2016) The global burden of viral hepatitis from 1990 to 2013: findings from the Global Burden of Disease Study 2013. Lancet 388(10049):1081–1088
5. WHO position paper on hepatitis A vaccines: June 2012-recommendations (2013). Vaccine 31(2):285–286
6. Ott JJ, Stevens GA, Groeger J, Wiersma ST (2012) Global epidemiology of hepatitis B virus infection: new estimates of age-specific HBsAg seroprevalence and endemicity. Vaccine 30:2212–2219 Epub 2012/01/26
7. Schweitzer A, Horn J, Mikolajczyk RT, Krause G, Ott JJ (2015) Estimations of worldwide prevalence of chronic hepatitis B virus infection: a systematic review of data published between1965 and 2013. Lancet 386(10003):1546–1555. https://doi.org/10.1016/S0140-6736(15)61412-X

8. Lozano R, Naghavi M, Foreman K, Lim S, Shibuya K, Aboyans V, Memish ZA (2012) Global and regional mortality from 235 causes of death for 20 age groups in 1990 and 2010: a systematic analysis for the global burden of disease study 2010. Lancet 380(9859):2095–2128
9. El-Shabrawi MH, Kamal NM (2013) Burden of pediatric hepatitis C. World J Gastroenterol 19(44):7880–7888
10. Razavi H, Elkhoury AC, Elbasha E, Estes C, Pasini K, Poynard T, Kumar R (2013) Chronic hepatitis C virus (HCV) disease burden and cost in the United States. Hepatology 57(6):2164–2170
11. Kamar N, Bendall R, Legrand-Abravanel F, Xia N-S, Ijaz S, Izopet J, Dalton HR (2012) Seminar hepatitis E. Lancet 379(9835):2477–2488
12. Institute of Medicine (2010) Hepatitis and liver cancer: a national strategy for prevention and control of hepatitis B and C. The National Academies Press, Washington, DC Available at: http://www.nap.edu/catalog/12793.html
13. Delgado-Borrego A, Smith L, Jonas MM, Hall CA, Negre B, Jordan SH, Ogrodowicz M, Raza R, Ludwig DA, Miller T, Lipshultz SE, Gonzalez-Peralta R, Chung RT (2012) Expected and actual case ascertainment and treatment rates for children infected with hepatitis C in Florida and the United States: epidemiologic evidence from Statewide and Nationwide Surveys. J Pediatr 161:915–921
14. Alter MJ, Kruszon-Moran D, Nainan OV, McQuillan GM, Gao F, Moyer LA, Kaslow RA, Margolis HS (1999) The prevalence of hepatitis C virus infection in the United States, 1988 through 1994. N Engl J Med 341(8):556–562
15. Khuroo MS, Khuroo MS, Khuroo NS (2016) Hepatitis E: discovery, global impact, control and cure. World J Gastroenterol 22(31):7030–7045
16. Wang FZ, Zhang GM, Shen LP, Liu JH, Zheng H, Wang F, Miao N, Sun XJ, Liang XF, Cui FQ (2017) Epidemiological characteristics of children aged 1-4 years without timely birth dose of hepatitis B vaccine vaccination in China, 2014. Zhonghua Liu Xing Bing Xue Za Zhi 38(1):32–36
17. Abdullah A, Hort K, Butu Y, Simpson L (2016) Risk factors associated with neonatal deaths: a matched case-control study in Indonesia. Glob Health Action 9(1):30445
18. Liu M, Cai H, Yi W (2013) Safety of telbivudine treatment for chronic hepatitis B for the entire pregnancy. J Viral Hepat 20(Suppl 1):65–70
19. Moyo B, Bloom K, Scott T, Ely A, Arbuthnot P (2017) Advances with using CRISPR/Cas-mediated gene editing to treat infections with hepatitis B virus and hepatitis C virus. Virus Res. pii: S0168-1702(16)30733-X
20. Jonas MM, Chang MH, Sokal E, Schwarz KB, Kelly D, Kim KM, Ling SC, Rosenthal P, Oraseanu D, Reynolds L, Thiry A, Ackerman P (2016) Randomized, controlled trial of entecavir versus placebo in children with hepatitis B envelope antigen-positive chronic hepatitis B. Hepatology 63(2):377–387
21. Murray KF, Szenborn L, Wysocki J, Rossi S, Corsa AC, Dinh P, McHutchison J, Pang PS, Luminos LM, Pawlowska M, Mizerski J (2012) Randomized, placebo-controlled trial of tenofovir disoproxil fumarate in adolescents with chronic hepatitis B. Hepatology 56(6):2018–2026
22. Hill A, Gotham D, Cooke G, Bhagani S, Andrieux-Meyer I, Cohn J, Fortunak J (2015 Apr) Analysis of minimum target prices for production of entecavir to treat hepatitis B in high- and low-income countries. J Virus Erad 1(2):103–110
23. Sarpel D, Baichoo E, Dieterich DT (2016) Chronic hepatitis B and C infection in the United States: a review of current guidelines, disease burden and cost effectiveness of screening. Expert Rev Anti-Infect Ther 14(5):511–521
24. Hagan LM, Yang Z, Ehteshami M, Schinazi RF (2013) All-oral, interferon-free treatment for chronic hepatitis C: cost-effectiveness analyses. J Viral Hepat 12:847–857
25. Hartwell D, Cooper K, Frampton GK, Baxter L, Loveman E (2014) The clinical effectiveness and cost-effectiveness of peginterferon alfa and ribavirin for the treatment of chronic hepatitis C in children and young people: a systematic review and economic evaluation. Health Technol Assess 65:i–xxii, 1–202
26. Soon IS, de Bruyn JC, Wrobel I (2013) Immunization history of children with inflammatory bowel disease. Can J Gastroenterol 27(4):213–216
27. Chu D, Yang JD, Lok AS, Tran T, Martins EB, Fagan E, Rousseau F, Kim WR (2013) Hepatitis B screening and vaccination practices in asian american primary care. Gut Liver 7(4):450–457
28. Cohen C, Holmberg SD, McMahon BJ, Block JM, Brosgart CL, Gish RG, London WT, Block TM (2011) Is chronic hepatitis B being undertreated in the United States? J Viral Hepat 18(6):377–383
29. Thiel, Thelma King (2015) Olivia and oliver: meet your miraculous liver – a coloring book. Kickstarter
30. Schwarz KB, Garrett B, Lee J, Thompson D, Thiel T, Alter MJ, Strathdee S (2008) Positive impact of a shelter-based hepatitis B vaccine program in homeless Baltimore and adolescents. J Urban Health 85:2
31. Valizadeh L, Zamanzadeh V, Bayani M, Zabihi A (2017) The social stigma experience in patients with hepatitis B infection: a qualitative study. Gastroenterol Nurs 40(2):143–150
32. Schwarzenberg SJ, Ling SC, Cloonan YK, Lin HS, Evon DM, Murray KF, Rodriguez-Baez N, Rosenthal P, Teckman J, Schwarz KB, Hepatitis B Research Network (HBRN) (2017) Health-related quality of life in pediatric patients with chronic hepatitis B living in the United States and Canada. J Pediatr Gastroenterol Nutr. [Epub ahead of print]
33. Suwantika AA, Yegenoglu S, Riewpaiboon A, Tu HA, Postma MJ (2013) Economic evaluations of hepatitis A vaccination in middle-income countries. Expert Rev Vaccines 12(12):1479–1494
34. Lawler EC (2017) Effectiveness of vaccination recommendations versus mandates: evidence from the

hepatitis A vaccine. J Health Econ 52:45–62 Epub 2017 Jan 18
35. Lahariya C, Paruthi R, Bhattacharya M (2016) How a new health intervention affects the health systems? Learnings from pentavalent vaccine introduction in India. Indian J Pediatr 83(4):294–299
36. Abahussin AA, Albarrak AI (2016) Vaccination adherence: review and proposed model. J Infect Public Health 9(6):781–789 Epub 2016 Sep 19
37. Schwarz KB, Garrett B, Alter MJ, Thompson D, Strathdee SA (2008) Seroprevalence of HCV infection in homeless Baltimore families. J Health Care Poor Underserved 19(2):580–587
38. Stene-Johansen K, Yaqoob N, Overbo J, Aberra H, Desalegn H, Berhe N, Johannessen A (2016) Dry blood spots a reliable method for measurement of hepatitis B viral load in resource-limited settings. PLoS One 11(11):e0166201
39. Hellmer N, Paxeus L, Magnius L, Enache B, Arnholm A, Johansson T, Bergstrom H (2014) Norder detection of pathogenic viruses in sewage provided early warnings of hepatitis A virus and norovirus outbreaks. Appl Environ Microbiol 80:6771–6781
40. Smith DB, Paddy JO, Simmonds P (2016) The use of human sewage screening for community surveillance of hepatitis E virus in the UK. J Med Virol 88(5):915–918
41. Kobayashi N, Oshiki M, Ito T, Segawa T, Hatamoto M, Kato T, Yamaguchi T, Kubota K, Takahashi M, Iguchi A, Tagawa T, Okubo T, Uemura S, Harada H, Motoyama T, Araki N, Sano D (2017) Removal of human pathogenic viruses in a down-flow hanging sponge (DHS) reactor treating municipal wastewater and health risks associated with utilization of the effluent for agricultural irrigation. Water Res 110:389–398
42. Ford N, Singh K, Cooke GS, Mills EJ, von Schoen-Angerer T, Kamarulzaman A, du Cros P (2012) Expanding access to treatment for hepatitis C in resource-limited settings: lessons from HIV/AIDS. Clin Infect Dis 54(10):1465–1472

Epidemiology of Viral Hepatitis A and E: A Global View

2

Kenrad E. Nelson and Brittany L. Kmush

Abstract

There are many similarities between the two human enterically transmitted hepatitis viruses, hepatitis A virus (HAV) and hepatitis E virus (HEV), in their epidemiology and the diseases they cause. However, important differences exist as well (Table 2.1). Both viruses are small, positive sense, single-stranded RNA viruses that replicate in the liver, causing similar symptoms and resulting in similar histopathology. Both viruses are non-enveloped when discharged from the liver into the biliary tree but also can be secreted into the bloodstream containing capsular material from the hepatocyte as a pseudomembrane. Both of these hepatitis viruses have been responsible for large epidemics and can be acquired from contaminated food. However, subclinical infection with HAV among infants and young children is very common especially in developing countries, but HEV infections typically occur as large waterborne epidemics in adolescents and adults in developing countries. Infants and young children have much lower rates of infection during these epidemics. A characteristic feature of HEV epidemics is a mortality of 1% or less in the general population but a mortality of 20% or higher among pregnant women. Sporadic infections from HEV occur among adults in industrialized countries from foodborne transmission. In contrast, clinically apparent hepatitis from HAV infections in developing countries is rare because of very high rates of subclinical infections among infants and young children resulting in high levels of immunity in the populations. Countries that have experienced the transition from low to higher levels of socioeconomic development have experienced an increasing number of hepatitis cases from HAV due to declining population immunity to the virus. The dynamic epidemiology of these two hepatitis viruses will be described in this chapter.

Keywords

Hepatitis A · Hepatitis E · Prevention · Vaccines · Viral hepatitis · Maternal mortality

K. E. Nelson (✉)
Department of Epidemiology, Bloomberg School of Public Health, Johns Hopkins University, Baltimore, MD, USA
e-mail: knelson3@jhu.edu; kenelson@jhsph.edu

B. L. Kmush
Department of Public Health, Food Studies, and Nutrition, Falk College of Sport and Human Dynamics, Syracuse University, Syracuse, NY, USA

M.-H. Chang, K. B. Schwarz (eds.), *Viral Hepatitis in Children*,
https://doi.org/10.1007/978-981-13-0050-9_2

Table 2.1 Comparative features of hepatitis A and E virus

	Hepatitis A	Hepatitis E
Virus family	*Picornaviridae*	*Hepeviridae*
Nucleic acid	Positive strand RNA	Positive strand RNA
Genomic size	7.5 kb	7.5 kb
Transmission	Person-to-person, fecal-oral, foodborne, blood	Fecal-oral, foodborne, blood
Incubation	2–5 weeks	3–7 weeks
Chronicity	None	Uncommon except in immune-compromised patients (transplant recipients, AIDS patients, etc.)
Reservoirs	Humans only	Gt. 1 and 2: humans
		Gt. 3 and 4: humans, swine, deer, mongoose, and other animals
Mortality	1–2%	1–2% in general population
		15–30% in pregnant women
Infection in young children	Very common	Rare
Subclinical infections in adults	Rare: 75–90% symptomatic	Common: 1–5% symptomatic
Severity of disease	Increases with age	Increases with age
Vaccine availability	Yes	Only in China
IGG protective	Yes	Not demonstrated

2.1 History and Discovery

Patients ill with jaundice have been reported throughout recorded history. Epidemics of jaundice have frequently accompanied military campaigns [1, 2]. However, the specific pathogens have been identified more recently. In 1909, McDonald suggested the hypothesis that a virus caused hepatitis, when he failed to implicate enteric bacteria as the cause [3]. In a study of an outbreak in 1930, Findlay and colleagues suggested that hepatitis was caused by a viral infection that was pathogenic only to humans [4]. Human transmission experiments were done in 1942 that documented that infection could occur after fecal-oral challenge. Studies in the 1960s found that the infection had an incubation period between 15 and 49 days and could be transmitted both by oral and parenteral routes [5, 6]. These studies also suggested that immunity after infection was long lasting and infectivity could be prevented with administration of immune serum globulin. In the 1960s, Krugman and colleagues documented that two hepatitis viral infections occurred in children at the Willowbrook State School in New York [6]. One had an incubation period of 15–50 days, and the other had an incubation period of 50–160 days. Subsequently, prisoners in Joliet, Illinois, were challenged orally with samples from the short incubation period-patients. Feinstone and colleagues studied filtered stools using immune electron microscopy (IEM). After convalescent serum was added to the filtered samples, they identified viral particles of hepatitis A virus [7]. A large waterborne epidemic involving nearly 30,000 persons occurred in Delhi, India, in December 1955–January 1956 [8]. Although it was believed that this was another epidemic caused by the enterically transmitted hepatitis agent, several unusual features challenged this hypothesis. First, the epidemic primarily involved adults but spared children. Second, the epidemic ended quickly with little or no secondary spread within households. Third, high mortality rates occurred among pregnant women. The overall mortality was under 1%, but it was over 20% among pregnant women. After the HAV was isolated, diagnostic reagents were developed. Samples stored from the Delhi outbreak tested negative for HAV. Nearly a decade later, Balayan studied a hepatitis outbreak in Afghanistan with similar features to the earlier Delhi outbreak. After filtering fecal samples from several jaundiced patients, he ingested the filtrate [9]. After 30 days, he developed symptoms of acute hepatitis. He found clumped HEV viral particles in his stool after it was mixed with convalescent sera from the Afghanistan patients and visualized by electron microscopy. The virus was subsequently sequenced and found to infect rhesus monkeys.

2.2 Virus Replication and Classification

2.2.1 Hepatitis A Virus

The hepatitis A virus is a positive sense, single-stranded, non-enveloped RNA virus in the *Picornaviridae* family. The RNA is 7.5 KB in length with a 5′ noncoding region, a single open reading frame coding a polyprotein, and a 3′ noncoding region. There are four genotypes that infect humans and three genotypes that infect only nonhuman primates but only one serotype. Infection with any of the genotypes causes similar symptoms [10]. However, the genotypes and sequences are sometimes useful as epidemiologic markers to trace the origin of an HAV strain associated with an outbreak. The virus replicates in gastrointestinal epithelial cells and hepatocytes. The viral genome is replicated using a negative sense strand intermediate. Oral challenge of monkeys with HAV is followed in a few days by detection of HAV antigen and negative strand viral genome in the lamina propria of cells in the small intestine [11]. This is followed by Kupffer cell positivity at 14 days and hepatic cell infection at 21 days. Viremia persists for 20–30 days after the incubation period of 15–45 days. The viremia declines with elevation of alanine aminotransferase (ALT) and other liver enzymes. Although HAV is not directly cytopathic, the virus can persist in the liver for 35–48 weeks after infection, because the type I interferon response to HAV infection is limited [12]. About 10% of patients have relapsing infection from HAV in the 6 months after the initial infection resolves [13]. This may be due in part to replication of virus remaining in the liver or to reinfection of the liver from virus in the bile that infects intestinal epithelial cells [12, 14]. These viruses complex with antibody and return to the liver as immune-complexed virus with IgA, which infects hepatocytes via the asialoglycoprotein receptor [14]. Although relapses from HAV occur, chronic hepatitis has not been reported.

Viruses contain the RNA genome, the VPg protein, and a capsid of the coat proteins VP1, VP2, and VP3 with icosahedral symmetry. The viral particles are released into the bile canaliculi and the blood. The viruses released into the bile do not contain an envelope. However, the viruses released into the blood contain portions of the liver cell membrane and are relatively more resistant to neutralizing antibodies [15].

2.2.2 Hepatitis E Virus

Hepatitis E viruses have been classified in the family *Hepeviridae*. These viruses are non-enveloped single-stranded RNA viruses. They are 7.2 kilobases in length with three open reading frames. Open reading frame (ORF)-1 codes for several enzymes for virus assembly, including a methyl transferase, cysteine protease, RNA helicase, and a RNA-dependent polymerase [16]. ORF-2 encodes the viral capsid. ORF-3 encodes several viral proteins and others that are used for viral exit from the hepatocyte [17]. The viruses replicate in hepatocytes and are released into the bile canaliculi. Some viral particles are also released into the sinusoidal bloodstream containing components of the hepatocyte as an envelope [18].

Five genotypes of HEV commonly infect humans, but there is only one serotype. Genotypes 1 and 2 only infect humans and are generally transmitted by fecally contaminated water. Genotype 3 and 4 strains have a zoonotic reservoir in swine, wild boar, deer, rabbits, and other animals [16]. Genotype 7 strains have been described recently with a reservoir in camels [19]. The animals harboring HEV genotype 3 and 4 strains have expanded in recent years to include goats, yak, moose, and cattle [20, 21].

Viruses in the *Hepeviridae* family have been isolated from a wide range of animals, in addition to those that infect humans. This information has resulted in a consensus classification of this family of viruses being published in 2014 [22]. This classification assigns the viruses into two genera, *Orthohepevirus*, including all mammalian and avian viruses, and *Piscihepevirus*, consisting of cutthroat trout virus. Species within the genus *Orthohepevirus* include *Orthohepevirus A* through *Orthohepevirus D*. *Orthohepevirus A* contains isolates from humans, pigs, wild boar, deer, mongoose, rabbit, and camels. *Orthohepevirus B* isolates include chicken and avian strains. *Orthohepevirus C* isolates include those from rats, bandicoots, shrew, ferret, and mink. *Orthohepevirus D* includes viruses from bats.

2.3 Global Epidemiology

The clinical features of HAV and HEV infections have many similarities. Infections with either virus are commonly clinically silent. However, asymptomatic persons infected with HAV are the critically important reservoir for spread within the population. The clinical and diagnostic issues of these two hepatitis viral infections are described in detail in other chapters of this book. The low infection rates among infants and young children with HEV infection contrast strikingly with the very high rates of HAV infections in this age group. In addition, the occurrence of chronic HEV infection among immune-compromised populations and the high mortality of pregnant women when infected with this virus provide marked contrasts to HAV infections.

2.3.1 Hepatitis A Virus

HAV infections are readily transmitted from person to person by fecal-oral exposures directly from fomites or contaminated food or water. The virus can also be transmitted by parenteral exposure to viremic carriers from injections or transfusions.

2.3.1.1 Global Prevalence

Hepatitis A infections are the most common cause of viral hepatitis globally. In developing countries with poor sanitation and hygiene, most infections occur among young children and are asymptomatic. Nearly 100% of the population has antibodies to HAV by 9 years of age, and clinical hepatitis among older children and adults is rare [23]. However, symptomatic hepatitis A among visitors from endemic areas is common. In areas with intermediate endemicity, clinical infections occur more commonly among older children and adults when 75–90% of infections are symptomatic [24]. In the United States, Western Europe, Australia, and a few other countries, the endemicity is low; these areas may experience isolated or community-wide foodborne outbreaks in adults and clinical hepatitis in high-risk populations, such as day-care center employees or families, injection drug users, men who have sex with men, or travelers to high endemic areas (Fig. 2.1).

Prior to the licensure and utilization of HA vaccines in the United States, the incidence of reported infection had cyclical peaks about every 10 years [25] (Fig. 2.2). There was regional variation in incidence with higher rates in Native Americans, Hispanics, and African Americans than Caucasians. In the 1988–1994 National Health and Nutritional Evaluation Survey in the United States, prior to the licensure of HAV vaccines, about a third of the population was antibody positive [25].

2.3.1.2 Modes of Transmission

Person to Person

HAV is commonly transmitted by person-to-person contact. Infants and young children are frequently the source in households, day-care centers, and hospitals because they are frequently asymptomatic and often have poor hygiene [26]. They often excrete the virus in their stool for longer periods and can contaminate the environment. The virus is resistant to heat and many chemicals and can retain infectivity on fomites.

Food- and Waterborne Transmission

Foodborne transmission is less common in the United States and Europe. However, large outbreaks occur periodically. An outbreak associated with contaminated pomegranate arils, which were imported into the United States from Turkey and infected 105 patients in 10 states, was

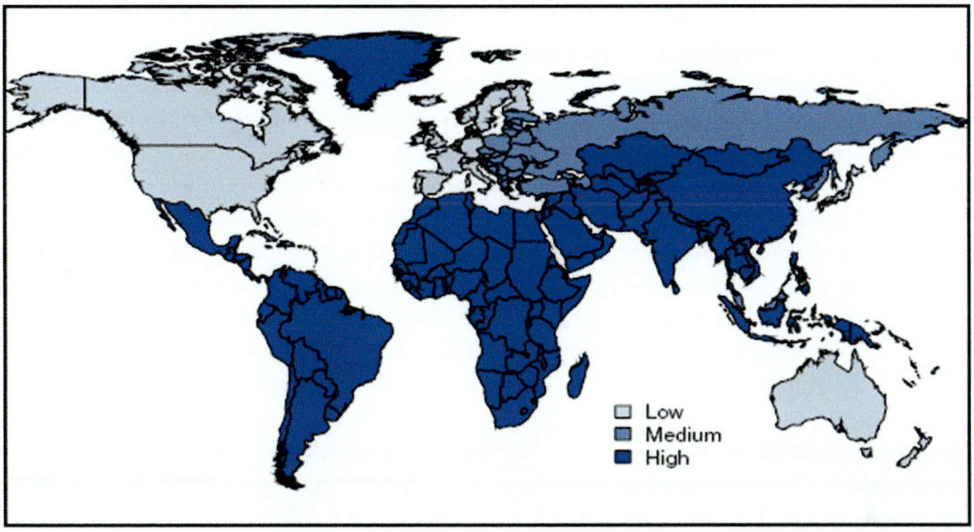

Fig. 2.1 Geographic distribution of hepatitis A endemicity, 2005* [39]
*For multiple countries, estimates of prevalence of antibody to hepatitis A virus (anti-HAV), a marker of previous HAV infection, are based on limited data and might not reflect current prevalence. In addition, anti-HAV prevalence might vary within countries by subpopulation and locality. As used on this map, the terms "high," "medium," and "low" endemicity reflect available evidence of how widespread infection is within each country rather than precise quantitative assessments. https://www.cdc.gov/mmwr/about.html
Springer Nature remains neutral with regard to jurisdictional claims in published maps and institutional affiliations

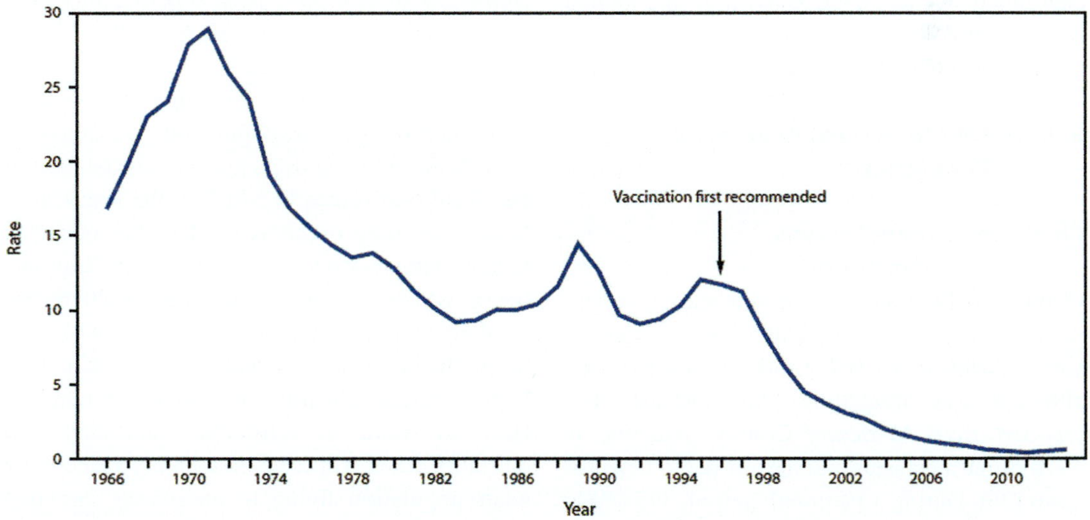

Fig. 2.2 Incidence* of reported acute hepatitis A cases – National Notifiable Diseases Surveillance System, United States, 1966–2013 [66]
*Rate per 100,000 population. Rate (number of cases) in 1971 (peak), 1996 (First Advisory Committee on Immunization Practice (ACIP) recommendation for hepatitis A vaccination), and 2011 (low) were 28.9 (59,606 cases), 11.7 (31,032 cases), and 0.4 (1.398 cases), respectively. https://www.cdc.gov/mmwr/about.html

reported in 2014 [27]. Other outbreaks involving contaminated green onions, frozen strawberries, oysters, sundried tomatoes, and other uncooked foods have been reported recently [28–33]. The source of the contamination is sometimes difficult to trace. It can include contaminated irrigation water, fertilizer, or infected agricultural workers or food handlers. Waterborne outbreaks are rare in developed countries but have been reported. An outbreak associated with infection from a public swimming pool at a camp in Louisiana was reported in 1992 [34].

Blood-Borne Transmission

Transmission of HAV by transfusion of blood products is rare in developed countries but has been reported [35]. Factor VIII or IX or pooled plasma concentrates that have been prepared from multiple donors have been reported to transmit HAV [36, 37]. The virus is resistant to solvent/detergent treatment.

Vertical Transmission

Vertical transmission has been reported rarely. One infant who acquired HAV from his mother was reported to be the source of an outbreak among hospital staff [38].

2.3.1.3 HAV Infections in Selected Populations

Child Care Centers, Schools, and Institutions

Outbreaks of HA among children, staff, and family members associated with day-care centers were reported in the 1970s and continue to occur, although less frequently. An outbreak was reported from Maricopa County, Arizona, in 1978 of an increasing number of acute hepatitis cases [26]. During a 10-month period, 398 (40%) of 1008 reported cases occurred in children, staff, or family members of children attending day-care centers. Typically, an infant in diapers who was asymptomatic would be the source case for a cluster of symptomatic hepatitis cases in the household or staff of the center. After this epidemiology was recognized, CDC developed guidelines to control day-care center outbreaks. If a day-care center employee or child develops hepatitis and is anti-HAV IgM positive, all day-care center children, employees, and family members are given hepatitis A vaccine (except for infants <12 months of age who should receive immunoglobulin). The same procedure is followed if two family members of a child attending a day-care center experience hepatitis A. Implementation of this strategy has substantially reduced the numbers of cases reported to be associated with day-care centers [39].

International Travelers

Hepatitis A is common among travelers from industrialized countries to high endemic countries. For this reason, HAV vaccine is recommended to protect travelers. Among American and European travelers, who have visited high endemic countries, the risk has been estimated to be 5 per 2000 person-months, which is similar to the risk of malaria acquisition [40, 41].

Illicit Drug Users

Outbreaks of HA have been reported in recent years among illicit drug users in the United States, Europe, and Australia. The anti-HAV IgG seroprevalence is higher among injection drug users than the general population. Transmission of HAV among drug users may include parenteral and fecal-oral routes [42–46]. In the last year, a large continuing outbreak of HAV has occurred among homeless persons in California. The outbreak, which started in San Diego in 2016, has resulted in more than 649 infections with 417 hospitalizations and 21 deaths to date [47]. This large outbreak illustrates the great potential for HAV to result in substantial morbidity and mortality when it spreads in a highly susceptible adult population living in unsanitary, crowded conditions.

Men Who Have Sex with Men (MSM)

Outbreaks of hepatitis A have been reported among MSM in the United States, Canada, Europe and Australia. MSM are an important, recently recognized risk group for HAV [48–52].

Occupation and Other Risk Groups

Health-care workers are frequently exposed to patients with acute hepatitis A. However, the virus levels in the stool of such patients may decline after they develop jaundice. However, health-care workers may also be exposed to patients with unapparent infections who are excreting virus. Exposure is likely frequent among nurses and other health-care workers on pediatric wards. Transmission of hepatitis A has been reported among pediatric ward employees [38, 39]. Since hepatitis A virus is excreted in the feces, pediatric health-care workers are exposed to blood and feces that might contain HAV.

Another population at risk of infection has been recognized recently. These are families who have adopted infants and children from international sites where HAV is highly endemic. A recent study reported 27 cases of acute hepatitis A among family members who adopted children from international sites [53]. A study in three international adoption clinics reported that 1–6% of adopted children were anti-HAV IgM positive. Recently, the ACIP has recommended that all household members and regular babysitters of newly arrived international adopted children should receive HAV vaccine [54, 55].

2.3.1.4 Prevention of Hepatitis A

Good hand hygiene among food handlers, cooks, kitchen workers, and agricultural employees is critical for the prevention of HA. In addition, transmission can be prevented with prophylaxis with either immune globulin or HAV vaccine.

Passive Prophylaxis

Immune globulin (Ig) is a sterile preparation from pooled human plasma that has been produced by cold ethanol fractionation [25]. Because of the high population seroprevalence of anti-HAV IgG, immune globulin pools contain protective antibodies. All components of the pool have tested negative for HBsAG, antibodies to HIV and HCV, and mini-pools were tested for HIV and HCV RNA by PCR amplification. A recent study of nine intramuscular Ig preparations found only two to have anti-HAV IgG potency greater than 100 IU/ml, which is the potency necessary for effective passive prophylaxis to prevent HAV [56]. Because the level of antibody to HAV in Ig preparations had decreased in recent years, the ACIP has recommended updated dosing instructions for Immune Globulin (Human) GamaSTAN S/D (the preparation available in the United States) to prevent hepatitis A [57]. The current recommended dosages of Ig (GamaSTAN S/D) for pre-exposure prophylaxis for persons who plan to travel to areas with high or intermediate HA endemicity are: up to 1 month of travel = 0.1 ml/kg body weight; up to 2 months = 0.2 ml/kg body weight; and longer than 2 months = repeat dose of 0.2 ml/kg every 2 months [57].

This is a change from the ACIP recommendations prior to September 2017 of 0.02 ml/kg body weight for 1–2 months prophylaxis and 0.06 ml/kg body weight for 3–5 months prophylaxis [39]. This larger dose recommendation tends to render the use of ISG for prophylaxis of HAV for travel impractical, since a 70 kg adult would need to be given 7.0 ml of ISG by IM injections. A preparation of high-dose HAV Ig (similar to HBiG) is needed but not yet available. Ig does not interfere with the immunogenicity of oral polio or yellow fever vaccine. However, Ig does interfere with the immune response of several live vaccines, including measles, mumps, rubella, and varicella vaccines [39]. Therefore, Ig should not be given with these vaccines or 2 weeks or less after MMR [39].

Hepatitis A Vaccine

After the epidemiology and clinical consequences of HAV became better understood, research to develop a vaccine commenced. Eventually, three inactivated vaccines were developed, shown to be highly effective and licensed. In a double-blind clinical trial in Thailand involving about 40,000 children who were 1–16 years of age and had high exposures to hepatitis A, an inactivated HAV vaccine (HAVRIX) was found to be 94% effective, safe, and well tolerated when given in 2 doses 1 month apart [58]. Another formalin-inactivated whole cell vaccine (VAQTA) was studied in approximately 1000 children in a community in New York with a high incidence of HAV and found 100% effective, immunogenic, and safe [59].

There are three inactivated HA vaccines available in the United States. Two are single antigen vaccines, HAVRIX, manufactured by GlaxoSmithKline, and VAQTA, manufactured by Merck & Co. The third vaccine, TWINRIX, is a bivalent vaccine containing both HAV and HBV antigens manufactured by GlaxoSmithKline. TWINRIX contains only half the antigen content of HAVRIX. These vaccines contain HAV antigens from viruses grown in cell culture, purified and inactivated with formalin exposure and absorbed to aluminum hydroxide [39]. They should be stored at 2–8 °C but not frozen. However, they maintain immunogenicity when stored at 37 °C. Both VAQTA and HAVRIX are available in two formulations, a lower dose for administration to persons 12 months to 18 years of age and a higher dose for persons over 18 years of age. The vaccines are licensed to be given in a two dose schedule, with the second dose administered 12–18 months after the first dose [39]. However, the antibody response after the first dose is usually quite good in a person with normal immune function [60]. The vaccines have reduced immunogenicity in AIDS patients with CD4+ cell counts below 200 cells/mm^3 and other immunocompromised conditions [39, 54, 61]. The levels of antibodies attained after natural infection are higher than after vaccine [62]. So testing for a postvaccination antibody response is not generally recommended.

In the United States, it is currently recommended by the CDC that all children receive HA vaccine at 1 year of age and a second dose at 12–18 months [39]. Either vaccine or Ig can be administered for postexposure prophylaxis [39]. A clinical trial was conducted among 1090 persons 2–40 years of age who were susceptible to HAV and had household or day-care center contact with a case of hepatitis A. The trial was designed as a non-inferiority trial. Symptomatic hepatitis A occurred in 25 (4.4%) of 565 recipients of hepatitis A vaccine and 17 (3.3%) of 522 recipients of Ig for a relative risk of 1.35 (95%CI: 0.70–2.67) [63]. The conclusion was that the HAV vaccine met the non-inferiority criterion when administered within 14 days of exposure. When prophylaxis can only be administered 14 days or more after exposure, Ig should be given. The advantages of HAV vaccine over Ig are that it induces active immunity with long-term protection and greater ease of administration. In persons with a household exposure, a secondary attack rate of 15–30% has been reported in the absence of prophylaxis [64]. The ACIP reviewed the data from the trial and recommended that a person exposed to HA should receive either a single antigen vaccine, within 14 days of exposure, or Ig at 0.02 ml/kg as soon as possible after exposure [55]. Persons over 40 years of age or infants should receive Ig because they have poor or absent responses to vaccine [55].

After these vaccines were licensed, the Advisory Committee on Immunization Practices (ACIP) of the US CDC made a series of recommendations, starting in 1996, when they recommended immunizing persons at high risk, such as travelers to high endemic areas, household contacts of a case, and medical personnel [25]. In 1999, the ACIP recommended immunizing children at age 2 years or older who lived in communities reporting an HAV incidence greater than 2 times the national average, i.e., over 20 cases per 100,000 population [25, 65]. In 2006, ACIP recommended immunizing all children at 1 year of age. In addition, they recommended vaccinating older children and adults at high risk of HAV infections, such as patients with chronic liver disease [39]. As a result of the implementation of these recommendations, focused primarily on immunizing children, there was a dramatic decline in the reported cases in all age groups (Fig. 2.3). The incidence declined from 17.7 cases per 100,000 population in 1996 to 0.4 cases per 100,000 in 2011 (Fig. 2.4) [66]. However, the remaining cases that were reported were more severe clinically, because selective immunization of high-risk adults was more difficult to implement [60].

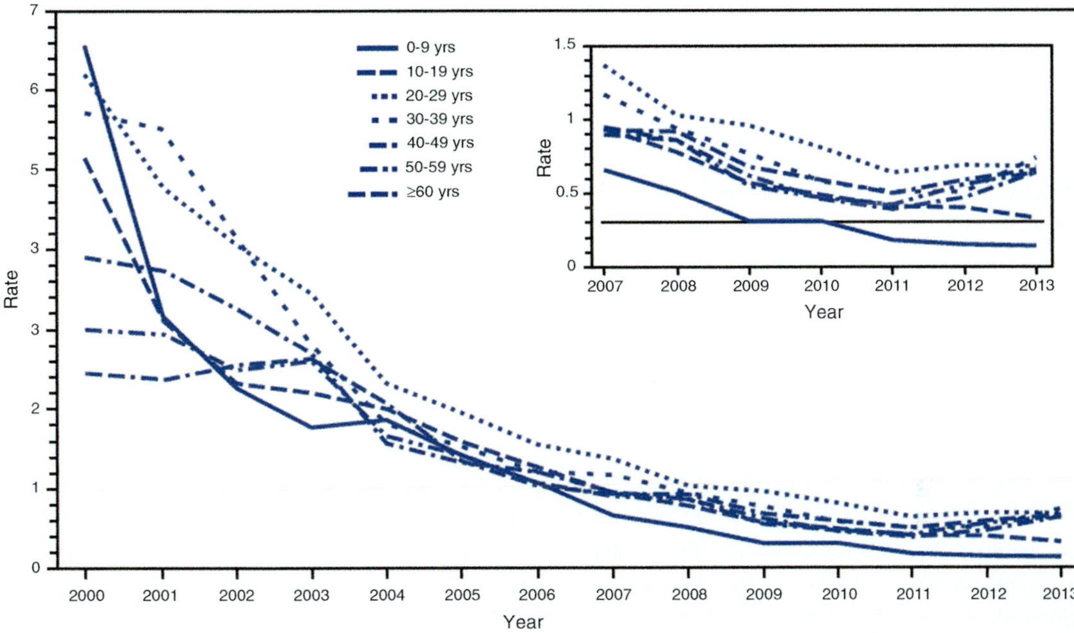

Fig. 2.3 Incidence* of reported acute hepatitis A cases, by age group – National Notifiable Diseases Surveillance System, United States, 2000–2013 [66]

*Rate per 100,000 population. https://www.cdc.gov/mmwr/about.html

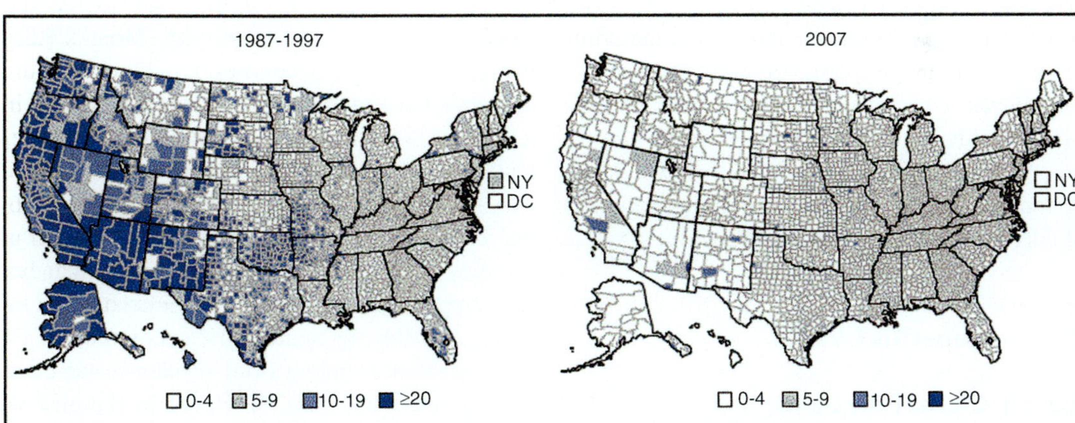

Fig. 2.4 Incidence* of reported acute hepatitis A cases, by county – National Notifiable Diseases Surveillance System, United States, 1987–1997** (pre-vaccine) and 2007 [66]

*Rate per 100,000 population; ** Annual average incidence. https://www.cdc.gov/mmwr/about.html

Global Issues in Hepatitis A Prevention

Several countries have experienced an increase in the reported cases of clinical hepatitis after improvement in sanitation and hygiene delayed the onset of infection to older ages, when most infections are symptomatic. Jacobsen and Koopman studied data on the age-related HAV seroprevalence in relation to the water quality index assessed by the United Nations and the Human Development Index (HDI) as a measure

Table 2.2 Epidemiological characteristics and genotype distribution of hepatitis E viruses that infect humans

Characteristics	Genotype 1	Genotype 2	Genotype 3	Genotype 4
Geographic location	Africa and Asia	Mexico, West Africa	Developed countries	China, Taiwan, Japan
Transmission route	Waterborne fecal-oral person-to-person	Waterborne fecal-oral	Foodborne	Foodborne
Groups at high risk for infection	Young adults	Young adults	Older adults (>40 years) and males Immunocompromised persons	Young adults
Zoonotic transmission	No	No	Yes	Yes
Chronic infection	No	No	Yes	No
Occurrence of outbreaks	Common	Smaller-scale outbreaks	Uncommon	Uncommon

From Centers for Disease Control and Prevention

of the standard of living in 159 countries [24]. They found that several countries, especially in Asia and South America, have experienced a transition from high to intermediate endemicity. These countries have experienced an increase in the rate of acute hepatitis and hospitalization from hepatitis. The public health dilemma faced by these countries is whether to include HAV vaccine in the routine childhood vaccination schedule. The WHO Scientific Advisory Group of Experts (SAGE) has recommended including HAV vaccine in the routine immunization schedules of transitional countries based upon a review of the incidence and morbidity of HAV and the cost-benefit of routine immunization [67]. A few countries have adopted routine immunization of children, including Israel and Argentina [68].

2.3.2 Hepatitis E Virus

2.3.2.1 Global Prevalence

Although these viruses cause infections in most countries as evidenced by seroprevalence data, the individual genotypes are somewhat restricted in their geographic distribution (Table 2.2). Genotype 1 viruses are endemic in Southern Asia, especially in the Indian subcontinent, and Africa, but they are not present in Europe or North America. Genotype 2 viruses have caused outbreaks only in Mexico and West Africa. Genotype 3 strains are endemic in Europe, North and South America, Central and Southern Japan, and Australia. Genotype 4 strains are found in China, Northern Japan, and India. Genotype 7 strains have been detected in camels and a camel owner in the Arabian Peninsula.

Seroprevalence data from various global populations indicate that HEV infections are common in every country where studies have been done (Fig. 2.5). However, it is difficult to compare the data from the different studies because serologic assays with differing sensitivity and specificity have been employed. Most studies from areas where genotypes 1 or 2 viruses are endemic have found seroprevalence below 5% in children under 10 years of age, which increases and peaks in the second and third decades of life (Figs. 2.6 and 2.7). Some studies have found men to have higher seroprevalence than women. Studies have differed concerning whether seroprevalence is higher in rural or urban populations. A study in South Africa reported 15.3% seroprevalence among rural residents and 6.6% among urban residents. However, in Bangladesh and India, the seroprevalence was higher among urban than rural residents. Outbreaks in rural areas may occur because of more localized contamination of the water supply.

2.3.2.2 Modes of Transmission

Waterborne Transmission

Epidemics of waterborne hepatitis from HEV are frequent during and after monsoon rains in the Indian subcontinent and South Asia. In addition,

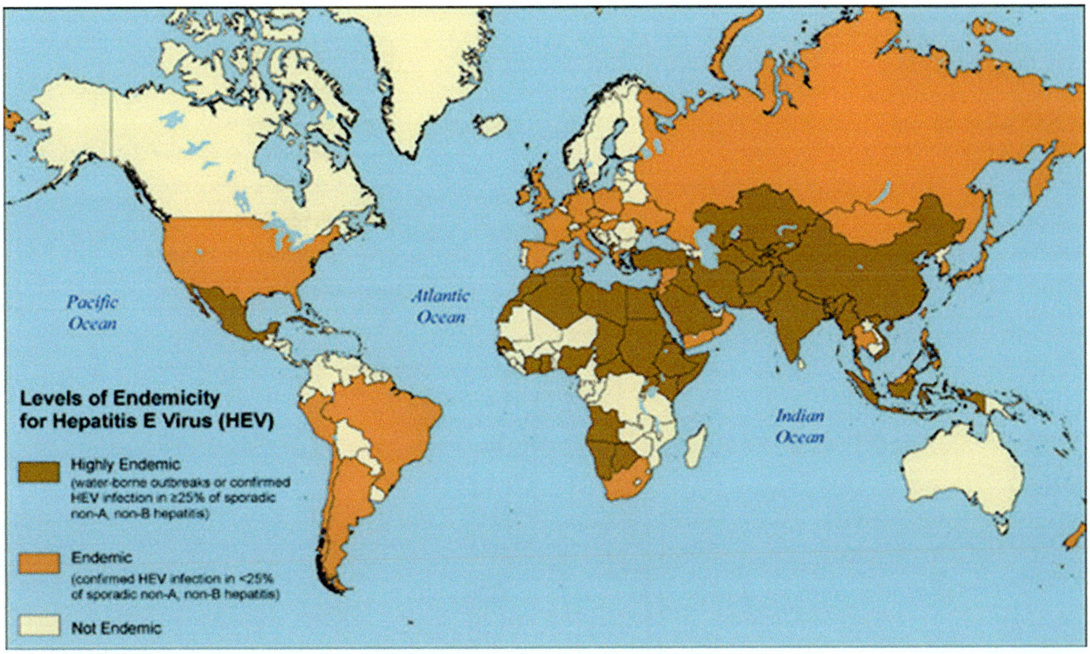

Fig. 2.5 Global distribution and levels of endemicity of hepatitis E virus (HEV). (From Centers for Disease Control and Prevention)

Springer Nature remains neutral with regard to jurisdictional claims in published maps and institutional affiliations

Fig. 2.6 Estimated seroprevalence of hepatitis E virus by age and global burden of disease region in 2005. (Reproduced with permission from Ref. [71])

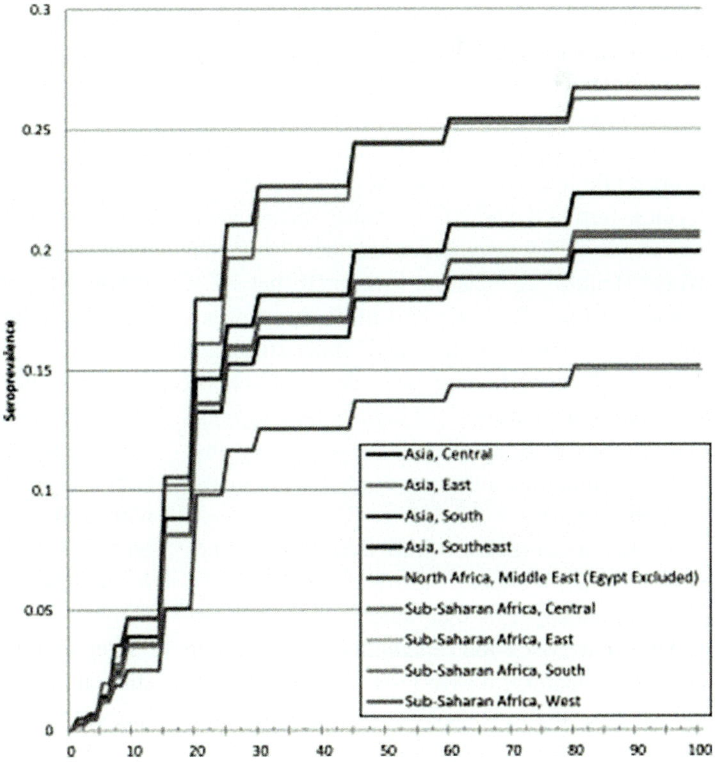

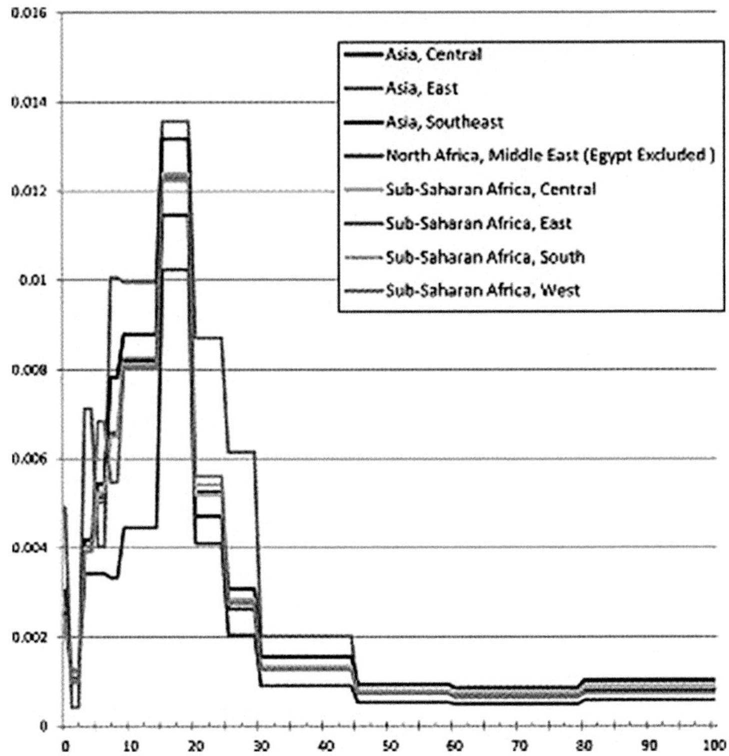

Fig. 2.7 Estimated incidence of hepatitis E virus by age and global burden of disease region in 2005. (Reproduced with permission from Ref. [71])

large outbreaks have been reported from sub-Saharan Africa in refugee populations when clean water is unavailable [69, 70]. These recurring epidemics commonly include thousands of cases and are associated with an overall mortality of about 1% but 10–25% mortality in pregnant women (Table 2.3). Pregnant women account for about a third of the overall mortality during these waterborne epidemics. Investigators from the World Health Organization estimated that HEV genotypes 1 and 2 caused 20.1 million symptomatic cases, 70,000 deaths, and 3000 stillbirths each year [71]. Verbal autopsy studies of general community populations of fatalities among pregnant women in Bangladesh have suggested that 9–20% of maternal mortality might be associated with HEV infection [72, 73].

An historical review of reported epidemics of jaundice with increased mortality among pregnant women suggests that waterborne outbreaks of HEV have occurred repeatedly since the late eighteenth century, at least [74]. These outbreaks involved populations in Western Europe as well as America but have been localized to South Asia and Africa during the most recent several decades.

A study from Dhaka, Bangladesh, found that sporadic cases of HEV infection were common in addition to large outbreaks [75]. Contaminated coastal water is an important source of accumulation of virus in shellfish. In addition, the use of river water for drinking or food preparation is common in some populations that could be responsible for endemic transmission of HEV [76].

Person to Person

Direct person-to-person transmission of HEV is unusual but does occur. In the large outbreak in Delhi in 1955 that included over 29,000 persons with acute hepatitis, there were few (if any) secondary cases and the outbreak ceased after 2 months. In contrast, another outbreak in Kitgum, Uganda, which lasted for over a year, had epidemiologic features characteristic of substantial person-to-person transmission [77]. In this outbreak, most cases occurred secondary to

Table 2.3 Morbidity and mortality from selected waterborne hepatitis E virus epidemics

Site	Years	Cases	Deaths: total	Deaths: pregnant women
Delhi, India	1954–1955	29,300	266	102
Bosnia, Yugoslavia	1964	4984	98	82
Kathmandu, Nepal	1973	10,000	118	30
Kashmir, India	1978–1979	20,000	600	436
Xinjiang, China	1986–1988	119,280	705	51
Shebeli, Somalia	1988–1989	11,413	346	48
Maharashtra, India	1989–1990	3580	50	32
Kanpur, India	1991	70,000	48	13
Islamabad, Pakistan	1993–1994	3458	8	4
Darfur, Sudan	2004	2621	45	19
Kitgum, Uganda	2007–2009	4789	72	13
Nellore, Andhra Pradesh, India	2008–2009	23,915	315	Unknown
Dhaka, Bangladesh	2008–2009	4751	18	4
Rajshahi, Bangladesh	2010	2162	12	3
Ichalkaranji/Kolhapur, Maharashtra, India	2012	5165	36	5
Refugee Camps, Upper Nile, South Sudan	2012–2013	10,055	214	22
Biratnagar, Morang, Nepal	2014	7000	17	2
Raipur, Chhattisgarh, India	2014	5000	31	12
Napak, Karamoja, Uganda	2013–2014	1498	32	18
Sambalpur, Odisha, India	2014–2015	3000	50	2
Refugee Camps, Gambella, Ethiopia	2014–2015	1117	21	2
Shimla/Solan, Himachal Pradesh, India	2015–2016	5000–10,000	22	3
Beria, South Sudan	2015–2016	2475	21	Unknown

Reproduced with permission from Ref. [146]

an index case in the household. There was also a high rate of infection in children under age 5 years, in marked contrast to most waterborne epidemics of HEV [78]. Epidemiologic data from Egypt indicate a high seroprevalence of IgG antibodies in young children, which is compatible with there being a high rate of person-to-person transmission, similar to hepatitis A virus [79]. Despite these unusual reports, most studies have found a low prevalence of HEV in young children and limited evidence of person-to-person transmission of HEV [80].

Foodborne Transmission

There is considerable evidence that the major means of transmission of genotypes 3 and 4 HEV in developed countries is through the consumption of contaminated food [16]. Nevertheless, it is often difficult to detect the specific food responsible for an infection of an individual patient because the incubation period is fairly long and the majority of infections are subclinical. However, several outbreaks have been reported where the food source was identified.

An early report from Japan concerned a person who developed acute hepatitis E after consuming sushi prepared from a Sitka deer he had hunted [81]. The virus from the sushi was identical to the virus isolated from him and his friend who had eaten the sushi [82]. In southern France, seven persons developed acute hepatitis E genotype 3 after consuming a sausage, *figatellu*, prepared from uncooked pig liver at two wedding parties [83]. Studies of the sausage identified HEV genotype 3 RNA identical to that recovered from the wedding guests. An outbreak in Australia involved 24 persons who developed acute hepatitis E after consuming pork liver pate [84]. An outbreak of 33 patients with acute hepatitis E was reported among the passengers on a worldwide ocean cruise [85]. This outbreak was associated with the consumption of raw shellfish.

Research in several countries has identified HEV RNA in commonly eaten foods. The most important reservoir for HEV globally is swine. Studies of pig feces in many countries have detected HEV RNA in a high proportion of animals, especially among 2–4-month-old animals. The infected pigs typically have viremia for 2–3 weeks but shed virus in their feces for 3–7 weeks [86]. In Europe and the United States, HEV genotype 3 strains are common. In China, pigs commonly excrete genotype 4 HEV in their feces [87]. Studies of pig liver for sale in grocery stores have detected HEV RNA in 6–11% of samples [88]. This finding has been replicated in European countries and China [87, 89, 90]. A study in Canada detected HEV genotype 3 RNA in strawberries that had been irrigated with water contaminated with pig manure from a neighboring farm [91]. HEV RNA has been detected in raw oysters [85, 92]. Contaminated food that is brought into the kitchen could contaminate surfaces or other food prior to cooking. Wild boar and deer are also a food reservoir of HEV that has been reported to be the source of hepatitis E in humans [93]. Other animals that have been found to be infected with HEV include rabbits, goats, mongeese, and camels [20, 94–99]. An infected camel transmitted HEV genotype 7 to his owner who was immunocompromised after having a liver transplant [19]. The patient developed chronic HEV infection. Subsequent studies of dromedary and Bactrian camels found serologic evidence of HEV infection to be common among both types of camels [94–96]. However, the importance of the camel reservoir in transmitting HEV to humans is unclear and has not been adequately studied. A recent report from China found HEV genotype 4 RNA in the milk of a cow [100]. The virus could be transmitted to cynomolgus monkeys by oral challenge, even after the milk was pasteurized but not after it had been boiled [100]. Additional research on the extent of the cow reservoir is important since these animals have not been considered a zoonotic source of human infection prior to this report. However, they are an important human food source [92, 101]. A serological study found anti-HEV IgG seroprevalence of 15% in cows in the United States. However, HEV RNA has not been detected in cows in the United States [102]. Research on the thermal inactivation of HEV in pork products has found it to be necessary to heat the food to an internal temperature of 71 °C for 20 minutes in order to completely inactivate HEV [103, 104]. Therefore, undercooked meat or smoked sausage could transmit HEV [105].

Transfusion and Parenteral Transmission

HEV can be transmitted by transfusion of blood products or by parenteral exposures from a viremic donor. Several epidemiologic factors favor the transmission of HEV by transfusion. First, HEV infections occur more frequently in adults. Second, infected persons usually are asymptomatic. Third, the infections involve the general population and are not concentrated in specific populations, such as injection drug users, men who have sex with men, or other groups. Therefore, it is not possible to reduce the risk by screening or excluding selected populations from donating blood.

Several transfusion-transmitted HEV infections were reported from northern Japan over a decade ago [106–109]. As a result of these reports, routine screening of blood donors from the Hokkaido area of Japan for HEV RNA was instituted in 2008 [110]. This screening identified 231 viremic donors among over two million donations [109]. A total of 19 transfusion-transmitted HEV infections have been detected in Japan during the last 15 years [106]. Studies in many countries have identified viremic donors at rates varying from 1 in 785 to 1 in 13,450 [109, 111]. A study of 225,000 blood donors in Southeastern UK detected 77 HEV RNA-positive donors [111]. Among 44 patients who had been transfused with these viremic donations, who could be followed, 18 developed HEV infection, of which 10 were persistent. These patients cleared long-standing infections after treatment with ribavirin or reducing their immunosuppressive therapy. Following this study, the UK blood services developed a policy of only transfusing patients with a transplant or a hematologic malignancy with blood that had screened negative for HEV RNA [112]. All blood is screened for HEV RNA prior to transfusion in Ireland at present [113].

Donations from 59,474 donors in Holland that were screened in pools of 96 and 192 samples detected 45 HEV RNA-positive donations. Although blood for transfusion in Holland is not routinely screened, donations for the production of solvent/detergent treatment (S/D) plasma are tested for HEV RNA. In 2013 and 2014, HEV RNA was detected in 1 of 762 donations intended for production of S/D plasma [114]. Blood donors in China are routinely screened for ALT. Donors with elevated ALT levels are more frequently positive for anti-HEV IgM, HEV antigen, or HEV RNA [115]. Despite the evidence that HEV viremic donors are common globally, few countries have adopted routine donor screening for HEV RNA.

Vertical Transmission

Transmission of HEV to the fetus during pregnancy or to the infant at birth from infected women has been reported [116, 117]. One study in Kashmir documented perinatal transmission of HEV to the infants of five of eight infected women [118]. Infant and cord blood samples had elevated ALT levels and anti-HEV IgG and HEV RNA; three had anti-HEV IgM. One infant was jaundiced. Two infected infants died, and HEV viremia resolved within 1 month in three infants. Another study of six infants born to mothers with hepatitis E in India reported three infants with plasma HEV RNA [117]. Chronic infection of infants infected at birth has not been reported. HEV RNA has been detected in the breast milk of a postpartum woman [119]. However, no data have been reported on the risk of transmission by breast feeding.

Occupational Transmission

Swine farmers, butchers, abattoir workers, and workers having contact with sewage have been reported to be at increased risk of HEV [120–123]. A study of wild boar hunters in Germany found these persons to have a high risk of HEV infection [123]. However, hunters who wore gloves when disemboweling and butchering the animals had lower HEV seroprevalence. A patient with acute hepatitis E acquired from a scalpel wound during surgery on a pig was reported recently [124].

2.3.2.3 HEV Infections in Selected Populations

Infants and Young Children

Most studies have found HEV infections and seroprevalence to be less common in young children. However, when infected, they can develop symptomatic acute hepatitis as well as asymptomatic infections [125].

Adolescents and Young Adults

Infections with HEV genotype 1 strains are most common in populations of young adults (Figs. 2.6 and 2.7) [71].

Middle-Aged and Older Adults

HEV infections are common in middle-aged and older adults, especially among persons infected with genotype 3 and 4 strains. HEV seroprevalence increases with age in populations where genotype 3 or 4 strains are endemic [16]. The highest seroprevalence is among older males in these countries. In a seroprevalence study of the NHANES repository, non-Hispanic blacks had a lower prevalence of antibodies to HEV, 15.3%, than Hispanics, 21.8%, or whites, 22.3% [126]. Lower anti-HEV seroprevalence in blacks was associated with single nucleotide polymorphisms linked to the e3 and e4 alleles of the apolipoprotein gene [127].

Pregnant Women

Pregnant women are at increased risk for infection, severe disease, and mortality from genotype 1 or 2 HEV infection [128]. Whether pregnant women who are infected with genotype 3 HEV may also have more severe infections is not clear [129]. Among 68 cases of HEV in Israel between 1993 and 2013, 9 were in pregnant women. The authors found an additional six cases of HEV infection during pregnancy from reports in the literature. The outcome in ten cases was favorable.

However, five cases had fulminant hepatitis, including two of the patients with locally acquired infection in Israel [129]. More data are needed on the natural history of autochthonous HEV infections in pregnant women in industrialized countries. However, acute hepatitis from HEV is uncommon in this population in developed countries.

Immunocompromised Populations

Patients who are immunocompromised are at risk for chronic HEV infections that can persist for years [130]. The majority of patients with chronic HEV have been reported among patients with solid organ transplants, who are receiving immunosuppressive drugs to prevent the rejection of their transplants [131]. However, chronic HEV infections have also been reported among patients with depressed immunity for other reasons, include HIV/AIDS and hematologic malignancy [132–134].

A review of data from 17 transplant centers in Europe found 85 solid organ transplant patients who had been infected with HEV after their transplant [135]. Fifty-six (65.9%) of these patients developed chronic hepatitis. Multivariate analysis found the use of tacrolimus, rather than cyclosporine, to prevent rejection was significantly associated with chronic HEV. Among the patients with chronic hepatitis, 18 (32.1%) achieved viral clearance after the dose of immunosuppressive therapy was reduced [135].

In addition to reducing the dose of immunosuppressive drugs, chronic HEV can be treated effectively with interferon or ribavirin. A retrospective review of 59 patients in several centers in France who had HEV infection after a transplant found that the infection cleared after they had received a median daily dose of 600 mg of ribavirin for an average of 3 months [136]. Although recurrence of the infection occurred in ten patients after ribavirin was stopped, they were retreated successfully.

2.3.2.4 Extrahepatic Symptoms

Although HEV replicates in the liver and mainly results in symptoms of acute hepatitis, some patients with chronic HEV have extrahepatic symptoms. The most frequently reported extrahepatic symptoms are neurological, including Guillain-Barre syndrome, neurologic amyotrophy, and encephalitis or meningitis [137]. Some patients have had evidence of extrahepatic replication of HEV. HEV RNA has been recovered from the cerebrospinal fluid of a patient with encephalitis; however, this is unusual [138]. Some patients with HEV infection have had acute pancreatitis, aplastic anemia, cryoglobulinemia, or acute membranous glomerulonephritis [138]. An HEV genotype 3 virus was isolated from a patient in the UK with chronic hepatitis that was sequenced and found to have a genetic insert of 151 nucleotides from the human ribosome protein [139]. This recombinant virus, the Kernow strain, was able to replicate effectively in several human hepatoma cell lines. This virus has been important for in vitro research in the biology of viral replication.

2.3.2.5 Prevention of Hepatitis E

Prevention of waterborne transmission of HEV in developing countries is quite difficult. WHO has estimated that more than 2.5 billion people in developing countries lack access to modern sanitation. However, physical and chemical methods can be utilized to disinfect water [71, 140]. Heat, ultraviolet radiation, and chlorination can be effective [141]. However, access to these methods is often limited during floods in poor countries.

Prevention of foodborne transmission is also challenging. However, persons who are at risk for chronic or severe acute infections should avoid eating high-risk food, such as undercooked pig liver, organ meats, liver pate, smoked sausage, or raw oysters. Despite these precautions, contamination can extend beyond these high-risk foods because of cross contamination in the kitchen or during transport.

Hepatitis E Vaccines

Two HEV vaccines have proved to be effective in clinical trials. The first vaccine was a submit vaccine that was tested in the Nepal military and found to be over 95% effective in preventing clinical hepatitis [142]. However, this vaccine was not licensed or produced after the trial. A second vaccine, Hecolin, was produced in China [143]. This vaccine is a subunit virus-like particle vaccine containing 239 amino acids that is produced in *E. coli*. The vaccine was found to be highly immunogenic and protected monkeys after challenge with HEV [144]. After satisfactory safety and immunogenicity studies in humans, a clinical trial in 112,604 persons between 16 and 65 years of age was completed in China [143]. The vaccine was given in three doses at baseline, 1 month, and 6 months. It was 100% effective in preventing clinical hepatitis in persons who received all three doses. A follow-up study after 4.5 years found the vaccine to have continued efficacy of 86.6% (95% confidence interval: 71–94%) in preventing hepatitis [145].

The vaccine is now licensed and available only in China. It could be very useful in preventing infection in high-risk patients such as pregnant women or immunosuppressed patients. However, additional data are needed to evaluate the efficacy of a shorter course of the vaccine given to subjects at high risk of severe morbidity or mortality.

2.4 Summary

Although the epidemiology and prevention tools and strategies for these two enterically transmitted hepatitis viruses differ, the implementation of currently available methods could reduce the morbidity and mortality from these infections considerably.

References

1. Cockayne EA (1912) Catarrhal jaundice, sporadic and epidemic, and its relation to acute yellow atrophy of the liver. QJM os6(1):1–29
2. Cuthbert JA (2001) Hepatitis A: old and new. Clin Microbiol Rev 14(1):38–58
3. McDonald S (1908) Acute yellow atrophy of the liver. Edin Med J 1:83–88
4. Findlay GM, Dunlop JL (1931) Observations on an epidemic of catarrhal jaundice. Trans R Soc Trop Med Hyg 25(1):7–28
5. Holmes AW, Wolfe L, Rosenblate H, Deinhardt F (1969) Hepatitis in marmosets: induction of disease with coded specimens from a human volunteer study. Science 165(3895):816–817
6. Krugman S, Giles JP, Hammond J (1967) Infectious hepatitis. Evidence for two distinctive clinical, epidemiological, and immunological types of infection. JAMA 200(5):365–373
7. Feinstone SM, Kapikian AZ, Purcell RH (1973) Hepatitis A: detection by immune electron microscopy of a virus-like antigen associated with acute illness. Science 182:1026–1028
8. Viswanathan R (1957) Infectious hepatitis in Delhi (1955–56). Indian J Med Res 45:1–29
9. Balayan MS, Andjaparidze AG, Savinskaya SS, Ketiladze ES, Braginsky DM, Savinov AP et al (1983) Evidence for a virus in non-A, non-B hepatitis transmitted via the fecal-oral route. Intervirology 20(1):23–31
10. Nainan OV, Xia G, Vaughan G, Margolis HS (2006) Diagnosis of hepatitis a virus infection: a molecular approach. Clin Microbiol Rev 19(1):63–79
11. Asher LV, Binn LN, Mensing TL, Marchwicki RH, Vassell RA, Young GD (1995) Pathogenesis of hepatitis A in orally inoculated owl monkeys (Aotus trivirgatus). J Med Virol 47(3):260–268
12. Lanford RE, Feng Z, Chavez D, Guerra B, Brasky KM, Zhou Y et al (2011) Acute hepatitis A virus infection is associated with a limited type I interferon response and persistence of intrahepatic viral RNA. Proc Natl Acad Sci U S A 108(27):11223–11228
13. Glikson M, Galun E, Oren R, Tur-Kaspa R, Shouval D (1992) Relapsing hepatitis A. Review of 14 cases and literature survey. Medicine (Baltimore) 71(1):14–23
14. Dotzauer A, Gebhardt U, Bieback K, Gottke U, Kracke A, Mages J et al (2000) Hepatitis A virus-specific immunoglobulin A mediates infection of hepatocytes with hepatitis A virus via the asialoglycoprotein receptor. J Virol 74(23):10950–10957
15. Feng Z, Hensley L, McKnight KL, Hu F, Madden V, Ping L et al (2013) A pathogenic picornavirus acquires an envelope by hijacking cellular membranes. Nature 496(7445):367–371
16. Hoofnagle JH, Nelson KE, Purcell RH (2012) Hepatitis E. N Engl J Med 367(13):1237–1244
17. Emerson SU, Nguyen H, Torian U, Purcell RH (2006) ORF3 protein of hepatitis E virus is not required for replication, virion assembly, or infection of hepatoma cells in vitro. J Virol 80(21):10457–10464
18. Yin X, Li X, Feng Z (2016) Role of envelopment in the HEV life cycle. Viruses 8(8):229
19. Lee GH, Tan BH, Chi-Yuan Teo E, Lim SG, Dan YY, Wee A et al (2016) Chronic infection with camelid hepatitis E virus in a liver transplant recipient who regularly consumes camel meat and milk. Gastroenterology 150(2):7.e3

20. Sanford BJ, Emerson SU, Purcell RH, Engle RE, Dryman BA, Cecere TE et al (2013) Serological evidence for a hepatitis e virus-related agent in goats in the United States. Transbound Emerg Dis 60(6):538–545
21. Meng XJ (2016) Expanding host range and cross-species infection of hepatitis E virus. PLoS Pathog 12(8):e1005695
22. Smith DB, Simmonds P, Jameel S, Emerson SU, Harrison TJ, Meng X et al (2014) Consensus proposals for classification of the family Hepeviridae. J Gen Virol 95(Pt 10):2223–2232
23. Jacobsen KH, Wiersma ST (2010) Hepatitis A virus seroprevalence by age and world region, 1990 and 2005. Vaccine 28(41):6653–6657
24. Jacobsen KH, Koopman JS (2005) The effects of socioeconomic development on worldwide hepatitis A virus seroprevalence patterns. Int J Epidemiol 34(3):600–609
25. Prevention of hepatitis A through active or passive immunization: recommendations of the advisory committee on immunization Practices (ACIP). MMWR Recomm Rep 45(RR-15):1–30 (1996)
26. Hadler SC, Webster HM, Erben JJ, Swanson JE, Maynard JE (1980) Hepatitis A in day-care centers. A community-wide assessment. N Engl J Med 302(22):1222–1227
27. Collier MG, Khudyakov YE, Selvage D, Adams-Cameron M, Epson E, Cronquist A et al (2014) Outbreak of hepatitis A in the USA associated with frozen pomegranate arils imported from Turkey: an epidemiological case study. Lancet Infect Dis 14(10):976–981
28. Wheeler C, Vogt TM, Armstrong GL, Vaughan G, Weltman A, Nainan OV et al (2005) An outbreak of hepatitis A associated with green onions. N Engl J Med 353(9):890–897
29. Bialek SR, George PA, Xia GL, Glatzer MB, Motes ML, Veazey JE et al (2007) Use of molecular epidemiology to confirm a multistate outbreak of hepatitis A caused by consumption of oysters. Clin Infect Dis 44(6):838–840
30. Hutin YJ, Pool V, Cramer EH, Nainan OV, Weth J, Williams IT et al (1999) A multistate, foodborne outbreak of hepatitis A. National hepatitis A investigation team. N Engl J Med 340(8):595–602
31. Dentinger CM, Bower WA, Nainan OV, Cotter SM, Myers G, Dubusky LM et al (2001) An outbreak of hepatitis A associated with green onions. J Infect Dis 183(8):1273–1276
32. Niu MT, Polish LB, Robertson BH, Khanna BK, Woodruff BA, Shapiro CN et al (1992) Multistate outbreak of hepatitis A associated with frozen strawberries. J Infect Dis 166(3):518–524
33. Donnan EJ, Fielding JE, Gregory JE, Lalor K, Rowe S, Goldsmith P et al (2012) A multistate outbreak of hepatitis A associated with semidried tomatoes in Australia, 2009. Clin Infect Dis 54(6):775–781
34. Mahoney FJ, Farley TA, Kelso KY, Wilson SA, Horan JM, McFarland LM (1992) An outbreak of hepatitis A associated with swimming in a public pool. J Infect Dis 165(4):613–618
35. Noble RC, Kane MA, Reeves SA, Roeckel I (1984) Posttransfusion hepatitis A in a neonatal intensive care unit. JAMA 252(19):2711–2715
36. Soucie JM, Robertson BH, Bell BP, McCaustland KA, Evatt BL (1998) Hepatitis A virus infections associated with clotting factor concentrate in the United States. Transfusion 38(6):573–579
37. da Silva SG, Leon LA, Alves G, Brito SM, Sandes Vde S, Lima MM et al (2016) A rare case of transfusion transmission of hepatitis A virus to two patients with haematological disease. Transfus Med Hemother 43(2):137–141
38. Rosenblum LS, Villarino ME, Nainan OV, Melish ME, Hadler SC, Pinsky PP et al (1991) Hepatitis A outbreak in a neonatal intensive care unit: risk factors for transmission and evidence of prolonged viral excretion among preterm infants. J Infect Dis 164(3):476–482
39. Advisory Committee on, Immunization Practices, Fiore AE, Wasley A, Bell BP (2006) Prevention of hepatitis A through active or passive immunization: recommendations of the Advisory Committee on Immunization Practices (ACIP). MMWR Recomm Rep 55(RR-7):1–23
40. Steffen R, Kane MA, Shapiro CN, Billo N, Schoellhorn KJ, van Damme P (1994) Epidemiology and prevention of hepatitis A in travelers. JAMA 272(11):885–889
41. Steffen R (1992) Risk of hepatitis A in travellers. Vaccine 10(Suppl 1):69
42. O'Donovan D, Cooke RP, Joce R, Eastbury A, Waite J, Stene-Johansen K (2001) An outbreak of hepatitis A amongst injecting drug users. Epidemiol Infect 127(3):469–473
43. Hutin YJ, Sabin KM, Hutwagner LC, Schaben L, Shipp GM, Lord DM et al (2000) Multiple modes of hepatitis A virus transmission among methamphetamine users. Am J Epidemiol 152(2):186–192
44. Spada E, Genovese D, Tosti ME, Mariano A, Cuccuini M, Proietti L et al (2005) An outbreak of hepatitis A virus infection with a high case-fatality rate among injecting drug users. J Hepatol 43(6):958–964
45. Harkess J, Gildon B, Istre GR (1989) Outbreaks of hepatitis A among illicit drug users, Oklahoma, 1984–87. Am J Public Health 79(4):463–466
46. Grinde B, Stene-Johansen K, Sharma B, Hoel T, Jensenius M, Skaug K (1997) Characterisation of an epidemic of hepatitis A virus involving intravenous drug abusers – infection by needle sharing? J Med Virol 53(1):69–75
47. Kushel M, Hepatitis A (2017) Outbreak in California – addressing the root cause. N Engl J Med
48. Cotter SM, Sansom S, Long T, Koch E, Kellerman S, Smith F et al (2003) Outbreak of hepatitis A among men who have sex with men: implications for hepatitis A vaccination strategies. J Infect Dis 187(8):1235–1240

49. Stokes ML, Ferson MJ, Young LC (1997) Outbreak of hepatitis A among homosexual men in Sydney. Am J Public Health 87(12):2039–2041
50. Henning KJ, Bell E, Braun J, Barker ND (1995) A community-wide outbreak of hepatitis A: risk factors for infection among homosexual and bisexual men. Am J Med 99(2):132–136
51. Centers for DC (1992) Hepatitis A among homosexual men – United States, Canada, and Australia. MMWR Morb Mortal Wkly Rep 41(9):4
52. Villano SA, Nelson KE, Vlahov D, Purcell RH, Saah AJ, Thomas DL (1997) Hepatitis A among homosexual men and injection drug users: more evidence for vaccination. Clin Infect Dis 25(3):726–728
53. Fischer GE, Teshale EH, Miller C, Schumann C, Winter K, Elson F et al (2008) Hepatitis A among international adoptees and their contacts. Clin Infect Dis 47(6):812–814
54. Rimland D, Guest JL (2005) Response to hepatitis A vaccine in HIV patients in the HAART era. AIDS 19(15):1702–1704
55. Advisory Committee on Immunization Practices (ACIP) Centers for Disease Control, and Prevention (2007) Update: Prevention of hepatitis A after exposure to hepatitis A virus and in international travelers. Updated recommendations of the Advisory Committee on Immunization Practices (ACIP). MMWR Morb Mortal Wkly Rep 56(41):1080–1084
56. Tejada-Strop A, Costafreda MI, Dimitrova Z, Kaplan GG, Teo C (2017) Evaluation of potencies of immune globulin products against hepatitis A. JAMA Intern Med 177(3):430–432
57. Nelson NP (2017) Updated dosing instructions for immune globulin (Human) GamaSTAN S/D for hepatitis A virus prophylaxis. MMWR Morb Mortal Wkly Rep 66(36):959–960
58. Innis BL, Snitbhan R, Kunasol P, Laorakpongse T, Poopatanakool W, Kozik CA et al (1994) Protection against hepatitis A by an inactivated vaccine. JAMA 271(17):1328–1334
59. Werzberger A, Mensch B, Kuter B, Brown L, Lewis J, Sitrin R et al (1992) A controlled trial of a formalin-inactivated hepatitis A vaccine in healthy children. N Engl J Med 327(7):453–457
60. Ly KN, Klevens RM (2015) Trends in disease and complications of hepatitis A virus infection in the United States, 1999–2011: a new concern for adults. J Infect Dis 212(2):176–182
61. Gouvea AF, De Moraes-Pinto MI, Ono E, Dinelli MI, Machado DM, Weckx LY et al (2005) Immunogenicity and tolerability of hepatitis A vaccine in HIV-infected children. Clin Infect Dis 41(4):544–548
62. Lemon SM, Murphy PC, Provost PJ, Chalikonda I, Davide JP, Schofield TL et al (1997) Immunoprecipitation and virus neutralization assays demonstrate qualitative differences between protective antibody responses to inactivated hepatitis A vaccine and passive immunization with immune globulin. J Infect Dis 176(1):9–19
63. Victor JC, Monto AS, Surdina TY, Suleimenova SZ, Vaughan G, Nainan OV et al (2007) Hepatitis A vaccine versus immune globulin for postexposure prophylaxis. N Engl J Med 357(17):1685–1694
64. Victor JC, Surdina TY, Suleimenova SZ, Favorov MO, Bell BP, Monto AS (2006) Person-to-person transmission of hepatitis A virus in an urban area of intermediate endemicity: implications for vaccination strategies. Am J Epidemiol 163(3):204–210
65. Prevention of hepatitis A through active or passive immunization: recommendations of the advisory committee on immunization practices (ACIP). MMWR Recomm Rep. 48(RR-12):1–37 (1999)
66. Murphy TV, Denniston MM, Hill HA, McDonald M, Klevens MR, Elam-Evans L et al (2016) Progress toward eliminating hepatitis A disease in the United States. MMWR Suppl 65(1):29–41
67. WHO position paper on hepatitis A vaccines – June 2012. Wkly Epidemiol Rec 87(28):261–276 (2012)
68. Dagan R, Leventhal A, Anis E, Slater P, Ashur Y, Shouval D (2005) Incidence of hepatitis A in Israel following universal immunization of toddlers. JAMA 294(2):202–210
69. Teshale EH, Howard C, Grytdal S (2010) A large outbreak of hepatitis E in northern Uganda. Emerg Infect Dis 16:126–129
70. Guthmann JP, Klovstad H, Boccia D, Hamid N, Pinoges L, Nizou JY et al (2006) A large outbreak of hepatitis E among a displaced population in Darfur, Sudan, 2004: the role of water treatment methods. Clin Infect Dis 42(12):1685–1691
71. Rein DB, Stevens G, Theaker J, Wittenborn JS, Wiersma ST (2012) The global burden of hepatitis E virus. Hepatology 55:988–997
72. Labrique AB, Sikder SS, Krain LJ, West KP Jr, Christian P, Rashid M et al (2012) Hepatitis E, a vaccine-preventable cause of maternal deaths. Emerg Infect Dis 18(9):1401–1404
73. Gurley ES, Halder AK, Streatfield PK, Sazzad HM, Huda TM, Hossain MJ et al (2012) Estimating the burden of maternal and neonatal deaths associated with jaundice in Bangladesh: possible role of hepatitis E infection. Am J Public Health 102(12):2248–2254
74. Teo CG (2012) Fatal outbreaks of jaundice in pregnancy and the epidemic history of hepatitis E. Epidemiol Infect:1–21
75. Sazzad HMS, Labrique AB, Teo C, Luby SP, Gurley ES (2017) Surveillance at private laboratories identifies small outbreaks of hepatitis E in Urban Bangladesh. Am J Trop Med Hyg 96(2):395–399
76. Yugo DM, Meng X (2013) Hepatitis E virus: foodborne, waterborne and zoonotic transmission. Int J Environ Res Public Health 10(10):4507–4533
77. Teshale EH, Grytdal SP, Howard C, Barry V, Kamili S, Drobeniuc J et al (2010) Evidence of person-to-person transmission of hepatitis E virus during a large outbreak in Northern Uganda. Clin Infect Dis 50(7):1006–1010

78. Patel RC, Kamili S, Teshale E (2015) Hepatitis E virus infections in children age 0–15, Uganda outbreak, 2007. J Clin Virol 73:112–114
79. Stoszek SK, Abdel-Hamid M, Saleh DA, El Kafrawy S, Narooz S, Hawash Y et al (2006) High prevalence of hepatitis E antibodies in pregnant Egyptian women. Trans R Soc Trop Med Hyg 100(2):95–101
80. Kmush B, Wierzba T, Krain L, Nelson K, Labrique AB (2013) Epidemiology of hepatitis E in low- and middle-income countries of Asia and Africa. Semin Liver Dis 33(1):15–29
81. Tei S, Kitajima N, Takahashi K, Mishiro S (2003) Zoonotic transmission of hepatitis E virus from deer to human beings. Lancet 362(9381):371–373
82. Takahashi K, Kitajima N, Abe N, Mishiro S (2004) Complete or near-complete nucleotide sequences of hepatitis E virus genome recovered from a wild boar, a deer, and four patients who ate the deer. Virology 330(2):501–505
83. Colson P, Borentain P, Queyriaux B, Kaba M, Moal V, Gallian P et al (2010) Pig liver sausage as a source of hepatitis E virus transmission to humans. J Infect Dis 202(6):825–834
84. Yapa CM, Furlong C, Rosewell A, Ward KA, Adamson S, Shadbolt C et al (2016) First reported outbreak of locally acquired hepatitis E virus infection in Australia. Med J Aust 204(7):274
85. Said B, Ijaz S, Kafatos G, Booth L, Thomas HL, Walsh A et al (2009) Hepatitis E outbreak on cruise ship. Emerg Infect Dis 15(11):1738–1744
86. Kanai Y, Tsujikawa M, Yunoki M, Nishiyama S, Ikuta K, Hagiwara K (2010) Long-term shedding of hepatitis E virus in the feces of pigs infected naturally, born to sows with and without maternal antibodies. J Med Virol 82(1):69–76
87. Geng Y, Wang C, Zhao C, Yu X, Harrison TJ, Tian K et al (2010) Serological prevalence of hepatitis E virus in domestic animals and diversity of genotype 4 hepatitis E virus in China. Vector Borne Zoonotic Dis 10(8):765–770
88. Feagins AR, Opriessnig T, Guenette DK, Halbur PG, Meng XJ (2007) Detection and characterization of infectious Hepatitis E virus from commercial pig livers sold in local grocery stores in the USA. J Gen Virol 88:912–917
89. Bouwknegt M, Lodder-Verschoor F, van DP, Rutjes SA, de RH (2007) Hepatitis E virus RNA in commercial porcine livers in The Netherlands. J Food Prot 70(12):2889–2895
90. Wenzel JJ, Preiss J, Schemmerer M, Huber B, Plentz A, Jilg W (2011) Detection of hepatitis E virus (HEV) from porcine livers in Southeastern Germany and high sequence homology to human HEV isolates. J Clin Virol 52(1):50–54
91. Brassard J, Gagne MJ, Genereux M, Cote C (2012) Detection of human food-borne and zoonotic viruses on irrigated, field-grown strawberries. Appl Environ Microbiol 78(10):3763–3766
92. Meng XJ (2011) From barnyard to food table: the omnipresence of hepatitis E virus and risk for zoonotic infection and food safety. Virus Res 161(1):23–30
93. Anheyer-Behmenburg HE, Szabo K, Schotte U, Binder A, Klein G, Johne R (2017) Hepatitis E Virus in Wild Boars and Spillover Infection in Red and Roe Deer, Germany, 2013–2015. Emerg Infect Dis 23(1):130–133
94. Woo PCY, Lau SKP, Teng JLL, Tsang AKL, Joseph M, Wong EYM et al (2014) New hepatitis E virus genotype in camels, the Middle East. Emerg Infect Dis 20(6):1044–1048
95. Rasche A, Saqib M, Liljander AM, Bornstein S, Zohaib A, Renneker S et al (2016) Hepatitis E virus infection in Dromedaries, North and East Africa, United Arab Emirates, and Pakistan, 1983–2015. Emerg Infect Dis 22(7):1249–1252
96. Woo PCY, Lau SKP, Teng JLL, Cao K, Wernery U, Schountz T et al (2016) New Hepatitis E Virus genotype in bactrian camels, Xinjiang, China, 2013. Emerg Infect Dis 22(12):2219–2221
97. Cossaboom CM, Córdoba L, Dryman BA, Meng X (2011) Hepatitis E virus in rabbits, Virginia. USA Emerg Infect Dis 17(11):2047–2049
98. Li TC, Saito M, Ogura G, Ishibashi O, Miyamura T, Takeda N (2006) Serologic evidence for hepatitis E virus infection in mongoose. Am J Trop Med Hyg 74(5):932–936
99. Izopet J, Dubois M, Bertagnoli S, Lhomme S, Marchandeau S, Boucher S et al (2012) Hepatitis E virus strains in rabbits and evidence of a closely related strain in humans, France. Emerg Infect Dis serial on the Internet
100. Huang F, Li Y, Yu W, Jing S, Wang J, Long F et al (2016) Excretion of infectious hepatitis E virus into milk in cows imposes high risks of zoonosis. Hepatology 64(2):350–359
101. Meng XJ (2013) Zoonotic and foodborne transmission of hepatitis E virus. Semin Liver Dis 33(1):41–49
102. Dong C, Meng J, Dai X, Liang J, Feagins AR, Meng X et al (2011) Restricted enzooticity of hepatitis E virus genotypes 1 to 4 in the United States. J Clin Microbiol 49(12):4164–4172
103. Feagins AR, Opriessnig T, Guenette DK, Halbur PG, Meng XJ (2008) Inactivation of infectious hepatitis E virus present in commercial pig livers sold in local grocery stores in the United States. Int J Food Microbiol 123(1–2):32–37
104. Barnaud E, Rogée S, Garry P, Rose N, Pavio N (2012) Thermal inactivation of infectious hepatitis E virus in experimentally contaminated food. Appl Environ Microbiol 78(15):5153–5159
105. Emerson SU, Arankalle VA, Purcell RH (2005) Thermal stability of hepatitis E virus. J Infect Dis 192(5):930–933
106. Satake M, Matsubayashi K, Hoshi Y, Taira R, Furui Y, Kokudo N et al (2017) Unique clinical courses of

transfusion-transmitted hepatitis E in patients with immunosuppression. Transfusion 57:280
107. Matsubayashi K, Nagaoka Y, Sakata H, Sato S, Fukai K, Kato T et al (2004) Transfusion-transmitted hepatitis E caused by apparently indigenous hepatitis E virus strain in Hokkaido. Jpn Transfus 44(6):934–940
108. Mitsui T, Tsukamoto Y, Yamazaki C, Masuko K, Tsuda F, Takahashi M et al (2004) Prevalence of hepatitis E virus infection among hemodialysis patients in Japan: evidence for infection with a genotype 3 HEV by blood transfusion. J Med Virol 74(4):563–572
109. Nelson KE (2014) Transmission of hepatitis E virus by transfusion: what is the risk? Transfusion 54(1):8–10
110. Sakata H, Matsubayashi K, Takeda H, Sato S, Kato T, Hino S et al (2008) A nationwide survey for hepatitis E virus prevalence in Japanese blood donors with elevated alanine aminotransferase. Transfusion 48(12):2568–2576
111. Hewitt PE, Ijaz S, Brailsford SR, Brett R, Dicks S, Haywood B et al (2014) Hepatitis E virus in blood components: a prevalence and transmission study in southeast England. Lancet 26
112. Tedder RS, Ijaz S, Kitchens S (2017) Hepatitis E Risks: pigs or blood-that is the question. Transfusion 57:267
113. Domanović D, Tedder R, Blümel J, Zaaijer H, Gallian P, Niederhauser C et al (2017) Hepatitis E and blood donation safety in selected European countries: a shift to screening? Euro Surveill 22(16)
114. Slot E, Hogema BM, Riezebos-Brilman A, Kok TM, Molier M, Zaaijer HL (2013) Silent hepatitis E virus infection in Dutch blood donors, 2011 to 2012. Euro Surveill 18(31):20550
115. Wang M, He M, Wu B, Ke L, Han T, Wang J et al (2017) The association of elevated alanine aminotransferase levels with hepatitis E virus infections among blood donors in China. Transfusion 57(2):273–279
116. Krain LJ, Atwell JE, Nelson KE, Labrique AB (2014) Fetal and neonatal health consequences of vertically transmitted hepatitis E virus infection. Am J Trop Med Hyg 90(2):365–370
117. Patra S, Kumar A, Trivedi SS, Puri M, Sarin SK (2007) Maternal and fetal outcomes in pregnant women with acute hepatitis E virus infection. Ann Intern Med 147(1):28–33
118. Khuroo MS, Kamili S (2003) Aetiology, clinical course and outcome of sporadic acute viral hepatitis in pregnancy. J Viral Hepat 10(1):61–69
119. Rivero-Juarez A, Frias M, Rodriguez-Cano D, Cuenca-Lopez F, Rivero A (2016) Isolation of hepatitis E virus from breast milk during acute infection. Clin Infect Dis 62(11):1464
120. Meng XJ, Wiseman B, Elvinger F, Guenette DK, Toth TE, Engle RE et al (2002) Prevalence of antibodies to hepatitis E virus in veterinarians working with swine and in normal blood donors in the United States and other countries. J Clin Microbiol 40(1):117–122
121. Vaidya SR, Tilekar BN, Walimbe AM, Arankalle VA (2003) Increased risk of hepatitis E in sewage workers from India. J Occup Environ Med 45(11):1167–1170
122. De Schryver A, De Schrijver K, François G, Hambach R, van Sprundel M, Tabibi R et al (2015) Hepatitis E virus infection: an emerging occupational risk? Occup Med (Lond) 65(8):667–672
123. Schielke A, Ibrahim V, Czogiel I, Faber M, Schrader C, Dremsek P et al (2015) Hepatitis E virus antibody prevalence in hunters from a district in Central Germany, 2013: a cross-sectional study providing evidence for the benefit of protective gloves during disembowelling of wild boars. BMC Infect Dis 15:440
124. Sarkar S, Rivera EM, Engle RE, Nguyen HT, Schechterly CA, Alter HJ et al (2015) An epidemiologic investigation of a case of acute hepatitis E. J Clin Microbiol 53(11):3547–3552
125. Verghese VP, Robinson JL (2014) A systematic review of hepatitis E virus infection in children. Clin Infect Dis 59(5):689–697
126. Kuniholm MH, Purcell RH, McQuillan GM, Engle RE, Wasley A, Nelson KE (2009) Epidemiology of hepatitis E virus in the United States: results from the Third National Health and Nutrition Examination Survey, 1988–1994. J Infect Dis 200(1):48–56
127. Zhang L, Yesupriya A, Chang M, Teshale E, Teo C (2015) Apolipoprotein E and protection against hepatitis E viral infection in American non-Hispanic blacks. Hepatology 62(5):1346–1352
128. Krain LJ, Nelson KE, Labrique AB (2014) Host immune status and response to hepatitis E virus infection. Clin Microbiol Rev 27(1):139–165
129. Lachish T, Erez O, Daudi N, Shouval D, Schwartz E (2015) Acute hepatitis E virus in pregnant women in Israel and in other industrialized countries. J Clin Virol 73:20–24
130. Kamar N, Rostaing L, Izopet J (2013) Hepatitis E virus infection in immunosuppressed patients: natural history and therapy. Semin Liver Dis 33(1):62–70
131. Kamar N, Selves J, Mansuy JM, Ouezzani L, Peron JM, Guitard J et al (2008) Hepatitis E virus and chronic hepatitis in organ-transplant recipients. N Engl J Med 358(8):811–817
132. Crum-Cianflone N, Curry J, Drobeniuc J, Weintrob A, Landrum M, Ganesan A et al (2012) Hepatitis E virus infection in HIV-infected persons. Emerg Infect Dis 18(3):502–506
133. Geng Y, Zhang H, Huang W, Harrison T J, Geng K, Li Z et al (2014) Persistent hepatitis e virus genotype 4 infection in a child with acute lymphoblastic leukemia. Hepat Mon 14(1):e15618
134. Kuniholm MH, Ong E, Hogema BM, Koppelman M, Anastos K, Peters MG et al (2016) Acute and chronic hepatitis E virus infection in human immunodeficiency virus-infected U.S. women. Hepatology 63(3):712–720

135. Kamar N, Garrouste C, Haagsma EB, Garrigue V, Pischke S, Chauvet C et al (2011) Factors associated with chronic Hepatitis in patients with Hepatitis E virus infection who have received solid organ transplants. Gastroenterology 140:1481
136. Kamar N, Izopet J, Tripon S, Bismuth M, Hillaire S, Dumortier J et al (2014) Ribavirin for chronic hepatitis E virus infection in transplant recipients. N Engl J Med 370(12):1111–1120
137. Dalton HR, Kamar N, van Eijk JJ, Mclean BN, Cintas P, Bendall RP et al (2016) Hepatitis E virus and neurological injury. Nat Rev Neurol 12(2):77–85
138. Kamar N, Bendall RP, Peron JM, Cintas P, Prudhomme L, Mansuy JM et al (2011) Hepatitis E virus and neurologic disorders. Emerg Infect Dis 17(2):173–179
139. Shukla P, Nguyen HT, Torian U, Engle RE, Faulk K, Dalton HR et al (2011) Cross-species infections of cultured cells by hepatitis E virus and discovery of an infectious virus-host recombinant. Proc Natl Acad Sci U S A 108(6):2438–2443
140. Hakim MS, Wang W, Bramer WM, Geng J, Huang F, de Man RA et al (2017) The global burden of hepatitis E outbreaks: a systematic review. Liver Int 37(1):19–31
141. Guerrero-Latorre L, Gonzales-Gustavson E, Hundesa A, Sommer R, Rosina G (2016) UV disinfection and flocculation-chlorination sachets to reduce hepatitis E virus in drinking water. Int J Hyg Environ Health 219(4–5):405–411
142. Shrestha MP, Scott RM, Joshi DM, Mammen MP, Joshi DM, Thapa GB, Thapa N et al (2007) Safety and efficacy of a recombinant hepatitis E vaccine. N Engl J Med 356(9):895–903
143. Zhu FC, Zhang J, Zhang XF, Zhou C, Wang ZZ, Huang SJ et al (2010) Efficacy and safety of a recombinant hepatitis E vaccine in healthy adults: a large-scale, randomised, double-blind placebo-controlled, phase 3 trial. Lancet 376(9744):895–902
144. Li SW, Zhang J, Li YM, Ou SH, Huang GY, He ZQ et al (2005) A bacterially expressed particulate hepatitis E vaccine: antigenicity, immunogenicity and protectivity on primates. Vaccine 23(22):2893–2901
145. Zhang J, Zhang XF, Huang SJ, Wu T, Hu YM, Wang ZZ et al (2015) Long-term efficacy of a hepatitis E vaccine. N Engl J Med 372(10):914–922
146. Nelson KE, Heaney CD, Labrique AB, Kmush BL, Krain LJ (2016) Hepatitis E: prevention and treatment. Curr Opin Infect Dis 29(5):478–485

3 Epidemiology of Viral Hepatitis B, C, and D: A Global View

Hwai-I Yang, Mei-Hsuan Lee, Jessica Liu, and Hui-Han Hu

Abstract

Viral hepatitis constitutes a great burden of public health in the world. In 2016, the World Health Assembly approved a global strategy to achieve elimination of this threat by 2030. To achieve this goal, countries and regions need to reduce incidence and mortality by 90% and 65%, respectively, by 2030. Five strategic directions have been proposed, with understanding the epidemiology of viral hepatitis being the first step toward elimination. Hepatitis B and C are responsible for 96% of all hepatitis mortality. Hepatitis D is an important cofactor of hepatitis B virus infection.

H.-I. Yang (✉)
Genomics Research Center, Academia Sinica, Taipei, Taiwan

Institute of Clinical Medicine, National Yang-Ming University, Taipei, Taiwan
e-mail: hiyang@gate.sinica.edu.tw

M.-H. Lee
Institute of Clinical Medicine, National Yang-Ming University, Taipei, Taiwan

J. Liu
Perinatal Epidemiology and Health Outcomes Research Unit, Division of Neonatology, Department of Pediatrics, Stanford University School of Medicine and Lucile Packard Children's Hospital, Palo Alto, CA, USA

California Perinatal Quality Care Collaborative, Palo Alto, CA, USA

H.-H. Hu
Genomics Research Center, Academia Sinica, Taipei, Taiwan

The World Health Assembly adopted the first *Global Health Sector Strategy on Viral Hepatitis, 2016–2021* in 2016, which has a vision of eliminating viral hepatitis as a public health problem. The targets for the year 2020 include a 30% reduction in new cases of chronic viral hepatitis B and C infections and a 10% reduction in viral hepatitis B deaths. By 2030 the global targets are to reduce new viral hepatitis infections by 90% and reduce mortality due to viral hepatitis by 65% (Fig. 3.1).

To achieve the 2030 goals, five strategic directions are proposed. These strategic directions include (1) information for focused action (what is the situation); (2) interventions for impact (what service should be delivered); (3) delivering for equity (how can these services be delivered); (4) financing for sustainability (how can the costs of delivering the package of services be met); and (5) innovation for acceleration (how can the trajectory of the response be changed). This strategy helps outline the priority actions to be taken by countries and by the World Health Organization (WHO), with respect to region-specific hepatitis epidemics, national priorities, and country contexts and taking national policies, jurisdiction, and legislation into consideration.

M.-H. Chang, K. B. Schwarz (eds.), *Viral Hepatitis in Children*,
https://doi.org/10.1007/978-981-13-0050-9_3

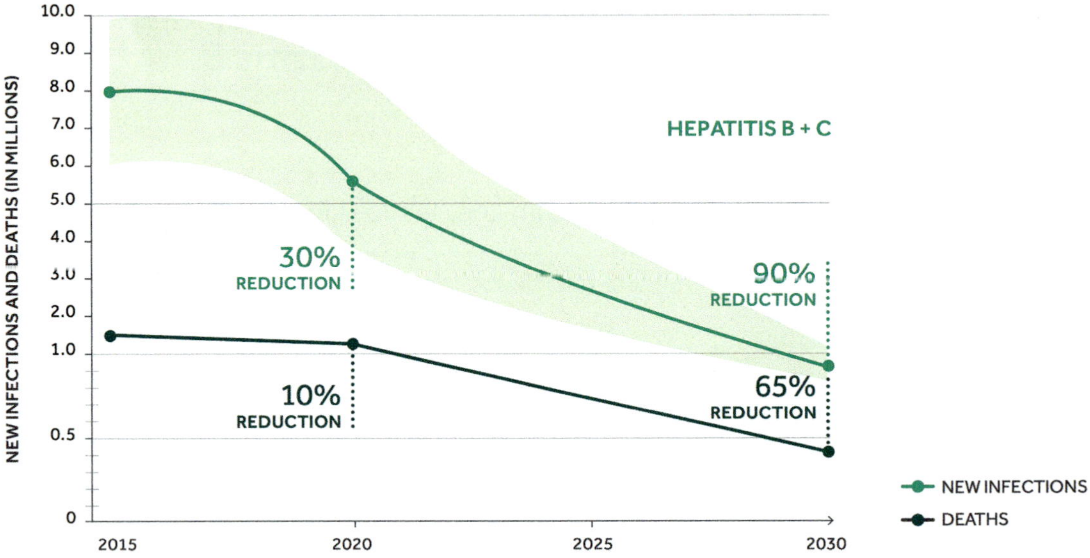

Fig. 3.1 World Health Organization (WHO) targets for reducing new cases of and deaths from chronic viral hepatitis B and C infection. (From WHO, global health sector strategy on viral hepatitis 2016–2021, June 2016)

Understanding the epidemiology of viral hepatitis is the first step toward elimination. A total of five hepatitis viruses have been identified, referred to as types A, B, C, D, and E, which caused 1.34 million deaths in the human population in 2015. The five hepatitis viruses are distinct with regard to modes of transmission, populations affected, and health outcomes (Fig. 3.2). Hepatitis A and E are typically caused by ingestion of contaminated food or water. Hepatitis B, C, and D usually occur as a result of parenteral contact with infected body fluids. All the hepatitis viruses can cause acute hepatitis, while only hepatitis B, C, and D viruses cause chronic hepatitis, which may progress to cirrhosis and primary liver cancer. Hepatitis B and C are of greatest concern as they are responsible for 96% of all hepatitis mortality. This chapter focuses on the epidemiology and global view of hepatitis B, C, and D.

3.1 Epidemiology and Global View of Hepatitis B

Hepatitis B virus (HBV) infection is a severe global health issue due to its geographically widespread distribution and its potential to cause advanced liver diseases such as cirrhosis and hepatocellular carcinoma (HCC). Understanding of the epidemiology and the natural history of HBV infection is necessary for disease prevention and intervention.

3.1.1 Global Distribution of HBV Infection

Worldwide estimates suggest that more than 2 billion people have been infected with HBV, and among them, 248 million are suffering from chronic HBV (CHB) infection, which is defined as being hepatitis B surface antigen (HBsAg)

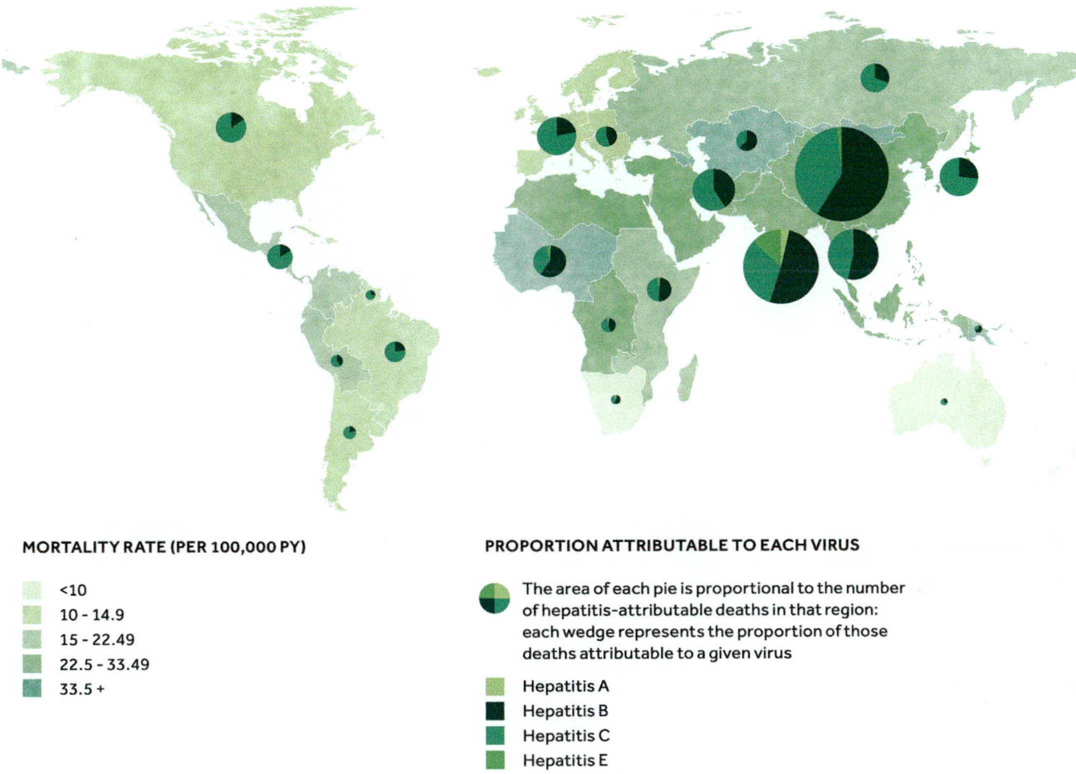

Fig. 3.2 Regional distribution of deaths from viral hepatitis. (From WHO, global health sector strategy on viral hepatitis 2016–2021, June 2016)

Springer Nature remains neutral with regard to jurisdictional claims in published maps and institutional affiliations

positive [1]. Globally, CHB infection accounts for approximately 30% of all cirrhosis and 53% of all HCC cases, [2] and 15–25% of CHB patients eventually die from these two advanced diseases [1]. In addition, it has been estimated that 600,000 deaths per year can be attributed to HBV infection [3].

The worldwide prevalence of HBsAg positivity is estimated to be 3.61% [1]. However, the prevalence varies greatly from one WHO region to another (Fig. 3.3). The highest prevalence can be found in most African (especially Sub-Saharan Africa), Western Pacific (including China, Taiwan, and most Pacific Islands), and Southeastern Asian regions, where the prevalence is as high as 8–15%. About 45% of HBV-infected individuals reside in these regions, and their lifetime risk of infection is more than 60%. The prevalence of HBsAg positivity is moderate in Eastern Mediterranean (including South-Central and Southwestern Asia), European (Southern and Eastern regions), and American (Central and Southern) regions, where prevalence rates range from 2% to 7%. Forty-three percent of HBV-infected individuals live in these regions, and their lifetime risk of infection is between 20% and 60%. The remaining 12% of HBV-infected individuals are located in low-prevalence areas, where the prevalence is less than 2%, and their lifetime risk of infection is less than 20%. These low-prevalence areas include the United States, Western Europe, and Australia [1, 4–6].

Over time, there has been an overall decrease in the prevalence of HBsAg positivity in most WHO regions and countries [4]. The Eastern Mediterranean region has seen a strong decrease in prevalence, while Eastern and Western Europe show stable high and low prevalences, respectively. Meanwhile,

A

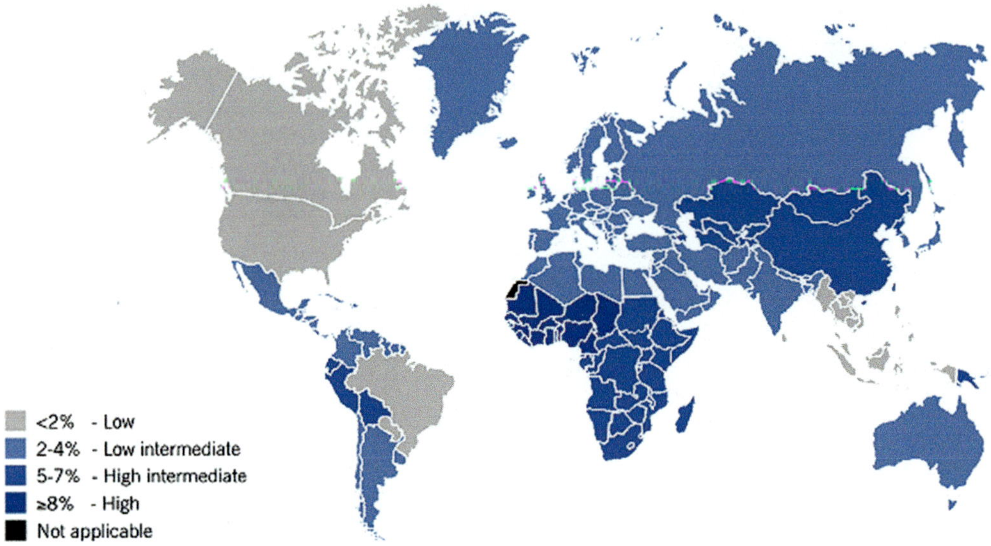

B

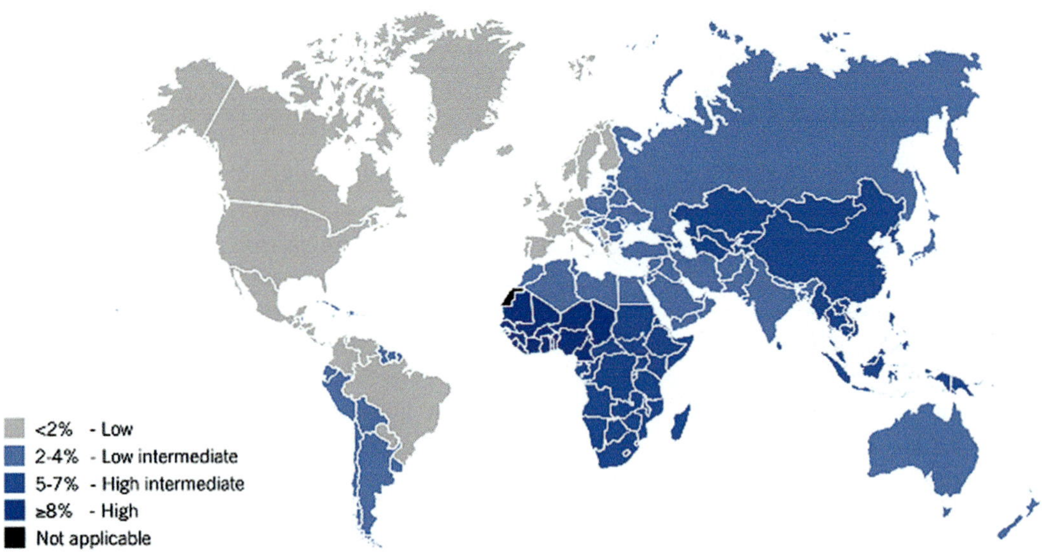

Fig. 3.3 Prevalence of chronic hepatitis B infection (**a**) in children 5–9 years old and (**b**) in adults 19–49 years old in 2005. (From WHO, guidelines for the prevention, care, and treatment of persons with chronic hepatitis B infection, March 2015)

Springer Nature remains neutral with regard to jurisdictional claims in published maps and institutional affiliations

Southeastern Asian and Western Pacific regions have seen low to medium reductions in prevalence, with the most prominent reductions occurring in China and Malaysia [1, 7]. However, there has been a notable increase in prevalence in African and Eastern European regions [1].

3.1.2 Global Distribution of HBV Genotypes

Due to the lack of a proofreading function in the HBV reverse transcriptase, transcription errors occur during viral replication, which result in different HBV genotypes, subgenotypes, mutants, and recombinants. To date, ten HBV genotypes, which are dispersed across different geographical regions, have been identified [8]. Genotype A is commonly found in Western and Sub-Saharan Africa, Northern and Northwestern Europe, North America, and India. Genotypes B and C are endemic to Asian regions. Genotype D is widespread in Africa, Eastern Europe, Mediterranean countries, the Middle East, Central Asia, and India. Genotype E is prevalent in Western Africa, while genotypes F and H are common in South and Central America. Genotype G is most predominant in France, Germany, Mexico, and the United States. Recently, genotype I was reported in Vietnam and Laos, and genotype J was identified on Japan's Ryukyu Islands [5, 6, 8–13].

In addition to different geographical distributions, HBV genotypes also have different impacts on disease and clinical progression, response to antiviral treatment, and prognosis [8]. Several studies have shown that HBV genotypes A and D have higher rates of progression from acute to chronic infection than genotypes B and C and that genotype A is significantly associated with chronicity [10, 14]. In Asian regions, it was reported that the rate of chronicity was higher in genotype B than in genotype C [15]. A Taiwanese study showed that the spontaneous HBV e antigen (HBeAg) seroconversion rate is higher in genotype B than in genotype C [16]. Regarding response rates to interferon treatment, they have been reported to be greater for genotypes A and B than for genotypes C and D, while genotype E is the most difficult to treat [17, 18]. For severe liver diseases, genotype C is widely accepted to be associated with higher risks of cirrhosis and HCC [19].

3.1.3 Transmission Routes and Risk of Chronic HBV Infection

There are two major routes of HBV transmission. Perinatal transmission, in which HBV is passed from infected mothers to their newborns, accounts for the majority of worldwide transmissions. It has been reported that 85% of infants born to HBeAg-seropositive mothers as well as mothers with high viral loads became chronically infected, while 32% of those born to HBeAg-seronegative mothers became chronically infected [20]. Another route of HBV transmission is horizontal transmission, which occurs through open wounds or scratches, blood transfusions, unprotected sexual contact, or risky behaviors such as sharing of unsterilized needles, tattooing, and body piercing during childhood or adulthood [4]. It has been widely reported that the probability of becoming chronically infected increases with decreasing age of first infection. Up to 90% of individuals with perinatal infections become chronically infected, while approximately 20–60% of individuals infected during early childhood become chronic carriers, and only 5–10% of infected adults become chronic carriers [21, 22]. Therefore, in endemic regions, 40–50% of chronic HBV infection originates from perinatal transmission. In areas with moderate endemicity, chronic HBV infection is usually caused by transmission during early childhood. In areas with low HBV prevalence, however, chronic HBV infection is typically acquired through transmission during adulthood [6, 23, 24].

3.1.4 Long-Term Consequences of Hepatitis B Virus Infection

Infection with the hepatitis B virus is a particularly serious threat to global public health, due to its widespread geographical distribution and its potential for serious clinical consequences such as cirrhosis, HCC, and liver-related death [24–26]. In addition, based on the comprehensive assessment of both epidemiological and mechanistic evidence, the International Agency for Research on Cancer (IARC) has notably also classified the HBV as a Group 1 human carcinogen with sufficient evidence to prove its causation of HCC [27]. In a landmark study of 22,707 Taiwanese men, men that were seropositive for HBsAg had a 223-fold increased risk of developing HCC, compared to non-infected men [25, 28]. Among individuals that are chronically infected with HBV, however, results from long-term prospective studies have shown that the progression of hepatitis B infection toward long-term clinical consequences is typically characterized by interactions between crucial viral, environmental, and host factors [29–32].

3.1.4.1 Cirrhosis

Specifically, risk factors that have been shown to affect progression of HBV-infected individuals to cirrhosis include age, male sex, viral genotypes, HBeAg serostatus, HBV DNA, HBsAg levels in the serum, and ALT levels [30, 31, 33, 34]. Studies from the Risk Evaluation of Viral Load Elevation and Associated Liver Disease/Cancer in HBV (REVEAL-HBV) study and other long-term prospective studies have shown that HBV DNA levels are a major driver of disease progression. Specifically, the risk for cirrhosis has been shown to increase with higher HBV DNA levels among HBV carriers, even after adjustment for age, sex, and other viral factors and stratification by sex, alcohol consumption, and cigarette smoking [33]. More recently, prediction models incorporating quantitative HBsAg levels have also been able to increase prediction accuracy for cirrhosis [31].

3.1.4.2 HCC

Many studies have examined cofactors of HBV-related HCC. Viral factors shown to affect progression to HCC include age, male sex, viral genotypes, HBeAg serostatus, HBV DNA, HBsAg levels in the serum, and seroclearance of HBeAg, HBV DNA, and HBsAg [29–32, 35–37]. An early study of individuals with chronic hepatitis B found that HBeAg seropositivity was associated with significantly increased risk for HCC, implying that active viral replication was a relevant determinant for HCC [37]. In a later landmark study, this was confirmed when a strong biological gradient of HCC risk was observed across serum HBV DNA levels. The corresponding relative risks with 95% confidence intervals were 1.0 (referent), 1.1 (0.5–2.3), 2.3 (1.1–4.9), 6.6 (3.3–13.1), and 6.1 (2.9–12.7), respectively, for serum HBV DNA levels of <300, 300–9999, 10,000–99,999, 100,000–999,999, and $\geq$ 1,000,000 copies/mL [38]. In addition, several studies in recent years have confirmed the role of quantitative HBsAg levels in predicting HCC risk, independent of conventional risk factors such as ALT and HBV DNA viral load. Specifically, higher serum HBsAg levels have been able to predict higher risk for HCC, even among individuals with low viral loads [31, 36]. Thus, as higher levels of seromarkers have been shown to predict higher HCC risk, it is important to also highlight the importance of the seroclearance of HBeAg, HBV DNA, and HBsAg, each of which has been shown to predict a decreased risk of HCC, while persistence of each is also predictive of an increased risk for HCC [32].

In addition to viral factors, studies have also shown that environmental factors such as a positive family history, increased alcohol consumption, and metabolic syndrome are also associated with increased risk for developing HCC [39–42]. Lastly, more recent studies have also focused on the role of host genetic factors in predicting a host's risk for HBV-related HCC. Notably, the role of the S267F variant on NTCP, the putative receptor for HBV, in modulating HBV infection and risk for HCC has been recently confirmed in the REVAL-HBV cohort [43].

3.1.5 The Era of Personalized Medicine

With the confirmation of a myriad of risk factors for HBV-related clinical outcomes such as cirrhosis and HCC, recent research has begun to focus on the establishment of risk calculation tools, which would allow for a personalized assessment of risk based on the clinical profile of each HBV-infected patient. Several tools have been created, both for the prediction of HBeAg, HBV DNA, and HBsAg seroclearance and for the prediction of cirrhosis and HCC [31, 44–49]. To date, only risk calculators for HCC have been robustly developed and externally validated in clinical settings. The easy-to-use REACH-B risk score is based on noninvasive clinical characteristics and has helped clinicians and HBV carriers to stratify their HCC risks according to their personal profiles, including age, sex, family history, alcohol consumption, serum ALT levels, HBeAg serostatus, serum HBV DNA, HBsAg levels, and HBV genotypes, and has recently been revised to incorporate quantitative HBsAg levels [48–50].

In conclusion, it is clear that infection with the hepatitis B virus poses a serious threat to global public health, and even with the availability of an effective vaccine and significantly low rates of new infection, high rates of chronic infection continue to plague highly endemic areas, and the long-term consequences of HBV infection are being seen with high rates of cirrhosis and HCC in HBV-endemic areas. With such robust and clinically applicable tools being developed through sound epidemiological research, the hope is that the dangerous consequences of HBV infection can be better anticipated, or even prevented, reducing the global disease burden resulting from the hepatitis B virus.

3.2 Epidemiology and Global View of Hepatitis C

Hepatitis C virus (HCV) is recognized as a major cause of chronic liver disease. Generally, liver cirrhosis occurs in 20 to 30% of patients with chronic HCV infection after two to three decades [51]. Once cirrhosis occurs, HCC develops in 1–4% of these patients per year [52]. In addition, HCV is estimated to be attributable for one third of HCC cases globally [53], representing a great public health burden. The transmission of HCV primarily occurs through blood contact.

3.2.1 Prevalence of HCV Infection

The global prevalence of HCV infection is estimated to be 2–3%, which equates to 130–180 million people living with HCV infection [54]. The seroprevalence of HCV has considerable geographical variation [55]. The estimated prevalence of HCV infection in economically developed countries is relatively low at 1–2% of the adult population, whereas it is up to 5–10% in less developed countries [56, 57]. Regions with the highest HCV prevalence include African, Eastern Mediterranean, Southeast Asian, and Western Pacific regions [56, 57], while areas with lower prevalence include the North American, Northern and Western European, and Australian regions. In Africa, countries with the highest HCV prevalence include Egypt and Cameroon, where the prevalence rates are reported to be higher than 10% [58, 59].

The estimated absolute number of individuals with HCV infection is 29.8 million in China, 18.2 million in India, 11.8 million in Egypt, 9.4 million in Pakistan, and 9.4 million in Indonesia [58]. Although many countries in Asia have a low to intermediate prevalence of HCV, highly endemic areas have at least 50% of people with HCV infection [60].

3.2.2 HCV Transmission Routes

3.2.2.1 Injection Drug Use

The prevalence of HCV infection among intravenous drug users ranges from 31% to 98% [61]. Illicit injection drug use is a primary transmission route for HCV infection in developed countries and accounts for approximately 60% and 80% of HCV infection in the United States [62] and Australia [63], respectively. For example, anti-HCV seroprevalence among injection drug users in the San Francisco Bay Area was higher with each decade of drug use, rising from 66.2% among subjects who had injected drugs for less than 10 years to 98.7% among those who had been injecting for 30 years or longer [64]. Drug users who had ever borrowed a needle had a 2.56 (95% CI = 1.2–5.5)-fold increased risk to be infected by HCV [65].

Sharing contaminated injection equipment among injection drug users was the main HCV transmission route. Injection drug users who never used syringe exchanges had a lower cumulative incidence of HCV than those who used the exchange (15% vs. 21–26%) [66]. Drug solutions mixed with a syringe previously used for injection, clean syringes drawing solutions from containers or filters previously used by HCV-infected injectors, or cleaning syringes, containers, or filters with contaminated rinse water may result in the cross-contamination of drug preparation and injection equipment [67].

3.2.2.2 Recipients of Blood and Blood Products

In the mid-1970s, it was discovered that the blood supply was contaminated with an unidentified agent causing posttransfusion non-A and non-B hepatitis [68]. Patients with hemophilia, thalassemia, cardiac surgery, or chronic renal disease had increased risk for posttransfusion hepatitis [69–71]. However, these days, posttransfusion hepatitis C has become relatively rare in developed countries. The incidence of transfusion-associated hepatitis from 1970 to 1998 decreased from 33% to nearly nonexistent HCV transmission due to effective blood donor screening [72]. One multicenter study conducted in Baltimore showed a reduction of posttransfusion hepatitis from 45 per 100,000 units transfused in 1985 to 3 per 100,000 units transfused in 1990 [73]. Compared to individuals who received a transfusion after 1992, patients who had a transfusion history or high volume of blood loss related to surgery before 1992 had a higher risk of being anti-HCV seropositive [74, 75].

HCV screening in blood products has not been feasible in developing countries, and receiving infected blood products remains a major source of HCV infection. Most of these countries are located in Africa and Asia, where blood safety is threatened by poverty, insufficient instruments and laboratory reagents, limited numbers of trained professionals, traditional cultural barriers, and difficulties in mobilizing volunteer donors [76, 77]. According to the Human Development Index (HDI), which ranks countries on the basis of life expectancy, literacy, and gross domestic product, countries with low HDI had 63% paid donors in their blood donor systems and only 51.3% of units screened for anti-HCV, compared with only 4% paid donors and nearly 100% of units screened for anti-HCV in countries with high HDI [78].

3.2.2.3 Unsafe Medical Injections

Unsafe medical injection, which is defined as the reuse of syringes or needles from patient to patient without sterilization, is also one of the primary modes of HCV transmission. Unsafe injections resulted in approximately 2.3–4.7 million HCV infections annually [79]. Transmission of HCV through contaminated injection equipment has been a major transmission source in most developing countries. One of the most well-known cases of unsafe medical injections was the massive Egyptian anti-schistosomal treatment campaign, later discontinued in the 1980s, which became the world's largest iatrogenic transmission of a blood-borne pathogen known to date and resulted in a large reservoir of chronic HCV infection and a high HCV seroprevalence [80]. More than 3 million injections were given per year to over 300,000 individuals between 1964 and 1969, and by the mid-1980s, the campaign had infected 10% of the entire adult population in Egypt with hepatitis C [80, 81].

Medical injection played an important role in the spread of HCV in the past. The age-specific prevalence is low in younger adults but is increased in older people [82–85], implying that the risk of infection was greatest around 30–50 years ago [86]. A community-based study found that the population attributable risk of medical injection for HCV infection was 57% [85]. Receiving injections by non-licensed practitioners was also more common in anti-HCV seropositives [87], suggesting that unlicensed or nonprofessional healthcare providers may have given medical injections without standard sterilization procedures.

3.2.2.4 Mother-to-Infant Transmission

In a landmark study in which HCV infection was observed in three generations of one family, vertical transmission of HCV was confirmed by molecular evolutionary method [88]. The mother-to-infant transmission rate ranges from 0.6% to 19.4% [89]. In the vast majority of cases, infants passively acquire the maternal antibody at birth. The antibody continues to be detectable in infants and then gradually clears by 12–18 months of age [90]. Testing for HCV RNA is generally used as a marker for the detection of HCV-infected infants [91]. Mothers with detectable HCV RNA or elevated serum HCV RNA levels had a higher likelihood to transmit HCV to their babies than those with undetectable HCV RNA [92]. There is also no obvious association between different HCV genotypes and the rate of vertical transmission [90, 93]. Moreover, there are no significant associations between mode of delivery and breastfeeding on HCV vertical transmission in HCV-infected mothers [94].

3.2.2.5 Sexual Transmission

Sexual transmission, which involves the exchange of bodily secretions or infected blood across mucosal surfaces, is one other possible mode of HCV transmission. Spouses with HCV-infected partners have a twofold higher risk of being HCV seropositive than spouses without HCV-infected partners [95]. In some studies, HCV genotypes were used to evaluate anti-HCV antibody-concordant couples, and the concordance rate was 50–82% in couples who both had detectable HCV RNA for HCV genotyping [95–97]. Moreover, among commercial sex workers, the prevalence of anti-HCV seropositivity ranged from 1% to 10% and was 2.9% to 13% among men who have sex with men [98]. The risk of HCV infection was highly correlated with the intensity of sexual exposures, including years of sexual exposure or numbers of sexual partners [99]. Similar to vertical transmission, individuals with high serum HCV RNA levels [100] or who were coinfected with HIV [101] had high rates of HCV transmission to their sexual partners. Partners of persons with chronic hepatitis C should be tested for anti-HCV and should be advised not to share percutaneous exposures to blood items.

3.2.2.6 Other Potential Risk Factors

There are several other biological routes associated with HCV transmission because of various human activities involving potential percutaneous exposure to blood or bodily fluids. These transmission routes include acupuncture [85], tattoos [102], cosmetic procedures [103], body piercings, commercial barbering, and religious or cultural practices such as circumcision [104].

3.2.3 Long-Term Consequences of HCV Infection

3.2.3.1 HCV Infection and Hepatic Diseases

The ability of HCV infection to increase the risk for liver-related outcomes is well documented, and clinical outcomes after HCV infection are highly variable. Among individuals with HCV infection, around 1.3–51% may develop liver cirrhosis and 0.1–5.3% may develop HCC over the course of 3.9–25 years [105, 106]. Based on the Risk Evaluation of Viral Load Elevation and Associated Liver Disease/Cancer in HCV (REVEAL-HCV) study cohort, the cumulative lifetime (30–75 years old) incidence of HCC for men and women is 23.7% and 16.7%, respectively [107]. Elevated serum levels of HCV RNA and alanine aminotransferase (ALT) increase the risk for HCC after long-term follow-up [108]. The lifetime risk for HCC is 3.6% for those who have had spontaneous viral clearance (undetectable HCV RNA) and 24.8% for those who have continued chronic HCV infection (detectable HCV RNA). In addition, for individuals with serum ALT levels ≦15 U/L, 16–45 U/L, and >45 U/L, the cumulative lifetime risk for HCC is 11.6%, 18.5%, and 34.3%, respectively [109]. Compared with other subtypes, individuals infected by HCV subtype 1b have further increased risk of HCC. The cumulative lifetime risk for HCC is 19.2% and 29.7% for subtypes non-1b and 1b ($p < 0.001$), respectively [110]. These seromarkers could also predict long-term development of HCC and had the potential to be used for risk stratification of HCV-infected patients in order to identify those in need of intensive care.

In order to integrate several important risk factors and predict the incidence of HCC, risk prediction models were developed for HCV-infected subjects [111]. Patients' risk profiles used in the prediction models include age, ALT, the ratio of aspartate aminotransferase to ALT, serum HCV RNA levels, the presence of cirrhosis, and HCV genotypes. Using patients' clinical profiles, risk scores are calculated, and the corresponding predicted risk for HCC can be determined. These risk prediction models are validated in another external HCV-infected community-based cohort, and results show the predictive accuracy of the prediction models to be around 70–73% [111]. In a hospital-based cohort that enrolled HCV-infected patients with antiviral treatment and compared their risk of HCC at baseline and after treatment using the risk prediction model [112], the authors found a significant reduction in the risk for HCC after treatment-induced RNA clearance. However, the risk for HCC did not change from baseline to after treatment among patients who did not experience treatment-induced RNA clearance. These findings suggest that the risk of HCC could be reduced with effective antiviral treatment.

3.2.3.2 HCV Infection and Extrahepatic Diseases

The large community-based prospective REVEAL-HCV study also found that patients with chronic hepatitis C infection, defined as having detectable serum HCV RNA, had increased risk of death from both hepatic and extrahepatic diseases, when compared to patients either seronegative for anti-HCV or seropositive for anti-HCV but with undetectable HCV RNA [113]. For example, HCV infection was reported to be associated with the incidence of cryoglobulinemia [114] and non-Hodgkin's lymphoma [114, 115].

Several studies have also shown that patients with HCV infection have a higher risk of diabetes mellitus than uninfected patients, suggesting that HCV may interfere with the insulin signaling pathway [116]. The National Health and Nutrition Examination Survey found that subjects with HCV infection have an increased likelihood of having diabetes, with an odds ratio of 3.8 (95% CI: 1.8 to 7.8), after controlling for potential risk factors [117]. Another large-scale study enrolled 10,975 subjects in an HBV- and HCV-endemic area and showed that the prevalence of HCV viremia was significantly different among diabetic and nondiabetic patients (6.9% vs. 4.5%, $p < 0.001$) [118]. Long-term follow-up studies have also showed that individuals seropositive for anti-HCV and HCV RNA have increased risk of developing diabetes [119].

Lastly, HCV infection is also associated with cardiovascular diseases. A large cross-sectional study found that patients with the presence of plaque and carotid intima media thickening, which are the early and asymptomatic signs of carotid atherosclerosis, had a twofold risk of being anti-HCV seropositive [120]. Another study, which was conducted using Australia's national registration database, found that 75,834 hepatitis C-diagnosed patients had a significantly increased risk of dying from cardiovascular diseases, compared to the general population [121]. In a similar retrospective study that compared 10,259 anti-HCV seropositive and 10,259 anti-HCV seronegative blood donors, anti-HCV seropositives had higher cardiovascular mortality rates, with a hazard ratio of 2.21 (95% CI: 1.41–3.46) [122]. In addition, a recent meta-analysis that included several observational studies found that HCV-infected patients have increased risks of cardiovascular-related mortality (OR = 1.65, 95% CI = 1.07–2.56), carotid plaques (OR = 2.27, 95% = 1.76–2.94), and cerebrovascular events (OR = 1.30, 95% CI = 1.10–1.55) [123]. Lastly, a community-based cohort study found that elevated serum HCV RNA levels increase the risk for cerebrovascular deaths, even after considering conventional risk factors. The dose-response relationship seen in this study

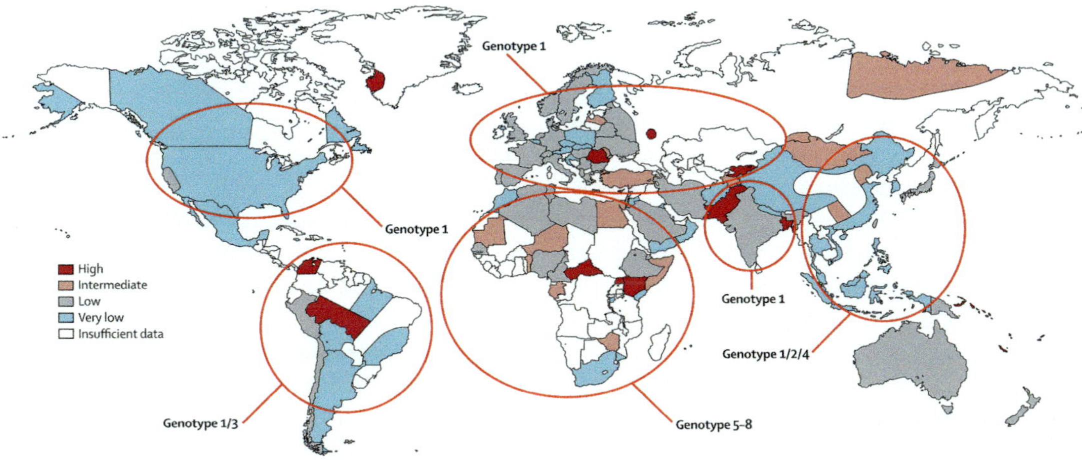

Fig. 3.4 Worldwide prevalence of HDV and the geographic distribution of its genotypes. (Reproduced with permission from Ref. [22])

Springer Nature remains neutral with regard to jurisdictional claims in published maps and institutional affiliations

supports a causal link between HCV infection and atherosclerotic changes [124].

3.3 Epidemiology and Global View of Hepatitis D

Hepatitis D virus (HDV) is the only member of the family *Deltaviridae* [125]. It appears to be a 36-nm spherical particle and consists of a circular RNA genome, a single HDV nucleocapsid antigen, and a lipoprotein envelope from HBV. HDV is a defective virus that requires HBV for its life cycle. Therefore, it is only possible to have coinfection or superinfection of HDV with HBV, which has been shown to cause a more severe disease than HBV mono-infection.

3.3.1 Geographical Distribution

The seroprevalence of antibodies against HDV (anti-HDV) in chronic HBV carriers demonstrates that HDV infection has a worldwide but nonuniform distribution. It is estimated that globally, 5% of HBsAg-seropositive individuals are coinfected with HDV, which corresponds to approximately 15–20 million people worldwide. High-prevalence areas include the Mediterranean, Middle East, and Central and Northern Asia, including Mongolia, Greenland, Sub-Saharan Africa, the Amazon basin, and some areas of the Pacific (Fig. 3.4). In some countries within these endemic areas, anti-HDV seropositivity is found in as many as 30% of CHB patients [126]. However, the prevalence of HDV is low in North America and Northern Europe, South Africa, and Eastern Asia. Interestingly, although there is a high HBV prevalence in Southeast Asia, HDV infection is relatively rare in areas other than Vietnam and the Pacific Islands. In the Amazon area, high HDV antibody prevalence rates have been found among children younger than 4 years [127].

The decline in the prevalence of HDV has been reported in Italy, Spain, Turkey, and Taiwan [128–132], mainly due to the availability of universal HBV vaccination, improvements in public health and hygiene, and increased awareness of transmission routes [133]. However, despite declining rates in some areas, some studies have reported an alarming prevalence of HDV infection in Northern California, Europe, Brazil, the Mediterranean Basin, and Vietnam, with rates ranging from 3.7% to 27.8% in CHB patients [134–138]. The epidemiology of HDV infection in children is similar with that in adults. Identical HDV strains in members from the same family had been reported, which highlights the importance of the intrafamilial spread of HDV in endemic areas [139, 140].

Eight major genotypes of HDV have been classified, based on the heterogeneity in viral genome sequences [141–143]. Genotype 1 is the most predominant, which presents throughout the world (Fig. 3.4). Genotype 2 is more commonly found in Eastern Asia such as Japan and Taiwan, while genotype 3 has been reported to cause outbreaks in Venezuela and Peru [144].

3.3.2 Transmission

HDV shares the same transmission routes with HBV: percutaneously or sexually through contacting infected blood or other body fluids of an infected person. Vertical transmission from mother to child is possible but considered to be rare [145]. Recent evidence showed a higher prevalence of HDV infection in patients aged 20–40 than the overall prevalence, implicating that sexual transmission might be a factor with higher importance in the spread of the disease than previously thought [136, 146]. Vaccination against HBV can prevent HDV coinfection. However, an increasing HDV prevalence has been observed in injection drug abusers [147] or in immigrants from areas where HDV is endemic.

3.3.3 Disease Progression and Long-term Consequences of HDV Infection

The risk of disease progression depends on the mode of infection. Coinfection with HBV and HDV usually results in mild, self-limited hepatitis and subsequent clearance of both viruses, with less than 10% of coinfected patients progressing to chronic HDV infection [144, 148]. However, some patients may develop severe fulminant hepatic failure [149]. Superinfection occurs when individuals with established chronic HBV are superinfected with HDV. Three phases are usually seen: acute, chronic, and late phases. The acute phase is characterized by high alanine aminotransferase (ALT) levels, active HDV replication, and suppression of HBsAg and HBV DNA. During the chronic phase, ALT levels decrease but may remain moderately elevated, HDV replication decreases, and HBV reactivation at low levels may occur. The late phase is characterized by reduced levels of both viruses or the replication of either virus that causes cirrhosis or HCC [150, 151]. Superinfection leads to chronic HDV in 70–90% of cases [150, 152] and can accelerate progression to a more severe disease than HBV mono-infected persons [153]. However, it is still unclear why HDV causes more severe hepatitis and a faster progression of fibrosis than HBV alone. It has been reported that superinfection of HDV may increase the risk of cirrhosis three times higher than those with HBV infection alone [149]. The association between HDV infection and HCC risk is controversial; some studies show that HDV infection is associated with increased risk of HCC, while others do not show an association [149, 154].

Several risk factors that affect disease progression of HDV infection have been identified. A Taiwanese study showed that among 194 patients with dual infection of HBV and HDV, 24 and 41 progressed to cirrhosis and HCC, respectively, during a median follow-up of 135 months. Older age, genotype 1 HDV, and genotype C HBV were found to be associated with adverse outcomes [155]. Another study from Italy tracked the course of 299 HDV-infected individuals for a mean period of 20 years. This study showed that persistent HDV replication was an important predictor of disease progression, which could lead to cirrhosis and HCC at annual rates of 4% and 2.8%, respectively. HDV replication was also the only predictor of liver-related mortality [156]. In addition, coinfection with other viruses such as HIV and HCV was shown to impact the course of HDV-related liver disease [157, 158].

HDV genotype can also influence outcomes of HDV infection. HDV genotype 1 has been shown to be associated with a higher incidence of acute liver failure following acute hepatitis D, a lower remission rate, and an increased incidence of adverse outcomes compared to genotype 2 [150,

155, 159]. Genotype 3 was reported to be associated with outbreaks of acute hepatitis D with a high incidence of fulminant hepatic failure in South America [160, 161].

3.3.4 Hepatitis D in Children

Although the incidence of HDV infection in children has decreased due to the implementation of the universal hepatitis B vaccination programs, there are still outbreaks reported in children in endemic areas of HBV infection [162].

HDV superinfection has profoundly modified the natural history of CHB in children, transforming a usually mild disease into progression toward severe hepatitis [163]. Severe cases of hepatitis, such as fulminant hepatic failure in children, are mainly caused by HDV superinfection [161]. One study in Turkey reported that although HDV infection was rare among HBV-infected children in the Western region of Turkey, all three children infected with HDV had biopsy-proven cirrhosis. In addition, there was a positive correlation between histological cirrhosis and the number of years following acute HDV infection [164]. Another Turkish study reported that 6 out of 206 children who had CHB were also infected with HDV. Among these children, three had cirrhosis, two had a moderate degree of hepatitis, and one had minimal inflammation [165]. However, a study from Taiwan found that high levels of HBV replication may result in the suppression of HDV and that HDV infection did not largely affect the natural course of HBV infection in Taiwanese children [139].

The baseline-event-anticipation score (BEA score) has been developed for predicting risk of liver-related morbidity or mortality (including decompensation, HCC, liver transplantation, and/or death) for patients with HDV infection and incorporates age, sex, region of origin, bilirubin, platelets, and international normalized ratio (INR) [166]. The accuracy of the BEA score was evaluated in two independent validation cohorts followed in Barcelona and Düsseldorf and may be used to assist with prognostication of HDV infection.

3.3.5 Seromarkers

The presence of HBsAg is a prerequisite for the diagnosis of HDV infection. Several seromarkers including HDV antigen (HDAg), anti-HDV, and HDV RNA may be used for the screening and diagnosis of HDV infection. Testing for serum HDAg in the acute phase may yield negative results, and repeat testing may be necessary [167]. In the chronic phase, as HDAg is complexed with high titers of anti-HDV, levels of HDAg are usually low.

Anti-HDV antibodies develop in every individual infected with HDV [126]. Low titers of anti-HDV may persist for years after recovery from infection and should not be used as an indication of active infection. Several commercial tests are available for total anti-HDV antibody. HDV RNA is an early and sensitive marker of acute HDV infection and is useful for assessing the resolution of HDV infection. However, there still is no standardized HDV RNA assay, and in-house assays can only be performed in specialized laboratories. In individuals seropositive for anti-HDV, the HDV RNA assay should be used for confirming active HDV infection. HDV genotyping may help to identify patients at increased risk of developing end-stage liver disease. However, its usage is not recommended in routine clinical practice.

3.4 Prevention and Treatment of Hepatitis B, C, and D

The hepatitis B vaccine is the most important tool for the prevention of hepatitis B virus infection. WHO recommends that all infants receive the hepatitis B vaccine within 24 hours after birth. Vaccination has reduced the rate of chronic infection to less than 1% among immunized children in countries in which 15% of children used to become chronic carriers. The implementation of a nationwide hepatitis B vaccination program in Taiwan in 1984 shows that vaccination of newborns has not only reduced the risk of infection but has also led to significant reduction in the incidence of childhood liver cancer [168, 169].

It is recommended by WHO that all children and adolescents younger than 18 years old who live in countries with low or intermediate endemicity and who are not previously vaccinated receive the vaccine. Some high-risk people, including those who frequently require blood or blood products, dialysis patients, recipients of solid organ transplantations, those who inject drugs, those with multiple sexual partners, household and sexual contacts of people with chronic HBV infection, those who will be travelling to endemic areas, and healthcare workers, are also recommended to be vaccinated. As the protection can last at least 20 years and is probably lifelong in those who complete vaccine series, WHO does not recommend booster vaccination for persons who have completed the three-dose vaccination schedule. In 2015, global coverage with the three doses of hepatitis B vaccine in infancy reached 84%. However, the coverage with the initial birth dose vaccination is still low at 39%.

In addition to vaccination, blood safety strategies such as screening of donated blood and blood components used for transfusion can prevent transmission of HBV. In 2013, 97% of blood donations were screened and quality assured worldwide; however, there exist gaps for improvement. Furthermore, eliminating unnecessary and unsafe injections and minimizing the number of partners and using barrier protective measures are also important strategies for protection against HBV transmission.

WHO also recommended the use of simple, noninvasive diagnostic tests to assess the stage of liver disease and eligibility for treatment; to prioritize treatment for those with most advanced liver disease and at greatest risk of mortality; the preferred use of the nucleos(t)ide analogues with a high barrier to drug resistance for first- and second-line treatment; lifelong treatment in those with cirrhosis; and regular monitoring for disease progression and toxicity of drugs and early detection of liver cancer.

As there is no vaccine for hepatitis C, the prevention of HCV infection depends mainly on reducing the risk of exposure in higher-risk populations and through sexual contact. Therefore, the provision of effective harm-reduction services to people who inject drugs, including sterile injecting equipment, and the promotion of correct and consistent use of condoms are important. Primary preventive interventions are also suggested for healthcare settings including testing of donated blood for hepatitis C, safe and appropriate use of healthcare injections, safe handling and disposal of sharps and waste, and training of health personnel.

For people infected with HCV, WHO recommends early and appropriate medical management including antiviral therapy if appropriate and regular monitoring for early diagnosis of chronic liver disease. The assessment for antiviral treatment should be implemented for all adults and children with chronic HCV infection. All patients with hepatitis C are recommended by WHO to be treated with direct-acting antivirals (DAA)-based regimens, except for a few specific groups of people in whom interferon-based regimens can still be used.

WHO does not have specific recommendations for hepatitis D. However, the WHO suggests that prevention of HBV transmission by hepatitis B immunization, safe injection practices, blood safety, and harm-reduction services with clean needles and syringes are effective in preventing HDV transmission. Currently, the vaccine against HBV is the method of choice to prevent HDV infection; however, it does not protect against HDV infection for those already infected with HBV. Passive immunoprophylaxis with hepatitis B immunoglobulin does not confer any protection against HDV infection, unless it controls the spread of HBV infection. In children, universal vaccination remains the fundamental method of prevention. It is prudent to check for adequate immunity to HBV after vaccination in children with household members known to have HDV infection, in order to inhibit intrafamilial transmission.

There is still no specific treatment for acute or chronic HDV infection. Although persistent HDV replication is the most important predictor of mortality and the need for antiviral therapy, the ultimate goal for eradication of HDV should be the clearance of HBsAg [170]. Oral antivirals against HBV showed little or no effect on HDV replication when used alone. Interferon-alpha-based therapy is the only drug effective against HDV [146, 171]. However, the overall rate of sustained virological response remains low, and most patients relapse after discontinuation of therapy. The optimal duration of therapy is not well defined, and more than 1 year of therapy may be necessary. Patients with fulminant hepatitis due to coinfection or superinfection with HDV did not respond to interferon-alpha therapy, and liver transplant is the only option for such patients [172]. New therapeutic agents and strategies for HDV infection are needed.

3.5 Summary

This chapter has provided a global view for hepatitis B, C, and D, in terms of worldwide distribution, transmission route, long-term consequences, and preventive measures.

References

1. Schweitzer A, Horn J, Mikolajczyk RT, Krause G, Ott JJ (2015) Estimations of worldwide prevalence of chronic hepatitis B virus infection: a systematic review of data published between 1965 and 2013. Lancet 386:1546–1555
2. Perz JF, Armstrong GL, Farrington LA, Hutin YJ, Bell BP (2006) The contributions of hepatitis B virus and hepatitis C virus infections to cirrhosis and primary liver cancer worldwide. J Hepatol 45:529–538
3. Mortality GBD, Causes of Death C (2015) Global, regional, and national age-sex specific all-cause and cause-specific mortality for 240 causes of death, 1990–2013: a systematic analysis for the Global Burden of Disease Study 2013. Lancet 385:117–171
4. Nelson NP, Easterbrook PJ, McMahon BJ (2016) Epidemiology of hepatitis B virus infection and impact of vaccination on disease. Clin Liver Dis 20:607–628
5. Te HS, Jensen DM (2010) Epidemiology of hepatitis B and C viruses: a global overview. Clin Liver Dis 14:1–21 vii
6. Liaw YF, Brunetto MR, Hadziyannis S (2010) The natural history of chronic HBV infection and geographical differences. Antivir Ther 15(Suppl 3):25–33
7. Ott JJ, Horn J, Krause G, Mikolajczyk RT (2016) Time trends of chronic HBV infection over prior decades – a global analysis. J Hepatol
8. Sunbul M (2014) Hepatitis B virus genotypes: global distribution and clinical importance. World J Gastroenterol 20:5427–5434
9. Allain JP (2006) Epidemiology of hepatitis B virus and genotype. J Clin Virol 36(Suppl 1):S12–S17
10. Liu CJ, Kao JH (2013) Global perspective on the natural history of chronic hepatitis B: role of hepatitis B virus genotypes A to J. Semin Liver Dis 33:97–102
11. McMahon BJ (2009) The influence of hepatitis B virus genotype and subgenotype on the natural history of chronic hepatitis B. Hepatol Int 3:334–342
12. Schaefer S (2007) Hepatitis B virus taxonomy and hepatitis B virus genotypes. World J Gastroenterol 13:14–21
13. Schaefer S (2007) Hepatitis B virus genotypes in Europe. Hepatol Res 37:S20–S26
14. Wai CT, Fontana RJ, Polson J, Hussain M, Shakil AO, Han SH, Davern TJ et al (2005) Clinical outcome and virological characteristics of hepatitis B-related acute liver failure in the United States. J Viral Hepat 12:192–198
15. Zhang HW, Yin JH, Li YT, Li CZ, Ren H, Gu CY, Wu HY et al (2008) Risk factors for acute hepatitis B and its progression to chronic hepatitis in Shanghai, China. Gut 57:1713–1720
16. Lin CL, Kao JH (2011) The clinical implications of hepatitis B virus genotype: recent advances. J Gastroenterol Hepatol 26(Suppl 1):123–130
17. Boglione L, D'Avolio A, Cariti G, Milia MG, Simiele M, De Nicolo A, Ghisetti V et al (2013) Sequential therapy with entecavir and PEG-INF in patients affected by chronic hepatitis B and high levels of HBV-DNA with non-D genotypes. J Viral Hepat 20:e11–e19
18. Shi YH (2012) Correlation between hepatitis B virus genotypes and clinical outcomes. Jpn J Infect Dis 65:476–482
19. Wong GL, Chan HL, Yiu KK, Lai JW, Chan VK, Cheung KK, Wong EW et al (2013) Meta-analysis: the association of hepatitis B virus genotypes and hepatocellular carcinoma. Aliment Pharmacol Ther 37:517–526
20. Beasley RP, Trepo C, Stevens CE, Szmuness W (1977) The e antigen and vertical transmission of hepatitis B surface antigen. Am J Epidemiol 105:94–98
21. Edmunds WJ, Medley GF, Nokes DJ, Hall AJ, Whittle HC (1993) The influence of age on the development of the hepatitis B carrier state. Proc Biol Sci 253:197–201
22. Hyams KC (1995) Risks of chronicity following acute hepatitis B virus infection: a review. Clin Infect Dis 20:992–1000
23. Chu CM, Hung SJ, Lin J, Tai DI, Liaw YF (2004) Natural history of hepatitis B e antigen to antibody seroconversion in patients with normal serum aminotransferase levels. Am J Med 116:829–834
24. Liaw YF, Chu CM (2009) Hepatitis B virus infection. Lancet 373:582–592

25. Beasley RP, Hepatitis B v (1988) The major etiology of hepatocellular carcinoma. Cancer 61:1942–1956
26. Lavanchy D (2004) Hepatitis B virus epidemiology, disease burden, treatment, and current and emerging prevention and control measures. J Viral Hepat 11:97–107
27. International Agency for Research on Cancer (2012) A review of human carcinogens: Part B – Biological agents, Lyon
28. Beasley RP, Hwang LY, Lin CC, Chien CS (1981) Hepatocellular carcinoma and hepatitis B virus. A prospective study of 22 707 men in Taiwan. Lancet 2:1129–1133
29. Bonino F, Piratvisuth T, Brunetto MR, Liaw YF (2010) Diagnostic markers of chronic hepatitis B infection and disease. Antivir Ther 15(Suppl 3):35–44
30. Chen CJ, Yang HI (2011) Natural history of chronic hepatitis B REVEALed. J Gastroenterol Hepatol 26:628–638
31. Lee MH, Yang HI, Liu J, Batrla-Utermann R, Jen CL, Iloeje UH, Lu SN et al (2013) Prediction models of long-term cirrhosis and hepatocellular carcinoma risk in chronic hepatitis B patients: risk scores integrating host and virus profiles. Hepatology 58:546–554
32. Liu J, Yang HI, Lee MH, Lu SN, Jen CL, Batrla-Utermann R, Wang LY et al (2014) Spontaneous seroclearance of hepatitis B seromarkers and subsequent risk of hepatocellular carcinoma. Gut 63:1648–1657
33. Iloeje UH, Yang HI, Su J, Jen CL, You SL, Chen CJ, Risk Evaluation Viral L (2006) Predicting cirrhosis risk based on the level of circulating hepatitis B viral load. Gastroenterology 130:678–686
34. Yu MW, Hsu FC, Sheen IS, Chu CM, Lin DY, Chen CJ, Liaw YF (1997) Prospective study of hepatocellular carcinoma and liver cirrhosis in asymptomatic chronic hepatitis B virus carriers. Am J Epidemiol 145:1039–1047
35. McMahon BJ, Alberts SR, Wainwright RB, Bulkow L, Lanier AP (1990) Hepatitis B-related sequelae. Prospective study in 1400 hepatitis B surface antigen-positive Alaska native carriers. Arch Intern Med 150:1051–1054
36. Tseng TC, Liu CJ, Yang HC, Su TH, Wang CC, Chen CL, Kuo SF et al (2012) High levels of hepatitis B surface antigen increase risk of hepatocellular carcinoma in patients with low HBV load. Gastroenterology
37. Yang HI, Lu SN, Liaw YF, You SL, Sun CA, Wang LY, Hsiao CK et al (2002) Hepatitis B e antigen and the risk of hepatocellular carcinoma. N Engl J Med 347:168–174
38. Chen CJ, Yang HI, Su J, Jen CL, You SL, Lu SN, Huang GT et al (2006) Risk of hepatocellular carcinoma across a biological gradient of serum hepatitis B virus DNA level. JAMA 295:65–73
39. Chen CL, Yang HI, Yang WS, Liu CJ, Chen PJ, You SL, Wang LY et al (2008) Metabolic factors and risk of hepatocellular carcinoma by chronic hepatitis B/C infection: a follow-up study in Taiwan. Gastroenterology 135:111–121
40. Chen CL, Yang WS, Yang HI, Chen CF, You SL, Wang LY, Lu SN et al (2014) Plasma adipokines and risk of hepatocellular carcinoma in chronic hepatitis B virus-infected carriers: a prospective study in Taiwan. Cancer Epidemiol Biomark Prev 23:1659–1671
41. Loomba R, Liu J, Yang HI, Lee MH, Lu SN, Wang LY, Iloeje UH et al (2013) Synergistic effects of family history of hepatocellular carcinoma and hepatitis B virus infection on risk for incident hepatocellular carcinoma. Clin Gastroenterol Hepatol 11:1636–1645 e1631–1633
42. Loomba R, Yang HI, Su J, Brenner D, Barrett-Connor E, Iloeje U, Chen CJ (2013) Synergism between obesity and alcohol in increasing the risk of hepatocellular carcinoma: a prospective cohort study. Am J Epidemiol 177:333–342
43. Hu HH, Liu J, Lin YL, Luo WS, Chu YJ, Chang CL, Jen CL et al (2016) The rs2296651 (S267F) variant on NTCP (SLC10A1) is inversely associated with chronic hepatitis B and progression to cirrhosis and hepatocellular carcinoma in patients with chronic hepatitis B. Gut 65:1514–1521
44. Liu J, Lee MH, Batrla-Utermann R, Jen CL, Iloeje UH, Lu SN, Wang LY et al (2013) A predictive scoring system for the seroclearance of HBsAg in HBeAg-seronegative chronic hepatitis B patients with genotype B or C infection. J Hepatol 58:853–860
45. Liu J, Tseng TC, Yang HI, Lee MH, Batrla-Utermann R, Jen CL, Lu SN et al (2014) Predicting HBsAg seroclearance in HBeAg-negative chronic hepatitis B patients: external validation of a scoring system. J Infect Dis
46. Liu J, Yang HI, Lee MH, Batrla-Utermann R, Jen CL, Lu SN, Wang LY et al (2014) Distinct seromarkers predict different milestones of chronic hepatitis B progression. Hepatology 60:77–86
47. Yang HI, Lee MH, Liu J, Chen CJ (2014) Risk calculators for hepatocellular carcinoma in patients affected with chronic hepatitis B in Asia. World J Gastroenterol 20:6244–6251
48. Yang HI, Sherman M, Su J, Chen PJ, Liaw YF, Iloeje UH, Chen CJ (2010) Nomograms for risk of hepatocellular carcinoma in patients with chronic hepatitis B virus infection. J Clin Oncol 28:2437–2444
49. Yang HI, Yuen MF, Chan HL, Han KH, Chen PJ, Kim DY, Ahn SH et al (2011) Risk estimation for hepatocellular carcinoma in chronic hepatitis B (REACH-B): development and validation of a predictive score. Lancet Oncol 12:568–574
50. Yang HI, Tseng TC, Liu J, Lee MH, Liu CJ, Su TH, Batrla-Utermann R et al (2016) Incorporating serum level of hepatitis B surface antigen or omitting level of hepatitis B virus DNA does not affect calculation of risk for hepatocellular carcinoma in patients with-

out cirrhosis. Clin Gastroenterol Hepatol 14:461–468 e462
51. Lauer GM, Walker BD (2001) Hepatitis C virus infection. N Engl J Med 345:41–52
52. Fattovich G, Stroffolini T, Zagni I, Donato F (2004) Hepatocellular carcinoma in cirrhosis: incidence and risk factors. Gastroenterology 127:S35–S50
53. Parkin DM (2006) The global health burden of infection-associated cancers in the year 2002. Int J Cancer 118:3030–3044
54. Hajarizadeh B, Grebely J, Dore GJ (2013) Epidemiology and natural history of HCV infection. Nat Rev Gastroenterol Hepatol 10:553–562
55. Lee MH, Yang HI, Jen CL, Lu SN, Yeh SH, Liu CJ, You SL et al (2011) Community and personal risk factors for hepatitis C virus infection: a survey of 23,820 residents in Taiwan in 1991-2. Gut 60:688–694
56. Lavanchy D, Purcell R, Hollinger FB, Howard C, Alberti A, Kew M, Dusheiko G et al (1999) Global surveillance and control of hepatitis C. J Viral Hepat 6:35–47
57. Madhava V, Burgess C, Drucker E (2002) Epidemiology of chronic hepatitis C virus infection in sub-Saharan Africa. Lancet Infect Dis 2:293–302
58. Lavanchy D (2011) Evolving epidemiology of hepatitis C virus. Clin Microbiol Infect 17:107–115
59. Friedt M, Gerner P, Lausch E, Trubel H, Zabel B, Wirth S (1999) Mutations in the basic core promotor and the precore region of hepatitis B virus and their selection in children with fulminant and chronic hepatitis B. Hepatology 29:1252–1258
60. Nguyen LH, Nguyen MH (2013) Systematic review: Asian patients with chronic hepatitis C infection. Aliment Pharmacol Ther 37:921–936
61. Memon MI, Memon MA (2002) Hepatitis C: an epidemiological review. J Viral Hepat 9:84–100
62. Alter MJ (1999) Hepatitis C virus infection in the United States. J Hepatol 31:88–91
63. Garner JJ, Gaughwin M, Dodding J, Willson K (1997) Prevalence of hepatitis C infection in pregnant women in South Australia. Med J Aust 167:470–472
64. Tseng FC, O'Brien TR, Zhang M, Kral AH, Ortiz-Conde BA, Lorvick J, Busch MP et al (2007) Seroprevalence of hepatitis C virus and hepatitis B virus among San Francisco injection drug users, 1998 to 2000. Hepatology 46:666–671
65. Hahn JA, Page-Shafer K, Lum P, Ochoa K, Moss AR (2001) Hepatitis C virus infection and needle exchange use among young injection drug users in San Francisco. Hepatology 34:180–187
66. Hagan H, McGough JP, Thiede H, Weiss NS, Hopkins S, Alexander ER (1999) Syringe exchange and risk of infection with hepatitis B and C viruses. Am J Epidemiol 149:203–213
67. De P, Roy E, Boivin JF, Cox J, Morissette C (2008) Risk of hepatitis C virus transmission through drug preparation equipment: a systematic and methodological review. J Viral Hepat 15:279–292
68. Feinstone SM, Kapikian AZ, Purcell RH, Alter HJ, Holland PV (1975) Transfusion-associated hepatitis not due to viral hepatitis type A or B. N Engl J Med 292:767–770
69. Allander T, Medin C, Jacobson SH, Grillner L, Persson MA (1994) Hepatitis C transmission in a hemodialysis unit: molecular evidence for spread of virus among patients not sharing equipment. J Med Virol 43:415–419
70. Pereira BJ, Milford EL, Kirkman RL, Levey AS (1991) Transmission of hepatitis C virus by organ transplantation. N Engl J Med 325:454–460
71. Khaja MN, Madhavi C, Thippavazzula R, Nafeesa F, Habib AM, Habibullah CM, Guntaka RV (2006) High prevalence of hepatitis C virus infection and genotype distribution among general population, blood donors and risk groups. Infect Genet Evol 6:198–204
72. Alter HJ, Houghton M (2000) Hepatitis C virus and eliminating post-transfusion hepatitis. Nat Med 6:1082–1086
73. Donahue JG, Munoz A, Ness PM, Brown DE, Yawn DH, McAllister HA, Reitz BA et al (1992) The declining risk of posttransfusion hepatitis C virus infection. N Engl J Med 327:369–373
74. Dubois F, Desenclos JC, Mariotte N, Goudeau A (1997) Hepatitis C in a French population-based survey, 1994: seroprevalence, frequency of viremia, genotype distribution, and risk factors. The Collaborative Study Group. Hepatology 25:1490–1496
75. Armstrong GL, Wasley A, Simard EP, McQuillan GM, Kuhnert WL, Alter MJ (2006) The prevalence of hepatitis C virus infection in the United States, 1999 through 2002. Ann Intern Med 144:705–714
76. Shan H, Wang JX, Ren FR, Zhang YZ, Zhao HY, Gao GJ, Ji Y et al (2002) Blood banking in China. Lancet 360:1770–1775
77. Tagny CT, Mbanya D, Tapko JB, Lefrere JJ (2008) Blood safety in Sub-Saharan Africa: a multi-factorial problem. Transfusion 48:1256–1261
78. Prati D (2006) Transmission of hepatitis C virus by blood transfusions and other medical procedures: a global review. J Hepatol 45:607–616
79. Kane A, Lloyd J, Zaffran M, Simonsen L, Kane M (1999) Transmission of hepatitis B, hepatitis C and human immunodeficiency viruses through unsafe injections in the developing world: model-based regional estimates. Bull World Health Organ 77:801–807
80. Frank C, Mohamed MK, Strickland GT, Lavanchy D, Arthur RR, Magder LS, El Khoby T et al (2000) The role of parenteral antischistosomal therapy in the spread of hepatitis C virus in Egypt. Lancet 355:887–891
81. Drucker E, Alcabes PG, Marx PA (2001) The injection century: massive unsterile injections

and the emergence of human pathogens. Lancet 358:1989–1992
82. Ishibashi M, Shinzawa H, Kuboki M, Tsuchida H, Takahashi T (1996) Prevalence of inhabitants with anti-hepatitis C virus antibody in an area following an acute hepatitis C epidemic: age-and area-related features. J Epidemiol 6:1–7
83. Shin HR (2006) Epidemiology of hepatitis C virus in Korea. Intervirology 49:18–22
84. Guadagnino V, Stroffolini T, Rapicetta M, Costantino A, Kondili LA, Menniti-Ippolito F, Caroleo B et al (1997) Prevalence, risk factors, and genotype distribution of hepatitis C virus infection in the general population: a community-based survey in southern Italy. Hepatology 26:1006–1011
85. Sun CA, Chen HC, Lu CF, You SL, Mau YC, Ho MS, Lin SH et al (1999) Transmission of hepatitis C virus in Taiwan: prevalence and risk factors based on a nationwide survey. J Med Virol 59:290–296
86. Wasley A, Alter MJ (2000) Epidemiology of hepatitis C: geographic differences and temporal trends. Semin Liver Dis 20:1–16
87. Wang CS, Chang TT, Chou P (1998) Differences in risk factors for being either a hepatitis B carrier or anti-hepatitis C+ in a hepatoma-hyperendemic area in rural Taiwan. J Clin Epidemiol 51:733–738
88. Tahara T, Toyoda S, Mukaide M, Hikiji K, Ohba K, Mizokami M (1996) Vertical transmission of hepatitis C through three generations. Lancet 347:409
89. Roberts EA, Yeung L (2002) Maternal-infant transmission of hepatitis C virus infection. Hepatology 36:S106–S113
90. Zanetti AR, Tanzi E, Paccagnini S, Principi N, Pizzocolo G, Caccamo ML, Damico E et al (1995) Mother-to-infant transmission of hepatitis C virus. Lancet 345:289–291
91. Dore GJ, Kaldor JM, McCaughan GW (1997) Systematic review of role of polymerase chain reaction in defining infectiousness among people infected with hepatitis C virus. Br Med J 315:333–337
92. Mast EE, Hwang LY, Seto DSY, Nolte FS, Nainan OV, Wurtzel H, Alter MJ (2005) Risk factors for perinatal transmission of hepatitis C virus (HCV) and the natural history of HCV infection acquired in infancy. J Infect Dis 192:1880–1889
93. Syriopoulou V, Nikolopoulou G, Daikos GL, Theodoridou M, Pavlopoulou I, Nicolaidou P, Manolaki N (2005) Mother to child transmission of hepatitis C virus: rate of infection and risk factors. Scand J Infect Dis 37:350–353
94. Tovo PA, Newell ML, Coll O, de Tejada BM, Lanari M, Bosi I, Papa I et al (2001) Effects of mode of delivery and infant feeding on the risk of mother-to-child transmission of hepatitis C virus. Br J Obstet Gynaecol 108:371–377
95. Tanaka K, Stuver SO, Ikematsu H, Okayama A, Tachibana N, Hirohata T, Kashiwagi S et al (1997) Heterosexual transmission of hepatitis C virus among married couples in southwestern Japan. Int J Cancer 72:50–55
96. Chayama K, Kobayashi M, Tsubota A, Koida I, Arase Y, Saitoh S, Ikeda K et al (1995) Molecular analysis of intraspousal transmission of hepatitis C virus. J Hepatol 22:431–439
97. Zylberberg H, Thiers V, Lagorce D, Squadrito G, Leone F, Berthelot P, Brechot C et al (1999) Epidemiological and virological analysis of couples infected with hepatitis C virus. Gut 45:112–116
98. Terrault NA (2002) Sexual activity as a risk factor for hepatitis C. Hepatology 36:S99–S105
99. Turner JM, Rider AT, Imrie J, Copas AJ, Edwards SG, Dodds JP, Stephenson JM (2006) Behavioural predictors of subsequent hepatitis C diagnosis in a UK clinic sample of HIV positive men who have sex with men. Sex Transm Infect 82:298–300
100. Thomas DL, Zenilman JM, Alter HJ, Shih JW, Galai N, Carella AV, Quinn TC (1995) Sexual transmission of hepatitis C virus among patients attending sexually transmitted diseases clinics in Baltimore-an analysis of 309 sex partnerships. J Infect Dis 171:768–775
101. van de Laar TJW, van der Bij AK, Prins M, Bruisten SM, Brinkman K, Ruys TA, van der Meer JTM et al (2007) Increase in HCV incidence among men who have sex with men in Amsterdam most likely caused by sexual transmission. J Infect Dis 196:230–238
102. Perez CM, Suarez E, Torres EA, Roman K, Colon V (2005) Seroprevalence of hepatitis C virus and associated risk behaviours: a population-based study in San Juan, Puerto Rico. Int J Epidemiol 34:593–599
103. Hwang LY, Kramer JR, Troisi C, Bull L, Grimes CZ, Lyerla R, Alter MJ (2006) Relationship of cosmetic procedures and drug use to hepatitis C and hepatitis B virus infections in a low-risk population. Hepatology 44:341–351
104. Habib M, Mohamed MK, Abdel-Aziz F, Magder LS, Abdel-Hamid M, Gamil F, Madkour S et al (2001) Hepatitis C virus infection in a community in the Nile Delta: risk factors for seropositivity. Hepatology 33:248–253
105. Tong MJ, el-Farra NS, Reikes AR, Co RL (1995) Clinical outcomes after transfusion-associated hepatitis C. N Engl J Med 332:1463–1466
106. Wiese M, Grungreiff K, Guthoff W, Lafrenz M, Oesen U, Porst H, East German Hepatitis CSG (2005) Outcome in a hepatitis C (genotype 1b) single source outbreak in Germany – a 25-year multicenter study. J Hepatol 43:590–598
107. Huang YT, Jen CL, Yang HI, Lee MH, Su J, Lu SN, Iloeje UH et al (2011) Lifetime risk and sex difference of hepatocellular carcinoma among patients with chronic hepatitis B and C. J Clin Oncol 29:3643–3650
108. Lee MH, Yang HI, Lu SN, Jen CL, Yeh SH, Liu CJ, Chen PJ et al (2010) Hepatitis C virus seromarkers and subsequent risk of hepatocellular carcinoma: long-term predictors from a community-based cohort study. J Clin Oncol 28:4587–4593
109. Lee MH, Yang HI, Yuan Y, L'Italien G, Chen CJ (2014) Epidemiology and natural history of hepa-

titis C virus infection. World J Gastroenterol 20:9270–9280
110. Lee MH, Yang HI, Lu SN, Jen CL, You SL, Wang LY, L'Italien G et al (2014) Hepatitis C virus genotype 1b increases cumulative lifetime risk of hepatocellular carcinoma. Int J Cancer 135:1119–1126
111. Lee MH, Lu SN, Yuan Y, Yang HI, Jen CL, You SL, Wang LY et al (2014) Development and validation of a clinical scoring system for predicting risk of HCC in asymptomatic individuals seropositive for anti-HCV antibodies. PLoS One 9:e94760
112. Rao HY, Li H, Chen H, Shang J, Xie Q, Gao ZL, Li J et al (2016) Real world treatment patterns and clinical outcomes of hcv treatment-naive patients in China: an interim analysis from the ccgenos study. J Gastroenterol Hepatol
113. Lee MH, Yang HI, Lu SN, Jen CL, You SL, Wang LY, Wang CH et al (2012) Chronic hepatitis C virus infection increases mortality from hepatic and extrahepatic diseases: a community-based long-term prospective study. J Infect Dis 206:469–477
114. Giordano TP, Henderson L, Landgren O, Chiao EY, Kramer JR, El-Serag H, Engels EA (2007) Risk of non-Hodgkin lymphoma and lymphoproliferative precursor diseases in US veterans with hepatitis C virus. JAMA 297:2010–2017
115. Su TH, Liu CJ, Tseng TC, Chou SW, Liu CH, Yang HC, Wu SJ et al (2016) Hepatitis C viral infection increases the risk of lymphoid-neoplasms: a population-based cohort study. Hepatology 63:721–730
116. Eslam M, Khattab MA, Harrison SA (2011) Insulin resistance and hepatitis C: an evolving story. Gut 60:1139–1151
117. Mehta SH, Brancati FL, Sulkowski MS, Strathdee SA, Szklo M, Thomas DL (2000) Prevalence of type 2 diabetes mellitus among persons with hepatitis C virus infection in the United States. Ann Intern Med 133:592–599
118. Huang JF, Dai CY, Hwang SJ, Ho CK, Hsiao PJ, Hsieh MY, Lee LP et al (2007) Hepatitis C viremia increases the association with type 2 diabetes mellitus in a hepatitis B and C endemic area: an epidemiological link with virological implication. Am J Gastroenterol 102:1237–1243
119. Lin YJ, Shaw TG, Yang HI, Lu SN, Jen CL, Wang LY, Wong KH et al (2016) Chronic hepatitis C virus infection and the risk for diabetes: a community-based prospective study. Liver Int
120. Ishizaka N, Ishizaka Y, Takahashi E, Tooda E, Hashimoto H, Nagai R, Yamakado M (2002) Association between hepatitis C virus seropositivity, carotid-artery plaque, and intima-media thickening. Lancet 359:133–135
121. Amin J, Law MG, Bartlett M, Kaldor JM, Dore GJ (2006) Causes of death after diagnosis of hepatitis B or hepatitis C infection: a large community-based linkage study. Lancet 368:938–945
122. Guiltinan AM, Kaidarova Z, Custer B, Orland J, Strollo A, Cyrus S, Busch MP et al (2008) Increased all-cause, liver, and cardiac mortality among hepatitis C virus-seropositive blood donors. Am J Epidemiol 167:743–750
123. Petta S, Maida M, Macaluso FS, Barbara M, Licata A, Craxì A, Cammà C (2016) Hepatitis C virus infection is associated with increased cardiovascular mortality: a meta-analysis of observational studies. Gastroenterology 150:145–155 e144
124. Lee MH, Yang HI, Wang CH, Jen CL, Yeh SH, Liu CJ, You SL et al (2010) Hepatitis C virus infection and increased risk of cerebrovascular disease. Stroke 41:2894–2900
125. Lai MM (1995) The molecular biology of hepatitis delta virus. Annu Rev Biochem 64:259–286
126. Wedemeyer H, Manns MP (2010) Epidemiology, pathogenesis and management of hepatitis D: update and challenges ahead. Nat Rev Gastroenterol Hepatol 7:31–40
127. Alvarado-Mora MV, Fernandez MF, Gomes-Gouvea MS, de Azevedo Neto RS, Carrilho FJ, Pinho JR (2011) Hepatitis B (HBV), hepatitis C (HCV) and hepatitis delta (HDV) viruses in the Colombian population – how is the epidemiological situation? PLoS One 6:e18888
128. Navascues CA, Rodriguez M, Sotorrio NG, Sala P, Linares A, Suarez A, Rodrigo L (1995) Epidemiology of hepatitis D virus infection: changes in the last 14 years. Am J Gastroenterol 90:1981–1984
129. Gaeta GB, Stroffolini T, Chiaramonte M, Ascione T, Stornaiuolo G, Lobello S, Sagnelli E et al (2000) Chronic hepatitis D: a vanishing disease? An Italian multicenter study. Hepatology 32:824–827
130. Huo TI, Wu JC, Lin RY, Sheng WY, Chang FY, Lee SD (1997) Decreasing hepatitis D virus infection in Taiwan: an analysis of contributory factors. J Gastroenterol Hepatol 12:747–751
131. Sagnelli E, Stroffolini T, Ascione A, Chiaramonte M, Craxi A, Giusti G, Piccinino F (1997) Decrease in HDV endemicity in Italy. J Hepatol 26:20–24
132. Degertekin H, Yalcin K, Yakut M (2006) The prevalence of hepatitis delta virus infection in acute and chronic liver diseases in Turkey: an analysis of clinical studies. Turk J Gastroenterol 17:25–34
133. Rizzetto M, Ciancio A (2012) Epidemiology of hepatitis D. Semin Liver Dis 32:211–219
134. Gish RG, Yi DH, Kane S, Clark M, Mangahas M, Baqai S, Winters MA et al (2013) Coinfection with hepatitis B and D: epidemiology, prevalence and disease in patients in Northern California. J Gastroenterol Hepatol 28:1521–1525
135. Ho E, Deltenre P, Nkuize M, Delwaide J, Colle I, Michielsen P (2013) Belgian association for the study of the L. Coinfection of hepatitis B and hepatitis delta virus in Belgium: a multicenter BASL study. Prospective epidemiology and comparison with HBV mono-infection. J Med Virol 85:1513–1517
136. Braga WS, Castilho Mda C, Borges FG, Leao JR, Martinho AC, Rodrigues IS, Azevedo EP et al (2012) Hepatitis D virus infection in the Western Brazilian

Amazon – far from a vanishing disease. Rev Soc Bras Med Trop 45:691–695
137. Amini N, Alavian SM, Kabir A, Aalaei-Andabili SH, Saiedi Hosseini SY, Rizzetto M (2013) Prevalence of hepatitis d in the eastern mediterranean region: systematic review and meta analysis. Hepat Mon 13:e8210
138. Dunford L, Carr MJ, Dean J, Nguyen LT, Ta Thi TH, Nguyen BT, Connell J et al (2012) A multicentre molecular analysis of hepatitis B and blood-borne virus coinfections in Viet Nam. PLoS One 7:e39027
139. Hsu HY, Chang MH, Chen DS, Lee CY (1988) Hepatitis D virus infection in children with acute or chronic hepatitis B virus infection in Taiwan. J Pediatr 112:888–892
140. Niro GA, Casey JL, Gravinese E, Garrubba M, Conoscitore P, Sagnelli E, Durazzo M et al (1999) Intrafamilial transmission of hepatitis delta virus: molecular evidence. J Hepatol 30:564–569
141. Radjef N, Gordien E, Ivaniushina V, Gault E, Anais P, Drugan T, Trinchet JC et al (2004) Molecular phylogenetic analyses indicate a wide and ancient radiation of African hepatitis delta virus, suggesting a delta virus genus of at least seven major clades. J Virol 78:2537–2544
142. Le Gal F, Gault E, Ripault MP, Serpaggi J, Trinchet JC, Gordien E, Deny P (2006) Eighth major clade for hepatitis delta virus. Emerg Infect Dis 12:1447–1450
143. Deny P (2006) Hepatitis delta virus genetic variability: from genotypes I, II, III to eight major clades? Curr Top Microbiol Immunol 307:151–171
144. Hadziyannis SJ (1997) Review: hepatitis delta. J Gastroenterol Hepatol 12:289–298
145. Zanetti AR, Ferroni P, Magliano EM, Pirovano P, Lavarini C, Massaro AL, Gavinelli R et al (1982) Perinatal transmission of the hepatitis B virus and of the HBV-associated delta agent from mothers to offspring in northern Italy. J Med Virol 9:139–148
146. Noureddin M, Gish R (2014) Hepatitis delta: epidemiology, diagnosis and management 36 years after discovery. Curr Gastroenterol Rep 16:365
147. Kucirka LM, Farzadegan H, Feld JJ, Mehta SH, Winters M, Glenn JS, Kirk GD et al (2010) Prevalence, correlates, and viral dynamics of hepatitis delta among injection drug users. J Infect Dis 202:845–852
148. Smedile A, Farci P, Verme G, Caredda F, Cargnel A, Caporaso N, Dentico P et al (1982) Influence of delta infection on severity of hepatitis B. Lancet 2:945–947
149. Farci P, Niro GA (2012) Clinical features of hepatitis D. Semin Liver Dis 32:228–236
150. Wu JC, Chen TZ, Huang YS, Yen FS, Ting LT, Sheng WY, Tsay SH et al (1995) Natural history of hepatitis D viral superinfection: significance of viremia detected by polymerase chain reaction. Gastroenterology 108:796–802
151. Hadziyannis SJ (1997) Hepatitis delta: an overview. In: Rizzetto M, Purcell RH, Gerin JL (eds) Viral hepatitis and liver disease. Edizioni Minerva Medica, Turin, pp 283–289
152. Hoofnagle JH (1989) Type D (delta) hepatitis. JAMA 261:1321–1325
153. Gheorghe L, Iacob S, Simionov I, Vadan R, Gheorghe C, Iacob R, Parvulescu I et al (2005) Natural history of compensated viral B and D cirrhosis. Rom J Gastroenterol 14:329–335
154. Kew MC (2013) Hepatitis viruses (other than hepatitis B and C viruses) as causes of hepatocellular carcinoma: an update. J Viral Hepat 20:149–157
155. Su CW, Huang YH, Huo TI, Shih HH, Sheen IJ, Chen SW, Lee PC et al (2006) Genotypes and viremia of hepatitis B and D viruses are associated with outcomes of chronic hepatitis D patients. Gastroenterology 130:1625–1635
156. Romeo R, Del Ninno E, Rumi M, Russo A, Sangiovanni A, de Franchis R, Ronchi G et al (2009) A 28-year study of the course of Hepatitis Delta infection: a risk factor for cirrhosis and hepatocellular carcinoma. Gastroenterology 136:1629–1638
157. Castellares C, Barreiro P, Martin-Carbonero L, Labarga P, Vispo ME, Casado R, Galindo L et al (2008) Liver cirrhosis in HIV-infected patients: prevalence, aetiology and clinical outcome. J Viral Hepat 15:165–172
158. Sheng WH, Hung CC, Kao JH, Chang SY, Chen MY, Hsieh SM, Chen PJ et al (2007) Impact of hepatitis D virus infection on the long-term outcomes of patients with hepatitis B virus and HIV coinfection in the era of highly active antiretroviral therapy: a matched cohort study. Clin Infect Dis 44:988–995
159. Wu JC, Choo KB, Chen CM, Chen TZ, Huo TI, Lee SD (1995) Genotyping of hepatitis D virus by restriction-fragment length polymorphism and relation to outcome of hepatitis D. Lancet 346:939–941
160. Casey JL, Brown TL, Colan EJ, Wignall FS, Gerin JL (1993) A genotype of hepatitis D virus that occurs in northern South America. Proc Natl Acad Sci U S A 90:9016–9020
161. Bensabath G, Hadler SC, Soares MC, Fields H, Dias LB, Popper H, Maynard JE (1987) Hepatitis delta virus infection and Labrea hepatitis. Prevalence and role in fulminant hepatitis in the Amazon Basin. JAMA 258:479–483
162. Borresen ML, Olsen OR, Ladefoged K, McMahon BJ, Hjuler T, Panum I, Simonetti J et al (2010) Hepatitis D outbreak among children in a hepatitis B hyper-endemic settlement in Greenland. J Viral Hepat 17:162–170
163. Farci P, Barbera C, Navone C, Bortolotti F, Vajro P, Caporaso N, Vegnente A et al (1985) Infection with the delta agent in children. Gut 26:4–7
164. Ozgenc F, Ecevit CO, Erdemir G, Sertoz R, Yagci RV (2013) Prevalence of hepatitis D co-infection in children with hepatitis B infection: cross-sectional

analyses from Western Turkey. Turk J Gastroenterol 24:345–348
165. Yuce A, Kocak N, Ozen H, Gurakan F (1996) Prevalence of antidelta in Turkish children with chronic hepatitis B infection. Arch Dis Child 75:355
166. Calle Serrano B, Grosshennig A, Homs M, Heidrich B, Erhardt A, Deterding K, Jaroszewicz J et al (2014) Development and evaluation of a baseline-event-anticipation score for hepatitis delta. J Viral Hepat 21:e154–e163
167. Aragona M, Macagno S, Caredda F, Crivelli O, Lavarini C, Maran E, Farci P et al (1987) Serological response to the hepatitis delta virus in hepatitis D. Lancet 1:478–480
168. Chang MH, Chen CJ, Lai MS, Hsu HM, Wu TC, Kong MS, Liang DC et al (1997) Universal hepatitis B vaccination in Taiwan and the incidence of hepatocellular carcinoma in children. Taiwan Childhood Hepatoma Study Group N Engl J Med 336:1855–1859
169. Chang MH, You SL, Chen CJ, Liu CJ, Lee CM, Lin SM, Chu HC et al (2009) Decreased incidence of hepatocellular carcinoma in hepatitis B vaccines: a 20-year follow-up study. J Natl Cancer Inst 101:1348–1355
170. Yurdaydin C (2012) Treatment of chronic delta hepatitis. Semin Liver Dis 32:237–244
171. Aziz S, Rajper J, Noor-ul-Ain W, Mehnaz A, Masroor M, Chang MH (2011) Interferon-alpha treatment of children and young adults with chronic hepatitis delta virus (HDV) infection. J Coll Physicians Surg Pak 21:735–740
172. Sanchez-Tapias JM, Mas A, Costa J, Bruguera M, Mayor A, Ballesta AM, Compernolle C et al (1987) Recombinant alpha 2c-interferon therapy in fulminant viral hepatitis. J Hepatol 5:205–210

Mother-to-Infant Transmission of Viral Hepatitis

4

Huey-Ling Chen

Abstract

Hepatitis virus infection is often initiated in infancy or childhood. Mother-to-infant transmission is an important transmission route for a large number of patients, with subsequent chronic hepatitis and associated long-term complications including cirrhosis, liver cancer, and mortality. In the past 30 years, measures to prevent mother-to-infant transmission have been investigated extensively especially in hepatitis B virus infection, including screening of pregnant women with HBsAg and/or HBeAg, neonatal immunization with HBV vaccines and hepatitis B immunoglobulin, and postimmunization surveillance for children with breakthrough infection. For up to 10% of infants born to HBsAg-/HBeAg-positive mothers, neonatal immunization may not offer effective protection, and these infants may become chronically infected. Recently, studies have shown that short-term antiviral therapy for HBV-infected pregnant women with a high viral load has effectively prevented mother-to-infant transmission. Mother-to-infant transmission of hepatitis C virus occurs in about 5% of HCV-infected mothers. Screening of pregnant women for HCV is still a controversial issue because no effective preventive measure is currently available. Surveillance of children born to HCV-infected mothers is recommended. Acute HAV and HEV infection in pregnant women is rare, but these infections should be considered when icteric illness occurs in pregnant women. HAV vaccination helps to decrease the susceptible population. Acute HEV infection in pregnant women frequently leads to fulminant hepatic failure, with a high mortality rate for the mother, fetus, and neonates. Most reported cases occurred in an endemic area. Safe drinking water, public health improvement, and newly developed HEV vaccines are effective measures to prevent infection. In conclusion, efforts toward interrupting mother-to-infant transmission of viral hepatitis will effectively improve maternal/fetal/neonatal outcomes, as well as preventing a large population in the world with chronic hepatitis and associated complications.

Keywords

Hepatitis · Pregnant women screening · HAV · HBV · HCV · HEV · Vaccination · Immunization · Antiviral therapy

H.-L. Chen (✉)
Department of Pediatrics, National Taiwan University College of Medicine and Children's Hospital, Taipei, Taiwan
e-mail: hueyling@ntu.edu.tw

M.-H. Chang, K. B. Schwarz (eds.), *Viral Hepatitis in Children*,
https://doi.org/10.1007/978-981-13-0050-9_4

4.1 Introduction

Neonates and infants whose livers are immature and whose immune systems are still developing are prone to infection by hepatitis viruses including hepatitis A virus (HAV), hepatitis B virus (HBV), hepatitis C virus (HCV), and hepatitis E virus (HEV) (Table 4.1). Some may develop acute hepatitis leading to neonatal mortality. But most importantly, many patients develop chronic infection that persists lifelong, causing subsequent chronic hepatitis and associated complications including cirrhosis, liver cancer, and mortality. Mother-to-infant transmission mainly occurs at three time points: intrauterine, peripartum, and the postnatal period. Preventive measures to interrupt mother-to-infant transmission have been investigated extensively in the past 30 years and have changed the epidemiology of viral hepatitis in the world. There are still challenges to improve the management of mother-to-infant transmission of viral hepatitis. This chapter will focus on the prevalence, risks, and management of mother-to-infant transmission of hepatitis viruses that cause chronic infection (HBV, HCV) and acute infection (HAV, HEV) of the host.

4.2 Mother-to-Infant Transmission of Hepatitis B Virus

Before the era of HBV immunization, it has been well recognized that most chronic hepatitis B infection is from mother-to-infant transmission. The earlier the age of infection, the higher the chance of becoming chronic infected. Approximately 50–90% of children infected before 1 year of age became chronic carriers [1]. Children born to HBsAg- and HBeAg-positive mothers have a 90% chance of becoming chronic HBsAg infected; children born to HBsAg-positive, HBeAg-negative mothers have a 10–40% chance of developing chronic infection [2–5]. Maternal HBV transmission is the major source of infection in those with chronic HBV infection and in hepatocellular carcinoma patients in endemic areas [6].

Table 4.1 Mother-to-infant transmission of various common types of viral hepatitis

	Rate of mother-to-infant transmission	Risk factors	Outcomes	Intervention	Children surveillance for infection
HAV	Rare	Maternal acute HAV before delivery	Self-limited	Isolation of index newborn and prevention of horizontal spread	IgM anti-HAV at birth
HBV	5–10% children born to HBeAg+ mothers; <0.5% children born to HBeAg- mothers in immunized children	HBeAg positivity; maternal viral load; maternal-fetal blood leakage; host factors	Chronic HBV infection; may develop acute/fulminant hepatitis in rare cases born to HBeAg- mothers	Maternal screening; maternal antiviral therapy since the 3rd trimester; neonatal immunization	HBsAg at 12mo or anytime when symptomatic
HCV	5%	Unknown	Resolving infection or chronic infection	Nil	Anti-HCV $\geq$ 18 mo or HCV RNA anytime when indicated
HEV	High (~100%) with maternal HEV RNA(+)	Endemic area, maternal acute symptomatic HEV infection	Neonatal mortality or acute resolving disease	Supportive medical care for acute hepatitis	IgM anti-HEV or HEV RNA
	Low (~0%) with maternal HEV RNA(−)				

Even after the implementation of universal immunization coverage, the majority of children with breakthrough HBV infection acquire infection from mother-to-infant transmission [7]. Despite optimal protection from HBIG at birth and 3–4 doses of HBV vaccines, HBV infection still occurs in children born to HBeAg-positive mothers, with infection rates ranged 5–10% [7–9]. Children born to HBeAg-negative mothers have a very low risk of HBV infection below 0.3% but may develop acute or fulminant hepatitis during infancy [7, 10].

Mother-to-infant transmission of HBV usually occurs in the perinatal period, or more precisely, during the intrauterine, peripartum, or postnatal period (Fig. 4.1). The majority of mother-to-infant transmission of HBV occurs during the peripartum period. Exposure of maternal blood through maternal-fetal hemorrhage or direct contact of newborns with infected maternal secretions and blood during labor is the most common route of transmission. Of note is that HBV infection has an incubation time of 30–180 days; therefore the infant who acquires HBV from his mother is usually detected as HBsAg-positive several months after viral transmission. In this regard, neonatal immunization starting after birth can prevent most mother-to-infant infection of HBV. There are several terms commonly used which are similar to "mother-to-infant transmission (MTIT)," including "mother-to-child-transmission (MTCT)" and "vertical transmission," although we consider the most appropriate term to be "mother-to-infant transmission (MTIT)" of HBV because the timing of transmission most likely occurs in the peripartum period. The prophylaxis strategies including maternal antiviral therapy and neonatal immunization both focus on preventing peripartum transmission. Horizontal transmission beyond 1 year of age is a rare event in children who have received immunoprophylaxis.

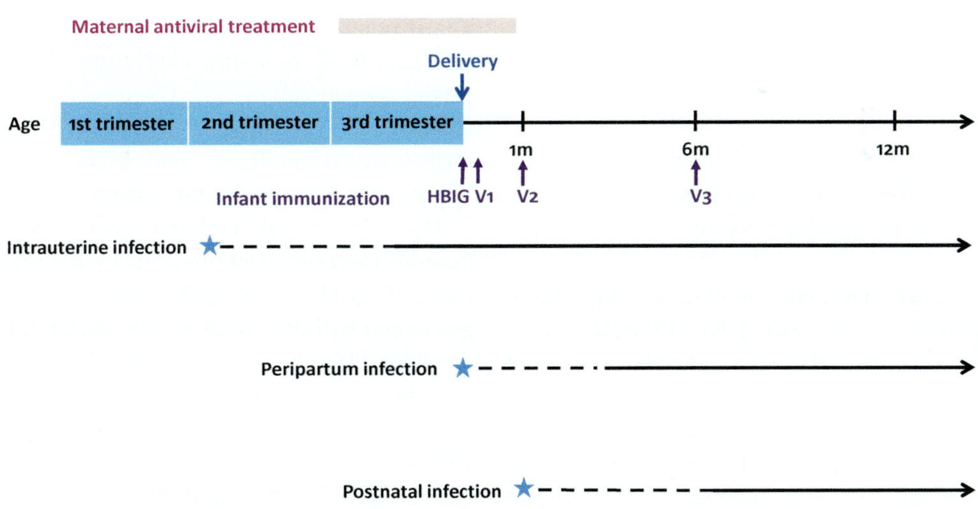

Fig. 4.1 Different timing (intrauterine, peripartum, postnatal) of mother-to-infant transmission of HBV. Intrauterine infection occurs in the second trimester or early third trimester, and the infant is detected to have positive HBsAg at the time of birth [11]. Most mother-to-infant transmission occurs at peripartum period during the process of labor. Therefore neonatal immunization and maternal antiviral treatment are effective in preventing HBV infection in children. Postnatal infection occurs after children are born and is a rare event in those receiving appropriate immunoprophylaxis

HBIG hepatitis B immunoglobulin
V1, V2, and V3: the first, second, and third doses of HBV vaccines

★ : Time of viral exposure

– – – – : incubation period

⟶ : time of infection (HBsAg positive)

Intrauterine infection occurs in a much lower frequency than peripartum infection. The fetus may contract HBV from leakage of maternal blood through the placenta and already has established HBV infection at the time of birth. The definition of intrauterine infection is HBsAg positivity in newborn's blood within 24 h of birth [11] which persists thereafter. However, because of the high sensitivity of current diagnostic tests, some children may have low levels of HBsAg positivity at birth but will not become chronically infected. It is noteworthy that positive HBV DNA detected in newborn blood or cord blood cannot be used as a reliable marker for intrauterine infection. It may merely represent exposure to maternal virus during the peripartum period or contamination of maternal blood at cord blood sampling.

Postnatal HBV infection in immunized children is rare but possible, especially in those infants who do not have an adequate immune response after neonatal immunization [12]. Nonresponders (anti-HBs < 10 mIU/mL) or low titer responders (10–100 mIU/mL) to HBV vaccination have been found to be related to host HLA alleles [13].

4.2.1 Risk Factors of Mother-to-Infant Transmission of Hepatitis B Virus

It is known that most mother-to-infant HBV transmission occurs in mothers with HBeAg positivity. Maternal HBV DNA levels have been known to be associated with increased rates of mother-to-infant transmission even using earlier methods of detection [14, 15]. Many recent studies with more sensitive methods for detection of viral load have documented that the higher maternal viral load, the higher the rate of children infected. The majority of reported cases of mother-to-infant HBV infection occurred in mothers with viral loads above 10^7–10^8 copies/mL. A few cases with maternal viral load at 10^6–10^7 copies/mL have been reported [16–20]. In a prospective study in Taiwan, there was a statistically significant risk of infants acquiring HBV infection when the maternal viral loads were above 10^7 copies/mL. Rates of infants with chronic HBV infection with maternal viral load levels of 5, 6, 7, 8, and 9 $\log_{10}$ copies/mL were 0.9% (95% confidence interval [CI], −0.9%–2.7%; $P = 0.334$), 2.6% (95% CI, −1.1%–6.2%; $P = 0.165$), 6.6% (95% CI, 0.5%–12.6%; $P = 0.033$), 14.6% (95% CI, 5.6%–23.6%; $P = 0.001$), and 27.7% (95% CI, 13.1%–42.4%; $P < 0.001$), respectively [17] (Fig. 4.2). Cases with maternal viral load at level of $10^{6\text{-}7}$ copies/mL may have additional risk factors to cause MTIT such as prematurity or maternal-fetal blood leakage [17].

Maternal-fetal hemorrhage of various causes including threatened abortion, threatened preterm labor, amniocentesis, and antepartum hemorrhage is an important risk factor for HBV transmission to the infant. Vacuum or forceps delivery and emergent cesarean section are also associated with increased mother-to-infant HBV transmission rates [21–25]. Breastfeeding does not increase infection rates in those infants with appropriate immunoprophylaxis, including hepatitis B immune globulin and hepatitis B vaccine [26–28]. It is recommended from the World Health Organization and Centers for Disease Control and Prevention of the United States that HBV-infected mothers can breastfeed their infants with neonatal immunization [29, 30].

Host factors of children also may affect immune responses and thus affect HBV infection rates. HLA-DR14-DR52 has been noted to be associated with low responsiveness to HBV vaccine [31–33].

Although HBV surface gene mutants in the *a*-determinant have been found in children after universal immunization [34, 35], with prevalence rates of 22.6% [36, 37], these mutants have not been found to affect vaccine efficacy. A trend of genotype shift has also been observed, with an increased percentage of HBsAg-positive children born to mothers with genotype C [38]. Whether this is related to higher risk of genotype C in mother-to-infant transmission or merely reflects higher maternal viral load is not clear.

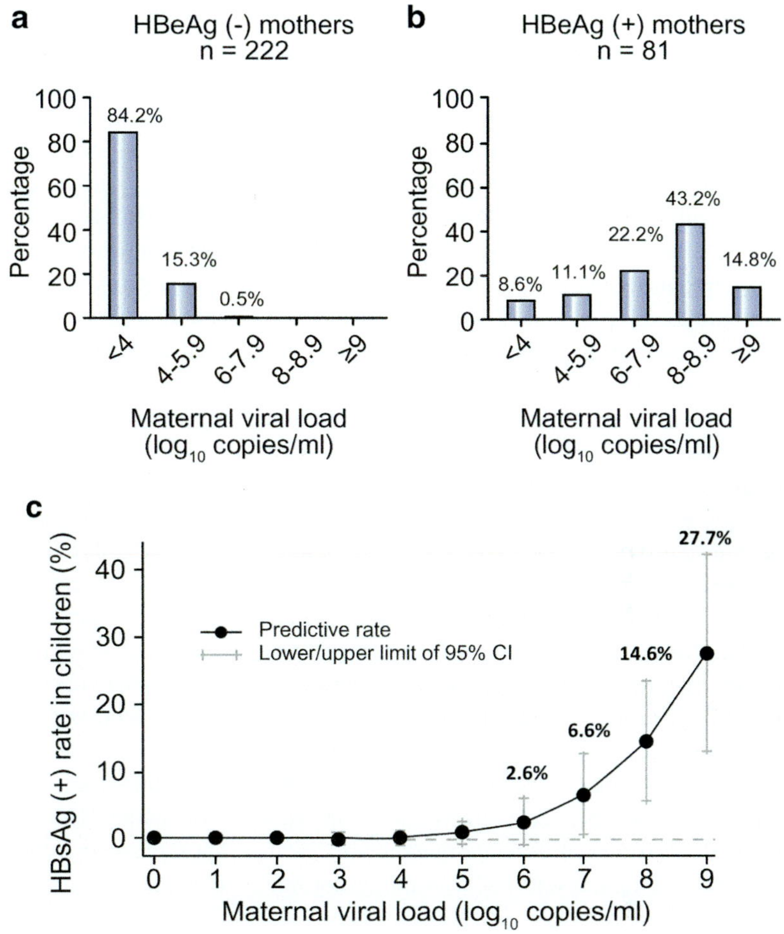

Fig. 4.2 (**a** and **b**) Viral load distribution in HBsAg mothers with HBeAg(−) and HBeAg(+); (**c**) predictive rates of children with HBV infection at various maternal HBV DNA levels. Significantly increased rates of infants with chronic HBV infection are observed with maternal viral load levels at 7, 8, and 9 $\log_{10}$ copies/mL ($P = 0.033$, $P = 0.001$, and $P < 0.001$, respectively). (Reproduced with permission from Ref. [17])

4.3 Mother-to-Infant Transmission of Hepatitis C Virus

Mother-to-infant transmission occurs in around 5% of mothers positive for anti-HCV and about 10% in mothers with HCV/HIV coinfection [39–41]. Maternal HIV coinfection has been the most important determinant of transmission, with an odds ratio of 2.56 in meta-analysis [40]. Mother-to-infant transmission is the major source of infection for childhood HCV infection in the era of effective blood product screening. The time of transmission may be intrauterine, intrapartum, or postnatal period.

Risk factors for mother-to-infant HCV transmission include high maternal viral load above 10^6 IU/mL [42–44], HIV coinfection [45, 46], prolonged labor, and use of internal fetal monitoring during labor [45]. The route of delivery has not been shown to influence the risk of vertical HCV transmission in meta-analysis [47], although one study has shown a reduced risk of transmission after cesarean delivery vs vaginal or emergent delivery [48]. Cesarean delivery is currently recommended only for obstetric indications in women with HCV infection [44, 47]. Breastfeeding was not found to carry an increased risk of mother-to-infant HCV infection [49].

There has been no apparent increased risk of obstetric complications in HCV-infected women during pregnancy and delivery. In a cohort study of 244 infants born to HCV-positive mothers, 4.7% (9/190) born to HCV RNA-positive mothers became infected, compared with 0/54 infants born to HCV RNA-negative mothers (P = 0.10).

Three infected children resolved their infection (became HCV RNA negative) [45]. In a prospectively followed group of 11 infants born to HCV-infected mothers, 2 were found to be infected. One of the two had hepatitis C virus RNA at the age of 1, 3, and 6 months, but not later. The other infant had hepatitis C virus RNA detectable at the age of 3 months and at 15, 18, and 24 months. In those infants born to HCV-infected mothers who did not develop chronic infection, maternally acquired anti-HCV gradually disappeared by the age of 6 months. The course of HCV-infected children may be characterized by fluctuating viral replication in chronic infection or viral clearance in acute infection [50]. It is notable that anti-HCV positivity before 12 months of age may be transplacental maternal antibody and cannot be used as a marker for diagnosing infant with mother-to-infant transmission of HCV.

The American Academy of Pediatrics recommends that infants born to HCV-infected mothers should be tested for anti-HCV at or after 18 months of age. For children positive for anti-HCV, an additional testing for HCV RNA (HCV viral load) is recommended. In infancy, HCV RNA is a more reliable marker for detecting infection than is anti-HCV antibody testing.

4.4 Mother-to-Infant Transmission of Hepatitis A Virus

HAV infection, which is endemic in many countries in the world, causes acute hepatitis or asymptomatic infection, but not chronic infection. Transmission of HAV is almost exclusively horizontal by the fecal-oral route. Acute hepatitis A accounts for <2% of hepatitis cases in pregnant women [51]. Mother-to-infant transmission of HAV is a rare event.

Acute hepatitis A in pregnancy has been generally considered as not leading to severe outcomes or complications. However, in a large case series, it was reported that 69% of pregnant women with acute hepatitis A infection had high rates of obstetric complications, including premature contraction, placental separation, premature rupture of membrane, and preterm labor. The newborns' outcomes were favorable [51].

Intrauterine infection of HAV has been reported to occur during as early as gestational age 13–20 weeks, with one case of fetal meconium peritonitis reported [52]. Acute hepatitis A in the late stage of pregnancy may cause infection of newborns. Infected newborns may develop self-limiting icteric hepatitis followed by recovery [53–55]. Transplacental-acquired maternal IgG antibodies are considered to have a protective role. In rare situations, transmission has been reported to occur in pregnant women infected 4 months prior to delivery; in that case, a mutated viral strain was identified [56]. An outbreak in a neonatal unit was reported from vertical transmission with horizontal spread [57]. Isolation of the HAV-infected newborn to prevent horizontal spread is recommended. Attendant healthcare personnel should be immunized for HAV.

The main measure to manage mother-to-infant HAV infection is to identify mothers with icteric illness or acute hepatitis who are positive with IgM anti-HAV. Once the mother is diagnosed with acute HAV, isolation of her newborn and appropriate infection control for the neonatal unit is required.

4.5 Mother-to-Infant Transmission of Hepatitis E Virus

Acute hepatitis E in pregnant women in endemic areas results in significant mortality in mothers, fetus, and newborns. Prevalence rates differ in different geographic areas. Most cases were reported in Asia, Africa, Latin America (genotype 1), sub-Saharan Africa, and Mexico (genotype 2), acquired via fecally contaminated water [58]. Zoonotic HEV strains (genotype 3 and 4) have more recently been identified in developed countries and in immunocompromised patients [59–61]. In India, HEV infection accounts for 60% of acute viral hepatitis in pregnant women [62].

In 55% of pregnant women, acute hepatitis E may results in fulminant hepatic failure (FHF). In pregnant women with FHF, the mortality was high (41%), as was the rate of intrauterine fetal death (58%) [62]. Women with HEV infection were more likely than those with other forms of viral hepatitis to have obstetric complications including antepartum hemorrhage, intrauterine fetal death, preterm delivery, and stillbirth [62]. The presence of systemic inflammatory response syndrome (SIRS) has been commonly observed in the fatal cases [63].

HEV infection is commonly transmitted from mother-to-fetus and causes high neonatal mortality. HEV infection in surviving infants is self-limiting with short-lasting viremia. In one study in India, 15/19 (78.9%) of newborns born to acute HEV-infected mothers had evidence of vertically transmitted HEV infection at birth (IgM anti-HEV or HEV RNA positive), and three had short-lasting IgG anti-HEV positivity because of transplacental antibody transmission. HEV-infected babies developed icteric or non-icteric hepatitis. Seven died in the first week of birth. All surviving babies had self-limiting disease, with HEV RNA undetected after 4–32 weeks of age [64].

These cases call attention to the importance of screening for HEV in pregnant women with icteric illness. The diagnosis of maternal and infant HEV infection relies largely on IgM anti-HEV and HEV RNA.

4.6 Pregnant Women Screening and Intervention

HBV Screening of pregnant women has been implemented in many countries together with universal neonatal immunization for many years. The screening for HBV infection is, mainly to select high-risk newborns for HBIG administration, in addition to three doses of HBV vaccines for all infants. There have been two types of maternal HBV screening: HBsAg alone or HBsAg with HBeAg (Table 4.2). The HBsAg/HBeAg strategy may increase the budget for pregnant women screening but saves costs of HBIG. Unfortunately total elimination of mother-to-infant HBV transmission has not yet been achieved in the high-risk group with maternal HBeAg positivity and high viral load despite optimal practice of universal immunization for more than two decades.

Table 4.2 Current pregnant women screening and universal infant hepatitis B virus (HBV) immunoprophylaxis strategies in different countries and a proposed maternal intervention/children surveillance program that can be linked to current strategy

	Pregnant women screening and intervention		Neonatal immunization		Surveillance of children with risk of breakthrough infection by HBsAg at 12–18 months	
Strategy type	HBsAg/HBeAg (high-risk group selection)	HBV DNA/AVT[b]	HBV vaccines to all infants	HBIG to high-risk group[c]	All children born to HBsAg + mothers	All children born to HBeAg + mothers
I	+/–	(+)	+	+	+	
II[a]	+/+	(+)	+	+		+
III	–/–	–	+	–	–	–

Examples of applied countries: strategy type I, USA, Italy, Korea; strategy type II, Taiwan, Singapore; strategy type III, Thailand

[a]In strategy type II, simultaneous or sequential HBsAg and HBeAg tests can be applied. For example, all pregnant women are screened with HBsAg and HBeAg at the same time, or all pregnant women are screened for HBsAg and with HBeAg tested only in those positive for HBsAg; the latter strategy is budget-saving

[b]HBV DNA testing and antiviral therapy (AVT) is a potential strategy for population-based pregnant women intervention that can be linked to current pregnant women screening, including HBV DNA test for high-risk group mothers and AVT for those who meet the criteria for intervention

[c]HBIG is given to high-risk group according to pregnant women screening strategy. In strategy I, HBIG is given to newborn born to all HBsAg(+) mothers; in strategy II, HBIG is given to newborn born to HBsAg(+)/HBeAg(+) mothers

In the recent decade, there have been increasing numbers of clinical trials using antiviral therapy (AVT) in pregnant women for prevention of mother-to-infant transmission of HBV, following the successful maternal intervention to prevent mother-to-infant HIV infection. The early trials used lamivudine (pregnancy category C) in high viral load mothers starting from late pregnancy, resulting in decreased rates but not totally prevention of infant HBV infection [65, 66]. Subsequently, since the wide application of category B antivirals including telbivudine and tenofovir, more studies of better quality have demonstrated a significant effect of AVT in preventing mother-to-infant HBV transmission. Because newer AVT can rapidly decrease maternal viral load in 8 weeks, most studies started AVT in pregnant women in the 3rd trimester (28–32 weeks of gestation), with an aim of reducing the maternal viral load to lower than 10^6 IU/mL at the time of delivery, which is considered a minimal risk to transmit HBV to newborns during the peripartum period [12, 18, 67–69].

The current recommendations for selecting pregnant women for maternal AVT are based on reported cases of mother-to-infant transmission and on related clinical trials of AVT in pregnant women. The cutoff of maternal HBV DNA levels eligible for pregnant women AVT of the clinical trials ranged from 6 to 8 $\log_{10}$ copies/mL (approximate 5.5–7.5 $\log_{10}$ IU/mL). Although the majority of infected children were born to mothers with viral load above 8 $\log_{10}$ copies/mL, few cases were reported to occur with maternal HBV DNA around 6 $\log_{10}$ copies/mL, possibly due to additional risk factors causing exposure of the infant to maternal blood or due to variations in laboratory methods used. The current recommendation from AASLD; ESPGHAN; APASL; Australian, UK, and NZ leaders; and the Society for Maternal-Fetal Medicine (SMFM) is to treat pregnant women with variable viral load cutoff levels: >200,000 IU/mL (AASLD, EASL), >6 $\log_{10}$ IU/mL (ESPGHAN), >6–7 $\log_{10}$ IU/mL (APASL), >7 $\log_{10}$ IU/mL (Australian, UK, and NZ leaders), and >6–8 $\log_{10}$ copies/mL (SMFM), respectively [70–75]. The lower the cutoff value, the larger the population of HBV-infected pregnant women is to be included in AVT treatment.

A systematic review and meta-analysis have shown that AVT improved HBV suppression and reduces mother-to-infant transmission in women with chronic HBV infection with a high viral load. The use of telbivudine (category B), lamivudine (category C), and tenofovir (category B) appears to be safe in pregnancy with no increased adverse maternal or fetal outcome [76]. Telbivudine and tenofovir have the advantage of category B and a shorter duration to achieve maternal viral reduction than lamivudine. Tenofovir has the advantage of minimal risk of drug resistance in long-term follow-up and no increase in the rates of birth defects (data of Antiretroviral Pregnancy Registry) when it was used starting since first/second or third trimester [77–79]. It is noted that since 2015, FDA has replaced the previously used pregnancy risk categories A, B, C, D, and X with narrative sections including pregnancy exposure registry and risk summary. The pregnancy letter category will be removed in updated drug labels.

For mothers with HIV/HBV coinfection, maternal AVT treatment with either lamivudine alone, tenofovir/lamivudine, or tenofovir/emtricitabine has resulted in desirable maternal HBV viral load reduction and may protect children from HBV infection when combined with neonatal HBIG and HBV vaccines after birth [80, 81].

Several issues should be discussed with the mothers before starting the AVT in pregnancy. It is noted that AVT in pregnant women may not completely eradicate mother-to-infant transmission, especially intrauterine infection, and in cases with poor immune response to HBV vaccines [12]. Multivariate analysis has revealed that children in the maternal TDF group had a lower risk (odds ratio 0.10) of infection compared to control group. The higher the maternal viral load, the higher the chance of children to be infected; therefore the use of AVT in pregnant mothers is more strongly recommended [17].

Safety for mothers and children is a great consideration for a wide application of this strategy. During the treatment course in pregnancy, most commonly reported side effects are gastrointestinal complaints such as nausea/vomiting or allergic reactions. Most are self-limited in 1–2 weeks, and very few cases reported intolerable side effects necessitating discontinuation of treatment. Another important issue is the time to stop maternal treatment after delivery, which may be closely related to postpartum maternal ALT elevations. In a control group of mothers with high viral loads who were not receiving AVT, the ALT level tended to elevate within 1–4 months postpartum, possibly due to hormonal changes after delivering the infants [12]. To prevent maternal ALT flares after delivery due to stopping AVT and potential liver injuries associated with viral load rebound, most of the AVT trials stopped the maternal drug 1–3 months after delivery. There have been conflicting reports of rates of maternal ALT flare between studies. One well-controlled and closely followed study showed a reduced frequency and extent of ALT elevation in the AVT group compared to controls [12]. A recent randomized controlled trial showed a higher rate of ALT elevation [69]. Another study showed no significant differences [82]. The discrepancy between studies mainly is the definition of ALT elevation or ALT flare and timing and frequency of follow-up. In general, there has been no severe adverse complication reported for the HBV mothers receiving this short-term AVT. Most ALT elevations postpartum are self-limited. For cases with ALT elevations during the period of AVT treatment, an option to continue AVT as a regular hepatitis case until HBeAg conversion may be considered. In patients with normal ALT during AVT but with ALT flare postpartum, reinitiating AVT for the mothers' own liver disease can be considered. These options should be carefully discussed with the mothers by the specialist.

The safety of infants born to mothers receiving AVT during pregnancy is an important consideration. Although the current trials have all shown no increase in the birth defects rates in the newborn, long-term follow-up data is lacking. Long-term follow-up of the children whose mothers received AVT during pregnancy should be done including effects on growth and development or other complications, the children's immune responses to vaccines, and rates of horizontal or occult HBV infection.

As for obstetric interventions, some studies have demonstrated a higher infection risk with amniocentesis especially in mothers with viral load above 7 $\log_{10}$ copies/mL [21] and a lower risk of infection with elective cesarean section compared with vaginal delivery or emergent cesarean section [25]. There are still controversies, and a routine recommendation for changing the obstetric procedure is not suggested [74]. According to the recommendation of SMFM, for HBV-infected women who have an indication for genetic testing and invasive testing (e.g., amniocentesis or chorionic villus sampling), counseling should include the fact that the risk for maternal-fetal transmission may increase with HBV viral load >7 $\log_{10}$ IU/mL. Cesarean delivery should not be performed for the sole indication for reduction of vertical HBV transmission [70].

Prenatal administration of HBIG to pregnant women to reduce mother-to-infant transmission has been evaluated in several studies in China. Pregnant women received multiple dosing of HBIG intravenously beginning at 28–32 weeks of gestation. A meta-analysis revealed that infants in the maternal HBIG group had a lower rate of HBsAg positivity (OR = 0.33, 95% CI, 0.21–0.51, $P < 0.01$, from 9 RCTs), but some adverse reactions have been reported [83]. This strategy is rarely adopted outside of China.

Although there is no evidence that breastfeeding increases HBV infection rates in immunized infants, breastfeeding was not recommended when mothers are using AVT, due to unpredicted drug exposure and effects in the newborns. It was recommended that breastfeeding be held during the first month when mothers are still on AVT and be resumed after stopping the drug. However, emerging evidence in HIV mother-infant pairs have shown negligible amounts of tenofovir excreted in breast milk (less than 3% of mother's serum concentration); <0.01% of therapeutic dose was absorbed in the newborn. Tenofovir was not detected in 94% of infant plasma samples, suggesting tenofovir can be used safely during breastfeeding with minimal infant drug exposure [74, 84, 85]. The other option is to consider stopping the AVT earlier than 4 weeks postpartum, which requires further studies to confirm safety for the mothers. The latest recommendations from AASLD, EASL, and Australian, UK, and NZ leaders have indicated that breastfeeding is not contraindicated for women under AVT [73–75]. With more evidence on data of infants' long-term safety, it is anticipated that the issue of breastfeeding for mothers on AVT will be clearer in the near future.

It is worth noticing that the strategy of screening pregnant women for HBV is closely linked to subsequent measures for interrupting mother-to-infant transmission, including selection of cases for AVT, newborn immunization strategies (selection of high risk newborns to receive HBIG), as well as screening of high-risk children for HBsAg positivity, as shown in Fig. 4.3 and Table 4.2. The cost-benefit of each strategy should be thoroughly considered based on each country's seroprevalence rate, mother-to-infant transmission rates, the budget available for screening, HBIG, vaccines, and laboratory tests. The high cost of HBV DNA testing of eligible mothers may have great financial impact on maternal screening, added on the subsequent AVT treatment cost. Budget-saving methods for population-based testing to select mothers eligible for treatment but not to over-expand the treatment population have been studied. The quantitative HBsAg level has been proposed to be an alternative method that will predict mother-to-infant transmission. Base on the prediction, AVT may be considered in pregnant women with an HBsAg level above 4–4.5 log10 IU/mL [86]. Alternatively, treatment can be given to all HBsAg-/HBeAg-positive women, without considering HBV DNA levels. This practice has been evaluated in a randomized controlled trial [87]. High viral load mothers (>10^6 copies/mL) are estimated to account for 80% of all HBeAg-positive mothers, and the rate may vary among different countries. This strategy may reduce the cost of HBV DNA but will expand the pregnant population to receive AVT. The benefit and risk of this practice remain to be confirmed (Table 4.2).

HCV There have been debates about screening of target groups vs universal screening of pregnant women with anti-HCV, because of lack of preventive measures for mother-to-infant transmission [47]. Prevalence of anti-HCV positivity in pregnant women varied among different countries and geographic areas and ranged from 0.1%–2.4%. In a nationwide survey in the United States during 2011 to 2014, the detection of HCV infection among women of childbearing age increased, and the proportion of infants born to HCV-infected mothers increased from 0.19% to 0.32%, indicating the population at risk for mother-to-infant transmission of HCV increased [88].

Due to the recent progress in direct-acting agents (DAA) for effective treatment and cure of HCV infection, screening and management strategies may evolve in the future. Currently, experience with any of these new DAAs in human pregnancy is lacking. Ribavirin is category X; sofosbuvir and ledipasvir are both category B drugs. Simeprevir monotherapy is a category C medication. Many new DAAs are expected to be available in the near future. The safety profiles of

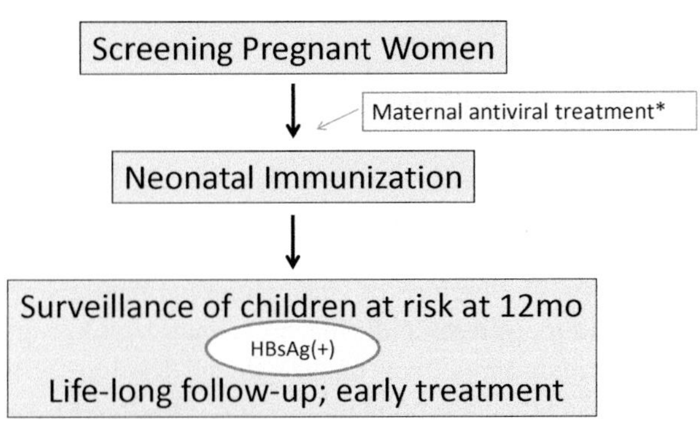

Fig. 4.3 Three steps to prevent and monitor mother-to-infant HBV transmission
***Maternal antiviral treatment is indicated in high risk group to prevent mother-to-infant transmission of HBV**

each drug will be carefully examined before evaluating a potential use in HCV in pregnancy [43].

For children born to mothers positive for HCV, postnatal surveillance for anti-HCV at or after age 18 months is indicated. HCV RNA is considered in children positive for anti-HCV or when testing at age 0–18 months is indicated.

HAV and HEV Identification of icteric hepatitis in pregnant women, especially in endemic areas of HAV and HEV infection, is most important. Zoonotic HEV strains should also be considered in non-endemic areas.

HAV vaccine is safe, effective, and widely applicable and should be given to all susceptible populations before pregnancy. Universal HAV vaccination in endemic countries may decrease the susceptible population of pregnant women and decrease the sources for horizontal infection [89].

The main measure to prevent HEV infection is to provide safe drinking water, which requires great efforts from the governments. Public health education and hand washing may decrease the chance of horizontal spread. Early detection of icteric illness and availability of medical care will improve the outcome of infected women and children. The newly developed HEV vaccines may decrease the disease burden in the future in applicable areas [90, 91]. Limited data regarding the safety and efficacy of HEV vaccines in pregnant women have been reported [92]. Further studies are warranted.

4.7 Summary

In summary, recent advances in preventing mother-to-infant transmission of HBV have several steps including pregnant women screening of HBsAg with or without HBeAg, pregnant women antiviral therapy in high viral load mothers, neonatal immunizations (HBIG and HB vaccines), and postimmunization surveillance of high-risk children at age 12 months. The HBV DNA cutoff, treatment, and follow-up protocol for maternal HBV AVT will be optimized, and long-term safety of mothers and children will be elucidated in future studies. A goal of global elimination of HBV will be anticipated with effective interruption of mother-to-infant transmission. For HCV infection, there have been controversies in whether to screen pregnant women for anti-HCV or not. For children born to mothers positive for HCV, postnatal surveillance for anti-HCV at age 18 months or older is indicated. Future development of safe and effective oral therapy for HCV infection will shed light on mothers and children infected with HCV. Safe drinking water and public health improvement are of great importance to prevent HAV and HEV infection. Universal HAV infection is effective in decreasing the population of susceptible pregnant women for acute HAV infection. The newly developed HEV vaccines may decrease the disease burden in endemic areas in the future.

References

1. Beasley RP (2009) Rocks along the road to the control of HBV and HCC. Ann Epidemiol 19(4):231–234
2. Beasley RP, Trepo C, Stevens CE, Szmuness W (1977) The e antigen and vertical transmission of hepatitis B surface antigen. Am J Epidemiol 105(2):94–98
3. Stevens CE, Neurath RA, Beasley RP, Szmuness W (1979) HBeAg and anti-HBe detection by radioimmunoassay: correlation with vertical transmission of hepatitis B virus in Taiwan. J Med Virol 3(3):237–241
4. Degli Esposti S, Shah D (2011) Hepatitis B in pregnancy: challenges and treatment. Gastroenterol Clin N Am 40(2):355–372 viii
5. Wong VC, Ip HM, Reesink HW, Lelie PN, Reerink-Brongers EE, Yeung CY et al (1984) Prevention of the HBsAg carrier state in newborn infants of mothers who are chronic carriers of HBsAg and HBeAg by administration of hepatitis-B vaccine and hepatitis-B immunoglobulin. Double-blind randomised placebo-controlled study. Lancet (London, England) 1(8383):921–926
6. Chang MH, Chen DS (2015) Prevention of hepatitis B. Cold Spring Harb Perspect Med 5(3):a021493
7. Chen HL, Lin LH, Hu FC, Lee JT, Lin WT, Yang YJ et al (2012) Effects of maternal screening and universal immunization to prevent mother-to-infant transmission of HBV. Gastroenterology 142(4):773–781
8. Kubo A, Shlager L, Marks AR, Lakritz D, Beaumont C, Gabellini K et al (2014) Prevention of vertical transmission of hepatitis B: an observational study. Ann Intern Med 160(12):828–835

9. Schillie S, Walker T, Veselsky S, Crowley S, Dusek C, Lazaroff J et al (2015) Outcomes of infants born to women infected with hepatitis B. Pediatrics 135(5):e1141–e1147
10. Tseng YR, Wu JF, Kong MS, Hu FC, Yang YJ, Yeung CY et al (2014) Infantile hepatitis B in immunized children: risk for fulminant hepatitis and long-term outcomes. PLoS One 9(11):e111825
11. Tang JR, Hsu HY, Lin HH, Ni YH, Chang MH (1998) Hepatitis B surface antigenemia at birth: a long-term follow-up study. J Pediatr 133(3):374–377
12. Chen HL, Lee CN, Chang CH, Ni YH, Shyu MK, Chen SM et al (2015) Efficacy of maternal tenofovir disoproxil fumarate in interrupting mother-to-infant transmission of hepatitis B virus. Hepatology 62(2):375–386
13. Yoon JH, Shin S, In J, Chang JY, Song EY, Roh EY (2014) Association of HLA alleles with the responsiveness to hepatitis B virus vaccination in Korean infants. Vaccine 32(43):5638–5644
14. Lee SD, Lo KJ, Wu JC, Tsai YT, Wang JY, Ting LP et al (1986) Prevention of maternal-infant hepatitis B virus transmission by immunization: the role of serum hepatitis B virus DNA. Hepatology (Baltimore, Md) 6(3):369–373
15. Lin HH, Chang MH, Chen DS, Sung JL, Hong KH, Young YC et al (1991) Early predictor of the efficacy of immunoprophylaxis against perinatal hepatitis B transmission: analysis of prophylaxis failure. Vaccine 9(6):457–460
16. Wiseman E, Fraser MA, Holden S, Glass A, Kidson BL, Heron LG et al (2009) Perinatal transmission of hepatitis B virus: an Australian experience. Med J Aust 190(9):489–492
17. Wen WH, Chang MH, Zhao LL, Ni YH, Hsu HY, Wu JF et al (2013) Mother-to-infant transmission of hepatitis B virus infection: significance of maternal viral load and strategies for intervention. J Hepatol 59(1):24–30
18. Han GR, Cao MK, Zhao W, Jiang HX, Wang CM, Bai SF et al (2011) A prospective and open-label study for the efficacy and safety of telbivudine in pregnancy for the prevention of perinatal transmission of hepatitis B virus infection. J Hepatol 55(6):1215–1221
19. Singh AE, Plitt SS, Osiowy C, Surynicz K, Kouadjo E, Preiksaitis J et al (2011) Factors associated with vaccine failure and vertical transmission of hepatitis B among a cohort of Canadian mothers and infants. J Viral Hepat 18(7):468–473
20. Zou H, Chen Y, Duan Z, Zhang H, Pan C (2012) Virologic factors associated with failure to passive-active immunoprophylaxis in infants born to HBsAg-positive mothers. J Viral Hepat 19(2):e18–e25
21. Yi W, Pan CQ, Hao J, Hu Y, Liu M, Li L et al (2014) Risk of vertical transmission of hepatitis B after amniocentesis in HBs antigen-positive mothers. J Hepatol 60(3):523–529
22. Lin HH, Lee TY, Chen DS, Sung JL, Ohto H, Etoh T et al (1987) Transplacental leakage of HBeAg-positive maternal blood as the most likely route in causing intrauterine infection with hepatitis B virus. J Pediatr 111(6 Pt 1):877–881
23. Xu DZ, Yan YP, Choi BC, Xu JQ, Men K, Zhang JX et al (2002) Risk factors and mechanism of transplacental transmission of hepatitis B virus: a case-control study. J Med Virol 67(1):20–26
24. Lin HH, Hsu HY, Chang MH, Hong KF, Young YC, Lee TY et al (1991) Low prevalence of hepatitis C virus and infrequent perinatal or spouse infections in pregnant women in Taiwan. J Med Virol 35(4):237–240
25. Pan CQ, Zou HB, Chen Y, Zhang X, Zhang H, Li J et al (2013) Cesarean section reduces perinatal transmission of hepatitis B virus infection from hepatitis B surface antigen-positive women to their infants. Clin Gastroenterol Hepatol 11(10):1349–1355
26. Beasley RP, Stevens CE, Shiao IS, Meng HC (1975) Evidence against breast-feeding as a mechanism for vertical transmission of hepatitis B. Lancet (London, England) 2(7938):740–741
27. Woo D, Cummins M, Davies PA, Harvey DR, Hurley R, Waterson AP (1979) Vertical transmission of hepatitis B surface antigen in carrier mothers in two West London hospitals. Arch Dis Child 54(9):670–675
28. Hill JB, Sheffield JS, Kim MJ, Alexander JM, Sercely B, Wendel GD (2002) Risk of hepatitis B transmission in breast-fed infants of chronic hepatitis B carriers. Obstet Gynecol 99(6):1049–1052
29. CDC (2015) Hepatitis B and C Infections. Available from https://www.cdc.gov/breastfeeding/disease/hepatitis.htm
30. WHO (1996) Hepatitis B and breastfeeding. Available from http://www.who.int/maternal_child_adolescent/documents/hepb_breastfeeding/en/
31. Hsu HY, Chang MH, Ho HN, Hsieh RP, Lee SD, Chen DS et al (1993) Association of HLA-DR14-DR52 with low responsiveness to hepatitis B vaccine in Chinese residents in Taiwan. Vaccine 11(14):1437–1440
32. Martinetti M, De Silvestri A, Belloni C, Pasi A, Tinelli C, Pistorio A et al (2000) Humoral response to recombinant hepatitis B virus vaccine at birth: role of HLA and beyond. Clin Immunol (Orlando, Fla) 97(3):234–240
33. Avanzini MA, Belloni C, De Silvestri A, Castellazzi AM, Marconi M, Moretta A et al (2003) Antigen-specific T cell response in infants after recombinant hepatitis B virus vaccination at birth: evaluation of T helper lymphocyte diversity. Clin Immunol (Orlando, Fla) 107(2):122–128
34. Carman WF, Van Deursen FJ, Mimms LT, Hardie D, Coppola R, Decker R et al (1997) The prevalence of surface antigen variants of hepatitis B virus in Papua New Guinea, South Africa, and Sardinia. Hepatology (Baltimore, Md) 26(6):1658–1666
35. Carman WF, Zanetti AR, Karayiannis P, Waters J, Manzillo G, Tanzi E et al (1990) Vaccine-induced escape mutant of hepatitis B virus. Lancet (London, England) 336(8711):325–329
36. Hsu HY, Chang MH, Ni YH, Chen HL (2004) Survey of hepatitis B surface variant infection in children 15

years after a nationwide vaccination programme in Taiwan. Gut 53(10):1499–1503
37. Hsu HY, Chang MH, Ni YH, Chiang CL, Chen HL, Wu JF et al (2010) No increase in prevalence of hepatitis B surface antigen mutant in a population of children and adolescents who were fully covered by universal infant immunization. J Infect Dis 201(8):1192–1200
38. Wen WH, Chen HL, Ni YH, Hsu HY, Kao JH, Hu FC et al (2011) Secular trend of the viral genotype distribution in children with chronic hepatitis B virus infection after universal infant immunization. Hepatology (Baltimore, Md) 53(2):429–436
39. La Torre A, Biadaioli R, Capobianco T, Colao MG, Monti M, Pulli F et al (1998) Vertical transmission of HCV. Acta Obstet Gynecol Scand 77(9):889–892
40. Benova L, Mohamoud YA, Calvert C, Abu-Raddad LJ (2014) Vertical transmission of hepatitis C virus: systematic review and meta-analysis. Clin Infect Dis 59(6):765–773
41. Dal Molin G, D'Agaro P, Ansaldi F, Ciana G, Fertz C, Alberico S et al (2002) Mother-to-infant transmission of hepatitis C virus: rate of infection and assessment of viral load and IgM anti-HCV as risk factors. J Med Virol 67(2):137–142
42. Wen JW, Haber BA (2014) Maternal-fetal transmission of hepatitis C infection: what is so special about babies? J Pediatr Gastroenterol Nutr 58(3):278–282
43. Kanninen TT, Dieterich D, Asciutti S (2015) HCV vertical transmission in pregnancy: new horizons in the era of DAAs. Hepatology (Baltimore, Md) 62(6):1656–1658
44. Dunkelberg JC, Berkley EM, Thiel KW, Leslie KK (2014) Hepatitis B and C in pregnancy: a review and recommendations for care. J Perinatol: official journal of the California Perinatal Association 34(12):882–891
45. Mast EE, Hwang LY, Seto DS, Nolte FS, Nainan OV, Wurtzel H et al (2005) Risk factors for perinatal transmission of hepatitis C virus (HCV) and the natural history of HCV infection acquired in infancy. J Infect Dis 192(11):1880–1889
46. Marine-Barjoan E, Berrebi A, Giordanengo V, Favre SF, Haas H, Moreigne M et al (2007) HCV/HIV co-infection, HCV viral load and mode of delivery: risk factors for mother-to-child transmission of hepatitis C virus? AIDS (London, England) 21(13):1811–1815
47. Cottrell EB, Chou R, Wasson N, Rahman B, Guise JM (2013) Reducing risk for mother-to-infant transmission of hepatitis C virus: a systematic review for the U.S. preventive services task force. Ann Intern Med 158(2):109–113
48. Gibb DM, Goodall RL, Dunn DT, Healy M, Neave P, Cafferkey M et al (2000) Mother-to-child transmission of hepatitis C virus: evidence for preventable peripartum transmission. Lancet (London, England) 356(9233):904–907
49. Lin HH, Kao JH, Hsu HY, Ni YH, Chang MH, Huang SC et al (1995) Absence of infection in breast-fed infants born to hepatitis C virus-infected mothers. J Pediatr 126(4):589–591
50. Ni YH, Lin HH, Chen PJ, Hsu HY, Chen DS, Chang MH (1994) Temporal profile of hepatitis C virus antibody and genome in infants born to mothers infected with hepatitis C virus but without human immunodeficiency virus coinfection. J Hepatol 20(5):641–645
51. Elinav E, Ben-Dov IZ, Shapira Y, Daudi N, Adler R, Shouval D et al (2006) Acute hepatitis a infection in pregnancy is associated with high rates of gestational complications and preterm labor. Gastroenterology 130(4):1129–1134
52. McDuffie RS Jr, Bader T (1999) Fetal meconium peritonitis after maternal hepatitis a. Am J Obstet Gynecol 180(4):1031–1032
53. Erkan T, Kutlu T, Cullu F, Tumay GT (1998) A case of vertical transmission of hepatitis a virus infection. Acta Paediatr (Oslo, Norway: 1992) 87(9):1008–1009
54. Tanaka I, Shima M, Kubota Y, Takahashi Y, Kawamata O, Yoshioka A (1995) Vertical transmission of hepatitis A virus. Lancet (London, England) 345(8946):397
55. Urganci N, Arapoglu M, Akyildiz B, Nuhoglu A (2003) Neonatal cholestasis resulting from vertical transmission of hepatitis A infection. Pediatr Infect Dis J 22(4):381–382
56. Fagan EA, Hadzic N, Saxena R, Mieli-Vergani G (1999) Symptomatic neonatal hepatitis a disease from a virus variant acquired in utero. Pediatr Infect Dis J 18(4):389–391
57. Watson JC, Fleming DW, Borella AJ, Olcott ES, Conrad RE, Baron RC (1993) Vertical transmission of hepatitis A resulting in an outbreak in a neonatal intensive care unit. J Infect Dis 167(3):567–571
58. Krain LJ, Atwell JE, Nelson KE, Labrique AB (2014) Fetal and neonatal health consequences of vertically transmitted hepatitis E virus infection. Am J Trop Med Hyg 90(2):365–370
59. Dalton HR, Bendall R, Ijaz S, Banks M (2008) Hepatitis E: an emerging infection in developed countries. Lancet Infect Dis 8(11):698–709
60. Nelson KE, Kmush B, Labrique AB (2011) The epidemiology of hepatitis E virus infections in developed countries and among immunocompromised patients. Expert Rev Anti-Infect Ther 9(12):1133–1148
61. Pischke S, Suneetha PV, Baechlein C, Barg-Hock H, Heim A, Kamar N et al (2010) Hepatitis E virus infection as a cause of graft hepatitis in liver transplant recipients. Liver Transpl 16(1):74–82
62. Patra S, Kumar A, Trivedi SS, Puri M, Sarin SK (2007) Maternal and fetal outcomes in pregnant women with acute hepatitis E virus infection. Ann Intern Med 147(1):28–33
63. Sahai S, Mishra V, Ganga D, Jatav OP (2015) Viral hepatitis in pregnancy – a study of its effect on maternal and foetal outcome. J Assoc Physicians India 63(1):28–33
64. Khuroo MS, Kamili S, Khuroo MS (2009) Clinical course and duration of viremia in vertically transmitted hepatitis E virus (HEV) infection in babies born to HEV-infected mothers. J Viral Hepat 16(7):519–523
65. Xu WM, Cui YT, Wang L, Yang H, Liang ZQ, Li XM et al (2009) Lamivudine in late pregnancy to prevent

perinatal transmission of hepatitis B virus infection: a multicentre, randomized, double-blind, placebo-controlled study. J Viral Hepat 16(2):94–103
66. van Zonneveld M, van Nunen AB, Niesters HG, de Man RA, Schalm SW, Janssen HL (2003) Lamivudine treatment during pregnancy to prevent perinatal transmission of hepatitis B virus infection. J Viral Hepat 10(4):294–297
67. Greenup AJ, Tan PK, Nguyen V, Glass A, Davison S, Chatterjee U et al (2014) Efficacy and safety of tenofovir disoproxil fumarate in pregnancy to prevent perinatal transmission of hepatitis B virus. J Hepatol 61:502
68. Zhang H, Pan CQ, Pang Q, Tian R, Yan M, Liu X (2014) Telbivudine or lamivudine use in late pregnancy safely reduces perinatal transmission of hepatitis B virus in real-life practice. Hepatology 60(2):468–476
69. Pan CQ, Duan Z, Dai E, Zhang S, Han G, Wang Y et al (2016) Tenofovir to prevent hepatitis B transmission in mothers with high viral load. N Engl J Med 374(24):2324–2334
70. Dionne-Odom J, Tita AT, Silverman NS (2016) #38: hepatitis B in pregnancy screening, treatment, and prevention of vertical transmission. Am J Obstet Gynecol 214(1):6–14
71. Sarin SK, Kumar M, Lau GK, Abbas Z, Chan HL, Chen CJ et al (2016) Asian-Pacific clinical practice guidelines on the management of hepatitis B: a 2015 update. Hepatol Int 10(1):1–98
72. Sokal EM, Paganelli M, Wirth S, Socha P, Vajro P, Lacaille F et al (2013) Management of chronic hepatitis B in childhood: ESPGHAN clinical practice guidelines: consensus of an expert panel on behalf of the European society of pediatric gastroenterology, hepatology and nutrition. J Hepatol 59(4):814–829
73. Terrault NA, Bzowej NH, Chang KM, Hwang JP, Jonas MM, Murad MH (2016) AASLD guidelines for treatment of chronic hepatitis B. Hepatology 63(1):261–283
74. Visvanathan K, Dusheiko G, Giles M, Wong ML, Phung N, Walker S et al (2016) Managing HBV in pregnancy. Prevention, prophylaxis, treatment and follow-up: position paper produced by Australian, UK and New Zealand key opinion leaders. Gut 65(2):340–350
75. Lampertico P, Agarwal K, Berg T, Buti M, Janssen HLA, Papatheodoridis G et al (2017) EASL 2017 clinical practice guidelines on the management of hepatitis B virus infection. J Hepatol 67(2):370–398
76. Brown RS Jr, McMahon BJ, Lok AS, Wong JB, Ahmed AT, Mouchli MA et al (2016) Antiviral therapy in chronic hepatitis B viral infection during pregnancy: a systematic review and meta-analysis. Hepatology 63(1):319–333
77. Heathcote EJ, Marcellin P, Buti M, Gane E, De Man RA, Krastev Z et al (2011) Three-year efficacy and safety of tenofovir disoproxil fumarate treatment for chronic hepatitis B. Gastroenterology 140(1):132–143
78. Chan HL, Chan CK, Hui AJ, Chan S, Poordad F, Chang TT et al (2014) Effects of tenofovir disoproxil fumarate in hepatitis B e antigen-positive patients with normal levels of alanine aminotransferase and high levels of hepatitis B virus DNA. Gastroenterology 146(5):1240–1248
79. APRSC Antiretroviral pregnancy registry international. Interim Report for 1 January through 31 January 2013. In. Wilmington: NC: Registry Coordinating Center 2012. Available from http://www.APRegistry.com
80. Sellier PO, Schnepf N, Amarsy R, Maylin S, Lopes A, Mazeron MC et al (2016) Short article: hepatitis B virus status in children born to HIV/HBV coinfected women in a French hospital: a cross-sectional study. Eur J Gastroenterol Hepatol 28(3):328–332
81. Wang L, Wiener J, Bulterys M, Wei X, Chen L, Liu W et al (2016) Hepatitis B virus (HBV) load response to 2 antiviral regimens, tenofovir/lamivudine and lamivudine, in HIV/HBV-coinfected pregnant women in Guangxi, China: the tenofovir in pregnancy (TiP) study. J Infect Dis 214(11):1695–1699
82. Nguyen V, Tan PK, Greenup AJ, Glass A, Davison S, Samarasinghe D et al (2014) Anti-viral therapy for prevention of perinatal HBV transmission: extending therapy beyond birth does not protect against post-partum flare. Aliment Pharmacol Ther 39(10):1225–1234
83. Shi Z, Li X, Ma L, Yang Y (2010) Hepatitis B immunoglobulin injection in pregnancy to interrupt hepatitis B virus mother-to-child transmission-a meta-analysis. Int J Infect Dis 14(7):e622–e634
84. Mugwanya KK, Hendrix CW, Mugo NR, Marzinke M, Katabira ET, Ngure K et al (2016) Pre-exposure prophylaxis use by breastfeeding HIV-uninfected women: a prospective short-term study of antiretroviral excretion in breast milk and infant absorption. PLoS Med 13(9):e1002132
85. Benaboud S, Pruvost A, Coffie PA, Ekouevi DK, Urien S, Arrive E et al (2011) Concentrations of tenofovir and emtricitabine in breast milk of HIV-1-infected women in Abidjan, cote d'Ivoire, in the ANRS 12109 TEmAA study, step 2. Antimicrob Agents Chemother 55(3):1315–1317
86. Wen WH, Huang CW, Chie WC, Yeung CY, Zhao LL, Lin WT et al (2016) Quantitative maternal hepatitis B surface antigen predicts maternally transmitted hepatitis B virus infection. Hepatology 64(5):1451–1461
87. Jourdain G, Ngo-Giang-Huong N, Cressey TR, Hua L, Harrison L, Tierney C et al (2016) Prevention of mother-to-child transmission of hepatitis B virus: a phase III, placebo-controlled, double-blind, randomized clinical trial to assess the efficacy and safety of a short course of tenofovir disoproxil fumarate in

women with hepatitis B virus e-antigen. BMC Infect Dis 16:393
88. Koneru A, Nelson N, Hariri S, Canary L, Sanders KJ, Maxwell JF et al (2016) Increased hepatitis C virus (HCV) detection in women of childbearing age and potential risk for vertical transmission – United States and Kentucky, 2011–2014. MMWR Morb Mortal Wkly Rep 65(28):705–710
89. Stuurman AL, Marano C, Bunge EM, De Moerlooze L, Shouval D. Impact of universal mass vaccination with monovalent inactivated hepatitis A vaccines – a systematic review. Hum Vaccin Immunother. 2017;13(3):724–36
90. Zhang J, Zhang XF, Huang SJ, Wu T, Hu YM, Wang ZZ et al (2015) Long-term efficacy of a hepatitis E vaccine. N Engl J Med 372(10):914–922
91. Shrestha MP, Scott RM, Joshi DM, Mammen MP Jr, Thapa GB, Thapa N et al (2007) Safety and efficacy of a recombinant hepatitis E vaccine. N Engl J Med 356(9):895–903
92. Wu T, Zhu FC, Huang SJ, Zhang XF, Wang ZZ, Zhang J et al (2012) Safety of the hepatitis E vaccine for pregnant women: a preliminary analysis. Hepatology (Baltimore, Md) 55(6):2038

Viral Hepatitis A in Children: Detection and Management

5

Palittiya Sintusek, Pattaratida Sa-nguanmoo, and Yong Poovorawan

Abstract

Hepatitis A virus (HAV) infection is one of the most common causes of acute viral hepatitis worldwide. HAV is transmitted mainly by person-to-person and spread by the fecal-oral route. Public health measures, including improved sanitation and hygiene, are the main factors leading to the reduction in the incidence of HAV infection in developing countries. The symptoms of HAV infection in children are varied, from asymptomatic to nonspecific (fever, lethargy) and to acute hepatitis and fulminant hepatitis. HAV infection is more severe in persons with underlying chronic liver disease. Because infection is usually spread silently by asymptomatic and very young children, outbreaks of infection commonly occur in diapered infants in childcare centers. When HAV infection occurs, public health organizations should be involved. Serological testing for IgM anti-HAV antibodies combined with molecular techniques for detecting HAV RNA are valuable techniques for the diagnosis of early-stage infection, leading to timely management of disease outbreaks. Advanced molecular techniques, including reverse transcription-polymerase chain reaction (RT-PCR), or real-time RT-PCR are very sensitive for the detection of HAV RNA and viral genotype by sequencing, either in suspected cases or in the environment as sources of infection. Treatment of acute hepatitis A is symptomatic. An HAV vaccine was licensed in 1995, which, in many countries, led to the recommendation for universal vaccination of young children, following which, the incidence of HAV infection has greatly reduced. Apart from rapid HAV detection and immunization programs, other strategies to prevent childhood outbreaks of HAV infection include health education, prevention of contact with the infection, improved sanitation campaigns, and post-exposure prophylaxis. Ideally, to eradicate HAV infection, universal immunization would be the goal.

Keywords

Viral hepatitis A · Outbreak · Childcare center · Post-exposure prophylaxis

P. Sintusek
Gastroenterology and Hepatology Unit, Department of Pediatrics, Faculty of Medicine, Chulalongkorn University, Bangkok, Thailand

Center of Excellence in Clinical Virology, Faculty of Medicine, Chulalongkorn University, Bangkok, Thailand

P. Sa-nguanmoo · Y. Poovorawan (✉)
Center of Excellence in Clinical Virology, Faculty of Medicine, Chulalongkorn University, Bangkok, Thailand
e-mail: Yong.P@chula.ac.th

M.-H. Chang, K. B. Schwarz (eds.), *Viral Hepatitis in Children*,
https://doi.org/10.1007/978-981-13-0050-9_5

5.1 Background

The incidence of hepatitis A virus (HAV) infection has declined in both Western and Eastern countries since the HAV vaccine became available in the 1990s [53, 131]. HAV vaccination programs aimed for universal immunization in children in many countries including the United States, [130] Latin America, Italy, Spain, Israel, [24] and Turkey [15]. Public health initiatives to improve hygiene, sanitation, and overall quality of life have reduced the likelihood of HAV transmission from the environment and have reduced the rate of infection. However, despite lowering the incidence of cases of hepatitis A, there have been continued outbreaks of infection, which have resulted in a significant public health problem [83, 99, 132]. To reduce and eliminate sporadic outbreaks of hepatitis from HAV infection, rapid diagnosis, management, and prevention of this disease with effective health and sanitation education and immunization are considered to be primary public health measures. This chapter will focus on the clinical presentation and laboratory profile of HAV-infected children, methods of HAV detection, management, and prevention of HAV infection including during outbreaks.

5.2 Clinical Manifestations of HAV Infection in Children

The clinical manifestations and severity of HAV infection increase with increasing age. Most infections in young children under the age of 6 years are asymptomatic, with the ratio of symptomatic to asymptomatic cases being 1:3 [46] to 1:13 [99] and the prevalence of asymptomatic cases being between 7% and 30% [21, 99]. The ratio of symptomatic to asymptomatic cases ranges from 1:1 to 1:3 [44] in primary school children, age 6–12 years old. Most of the infections in adolescents and young adults are symptomatic [66] with symptoms varying from mild, icteric (jaundiced), and non-icteric to fulminant hepatitis (Fig. 5.1). Immunocompromised patients and those patients with chronic liver diseases and cirrhosis are at increased risk of severe disease and death from fulminant HAV infection [17, 125]. There have been no cases of chronic HAV infection or congenital HAV infection reported so far [120, 121]. IgG anti-HAV antibodies that cross the placenta may provide protection to the infant after delivery; however, HAV infection in pregnant women can precipitate preterm labor [120, 121].

5.2.1 The Clinical Spectrum of HAV Infection: Asymptomatic Cases

In asymptomatic cases, HAV infection is divided into subclinical and inapparent categories [22].

Subclinical infections are characterized as having biochemical changes consistent with hepatitis but without clinical symptoms.

Inapparent infections can be identified by positive serological findings for HAV with normal liver biochemistry profiles.

The prognosis for asymptomatic patients is good. However, asymptomatic individuals with HAV infection may spread the infection to others and may cause an outbreak of the disease.

5.2.2 The Clinical Spectrum of HAV Infection: Symptomatic Cases

In symptomatic cases of HAV infection, typical clinical manifestations are either icterus (jaundice) or without icterus. Atypical manifestations of HAV infection also occur, as well as extrahepatic manifestations.

5.2.3 Typical Manifestations of Symptomatic HAV Infection

Typical HAV infection has a clinical course that may be divided into three phases: the incubation phase, which is usually 4 weeks (range 2–7 weeks), the symptomatic period of infection (2 weeks–6 months), and the convalescent phase.

Typical clinical features of HAV infection follow the incubation phase, 2–7 weeks following

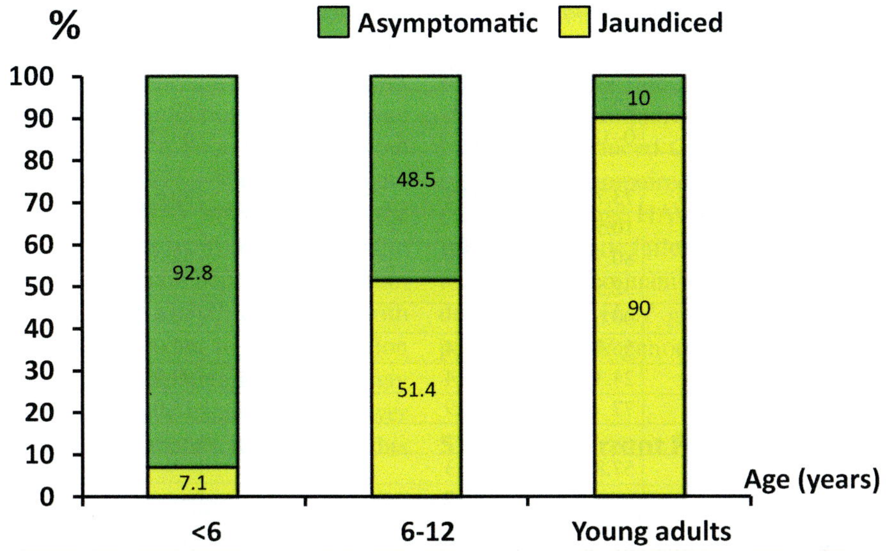

Fig. 5.1 Ratio of jaundiced and asymptomatic hepatitis A virus (HAV) infection in children during three outbreaks in Thailand [99, 125]

contact with HAV. The prodromal symptoms, or nonspecific symptoms, of viral infection include fever, malaise, headache, myalgia, arthralgia, rash, and nonspecific gastrointestinal symptoms (nausea, anorexia, vomiting, abdominal discomfort, and diarrhea) that may last from several days to a week, followed by jaundice, dark urine, pale stools, right upper quadrant pain, and pruritus.

The clinical symptoms of rash and arthralgia in HAV infection have been shown to be due to immune complex deposition [26, 51, 52] and are found in between 7% and 8.8% [12] and 19% of cases, respectively [117, 121, 129]. The prodromal symptoms usually diminish when jaundice appears. The clinical findings in the convalescent period can persist for 2 weeks to several months, but typically last for less than 3 months, and nearly all patients return to normal within 6 months [121].

The most common prodromal symptoms of HAV infection are dark urine and gastrointestinal symptoms that include vomiting, abdominal pain, and diarrhea [15, 64, 121]. In a study of HAV infection in children, published in 2014 [15], there was a significantly different incidence of abdominal pain, jaundice, dark urine, arthralgia, myalgia, pale stools, and pruritus in older, compared with younger, child age groups [15]. In the same study, it was reported that the most frequent physical findings of HAV infection in children were hepatomegaly and jaundice [15]. These common and well-recognized clinical presentations in children will lead the physician to suspect HAV infection in a newly presenting index case, especially in endemic areas with a high incidence of HAV infection (Table 5.1).

Laboratory findings associated with HAV infection include marked elevation of serum aspartate aminotransferase (AST) and alanine aminotransferase (ALT) up to 500–5000 IU/dL with raised ALT predominating and preceding an elevation in serum bilirubin, which may exceed more than 171 μmol/L [54]. Serum aminotransferase levels usually return to normal within 1 month after the onset of jaundice.

5.2.4 Atypical Manifestations of Symptomatic HAV Infection

In a recent study from Turkey [135], an atypical presentation was present in 12.8% of HAV-infected children, with symptoms including relapsing hepatitis, recurrent HAV infection,

extracorporeal liver support system (extracorporeal bilirubin elimination) [67]. The possibility that HAV infection may trigger cholestatic disorders in genetically predisposed individuals has been demonstrated by a published case [67] of a patient who had prolonged cholestatic HAV infection and the presence of two pro cholestatic gene polymorphisms, the c.3084 [GG] variant within the gene encoding the hepatic canalicular bile salt transporter *ABCB11* and the c.711 [AT] variant of the phosphatidylcholine floppase *ABCB4*.

5.2.9 Autoimmune Hepatitis (AIH)

The pathogenesis of autoimmune hepatitis (AIH) in HAV-infected patients is unclear, but HAV is a potential trigger of AIH [62, 94, 126] in patients with a genetic predisposition [48]. Furthermore, a recently reported study [1] detected seropositive autoantibodies of AIH in 63% of patients with HAV infection; this finding might support an immunological basis for the pathogenesis of HAV [1] or might be nonspecific epiphenomena similar to what occurs in patients with HBV, HCV, Wilson's disease, and nonalcoholic fatty liver disease (NAFLD). For patients who present with acute HAV infection with persistent, abnormal aminotransferases for more than 1 or 2 months, markers of HAV infection should be investigated, including serum viral antigen, HAV RNA, or HAV IgM antibodies. In the absence of evidence of HAV persistence, AIH should be suspected and investigated including liver biopsy for the histopathological confirmation, as this condition requires immunosuppressive treatments as soon as possible [49, 118].

5.2.10 Extrahepatic Manifestations of HAV Infection

Rare extrahepatic manifestations of HAV infection include acute kidney injury [20, 57, 137], autoimmune hemolytic anemia [16, 71, 77], aplastic anemia and red cell aplasia [16], immune thrombocytopenia [72], lupus-like syndrome [114], acute pancreatitis [8], hemophagocytic syndrome [111], encephalitis [47], transverse myelitis [61], and Guillain-Barré syndrome [18].

5.3 Transmission and Diagnosis of HAV Infection

HAV is a non-enveloped, single-stranded RNA virus of the *Picornaviridae* family. This virus is transmitted mainly by the fecal-oral route via person-to-person contact and ingestion of contaminated water, ice [100], or food [132], especially uncooked shellfish [36], including oysters, clams, and mussels. As a result, important sources of infection are childcare centers [99] and food-borne or waterborne outbreaks [100].

Following viral access into the human body, the virus migrates from the gastrointestinal (GI) tract to the bloodstream to the liver and replicates in hepatocytes. The HAV is then secreted into the biliary system and shed into the stool [81, 91]. Viral particles can be detected in the blood in the viremic state and in stool after viral excretion. The peak infectivity of hepatitis A correlates with the greatest viral load in the stool, where HAV antigen can be detected 2 weeks before the onset of jaundice or elevation of liver enzymes. Urine and saliva may also have detectable HAV RNA and IgM HAV antibodies [2, 105] during this time.

HAV was first visualized in human fecal samples by electron microscopy [65] and in the serum and liver of marmosets infected with human HAV [102]. In clinical practice, acute HAV is diagnosed by detecting the presence of HAV-specific IgM antibodies using routine serologic testing; HAV RNA is detected using molecular techniques. Cell culture is used to identify HAV from individual samples or from the environment during the investigation of outbreaks of HAV infection.

5.4 Methods Used for HAV Identification

The definitive diagnosis of acute HAV infection depends not only on the clinical presentation of hepatitis but also on the identification of HAV by direct visualization by electron microscopy or examination of changes in liver biopsies by light microscopy, serologic testing for virus or antibodies to HAV, or molecular techniques for detection of HAV RNA. These detection methods for HAV infection are crucial, especially in situations where HAV infection outbreaks are being investigated. Before the development of modern serology and molecular diagnosis, former diagnostic methods relied on infectivity assays in cell culture, with the disadvantage of time-consuming procedures that required 2–4 weeks before a result was obtained. Recently, molecular detection methods have been developed that include specific RT-PCR and real-time RT-PCR, which can detect early HAV infection, improving the prevention and control of disease outbreaks.

5.4.1 Immuno-electron Microscopy (IEM)

IEM was the first technique used to detect the HAV [83]. HAV particles were visualized in fecal suspensions obtained from infected human volunteers. The IEM and reactive antigen aggregation method were performed by using homologous antibody coats [65]. As a result, the coated or aggregated antigen can be visualized by EM [65].

5.4.2 Immunofluorescence (IF) Assay

Immunofluorescence (IF) is another commonly used method to detect HAV, which has been used for several decades. Before the development of the IF technique, hepatitis A antigen (HA-Ag) was demonstrated in nonhuman primate liver biopsies [85, 97] and from infected cell culture [6, 27]. The technique of IF uses anti-HAV immunoglobulin G (IgG) conjugated to fluorescein isothiocyanate (FITC) and visualized using fluorescence microscopy.

5.4.3 Immunohistochemistry (IHC)

The technique of immunohistochemistry (IHC) uses a primary antibody to HAV and a secondary antibody that is conjugated to a chromogenic label that can be visualized by light microscopy. This technique can be used to detect HAV in routine formalin-fixed, paraffin-embedded diagnostic liver tissue samples.

5.4.4 Identification of Antibodies to HAV

Commercial assays are routinely used in clinical diagnostic laboratories to detect serum IgM and IgG antibodies to HAV. The most commonly used serological diagnostic techniques include radioimmunoassay [78], immune adherence hemagglutination (IAHA) [110], and enzyme-linked immunosorbent assay (ELISA) [40]. In 1995, [116] first described the detection of IgM antibodies to HAV as a diagnostic marker of acute HAV infection and noted the levels of these serum antibodies can rise after the end of incubation period, or 5 days following the onset of symptoms, and can persist for up to 6 months (Fig. 5.2). However, ELISA typically does not detect lower concentrations of serum antibodies to HAV that exist 4–6 months following acute HAV infection. The sensitivity and specificity of current commercial ELISA kits used worldwide for the detection of current or recent HAV infection are greater than 98% [98]. Serum IgM anti-HAV antibodies can initially can be detected about 1 week before the onset of symptoms [66]. IgG antibodies are produced later and persist for a lifetime, and for this reason, serum IgG anti-HAV antibodies can be used to detect and monitor immunity to HAV from past infection or vaccination. However, ELISA does not detect the presence of HAV neutralizing antibodies, which require detection by a neutralization assay [76].

For outbreaks of HAV infection occurring in children, asymptomatic children can be difficult to detect as the serum IgM anti-HAV antibodies may be negative during the incubation period. Serial testing for antibodies to HAV is important but is costly and requires blood sampling by venipuncture. Alternative specimens, such as urine and saliva analyzed by molecular techniques, may provide useful diagnostic samples. However, rapid and sensitive assays remain

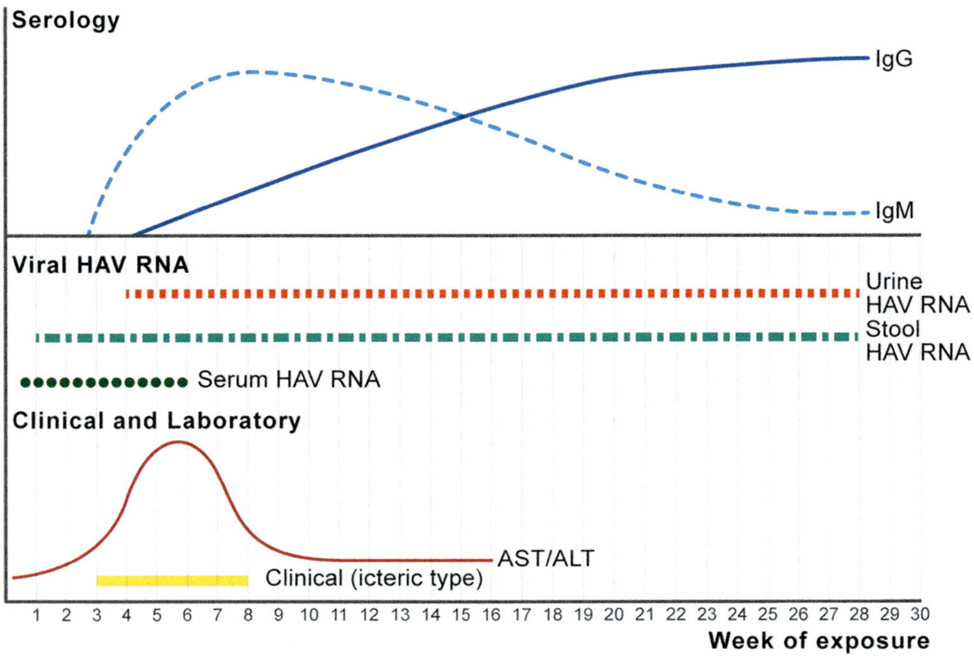

Fig. 5.2 Timeline for hepatitis A virus infection with clinical manifestations and laboratory diagnosis (Modified from [2, 5, 55, 56, 80, 81, 105]). *IgG* immunoglobulin G, *IgM* immunoglobulin M, *HAV* hepatitis A virus, *RNA* ribonucleic acid, *ALT* alanine aminotransferase, *AST* aspartate aminotransferase

important, particularly when outbreaks of infection occur in children, and so molecular diagnostic methods are recommended to increase the detection rate of HAV infection, with techniques that can be applied to various samples, including serum, stool, food, and environment samples [91]. The current diagnostic molecular techniques for HAV infection are described below.

5.4.5 Reverse Transcription-Polymerase Chain Reaction (RT-PCR)

HAV RNA can be extracted from clinical or environmental samples by using proteinase K digestion, followed by guanidinium thiocyanate phenol-chloroform extraction or using a commercially available RNA extraction kit. RNA is then converted to cDNA by specific or random primers, with primer pairs spanning the desired specific HAV genomic region. This technique has been reported to have been used in various sample types, including serum [122], sewage [70], and shellfish [88]. However, the efficacy of RT-PCR can be reduced if there are nucleic acid inhibitors in the tested material [91].

5.4.6 Real-Time RT-PCR

The use of the technique of real-time RT-PCR is believed to overcome the effects of nucleic acid inhibitors [109]. This technique is very sensitive and specific, reliable, reproducible, and less time-consuming and included refinements in use including the molecular beacon [134]. TaqMan [23] and SYBR Green [14] have all been applied to the detection of HAV RNA in diagnostic samples.

5.4.7 Cell Culture to Detect HAV

This diagnostic method has been used mainly to distinguish between the infectious and noninfectious virus in both specimens and patients and is a practical approach to monitor the safety of food and environmental samples and to study the molecular epidemiology of HAV. This method can be used to evaluate the efficacy of disinfection to remove HAV in food and water. For patients with the prolonged shedding of HAV RNA, this method can prove whether patients are contagious and require isolation. Although there are many culture methods described for the detection of HAV [35, 41], the disadvantages of these traditional culture methods are that HAV is not cytopathic in infected cells and grows slowly in cell culture making it an extremely time-consuming and expensive diagnostic method.

5.4.8 HAV Genotyping

Identification of the HAV genotype by sequencing has been reported to include phylogenetic analysis of the VP1/P2B region, supported by information derived from the GenBank database (National Center for Biotechnology Information, Bethesda, MD). Recently, a rapid, online HAV genotyping tool (National Institute for Public Health and the Environment, Ministry of Health, Welfare, and Sport, Bilthoven, The Netherlands) has become available on http://www.rivm.nl/mpf/hav/typingtool/.

5.4.9 HAV Recombinant Studies

Although not routinely used in the diagnosis of HAV infection, there have been some recent reports on the value of HAV recombinant studies in the detection of infection in disease outbreaks [89]. Genetic analysis of selected genome regions of HAV has shown that four distinct human HAV genotypes can be found worldwide (I, II, III, and VII). Analysis using full-length VP1 sequences revealed that human strain 9F94 has a close genetic relation with strain SLF-88 (sub-genotype VII). Capsid recombination can play a significant role in shaping the genetic diversity of HAV and may have important implications for the control of HAV infection. These techniques are not currently used in clinical diagnosis [9].

5.4.10 Application of HAV Detection in Clinical Practice

HAV can be identified in serum, saliva, stool, urine, water, and food. In suspected acute HAV infection, physicians use the detection of serum HAV IgM as the "gold standard" for diagnosis. Viremia occurs soon after infection and usually persists for a week after the initial clinical presentation [100]. Typically, HAV IgM becomes detectable 5–10 days before the onset of symptoms and declines to undetectable levels within 6 months following infection [84]. However, in asymptomatic children under 6 years old, early detection is crucial to prevent disease transmission to others, especially when an outbreak occurs. In 2004, a study by V.S. de Paula and colleagues [28] showed that 12–13% of primary school and daycare children could have negative HAV IgM serology but positive HAV RNA in serum. Poovorawan and colleagues found that the combination of HAV RNA and anti-HAV IgM detection could increase the diagnostic yield by 7.2% in the early phase of the acute infection [100]. As a result, the use of both serum IgM anti-HAV antibody and HAV RNA is valuable in epidemic and infection outbreak situations in children and may lead to more effective control.

For the diagnosis of HAV infection in children, alternative samples have been proposed for diagnoses, such as urine, saliva, and stool. A recent study has shown that HAV RNA could be detected in 67.7%, 52.3%, 12.3%, and 8.7% of serum, stool, urine, and saliva specimens, respectively, using RT-PCR [56]. This study has demonstrated the limitations of detecting HAV RNA in urine and saliva [56]. However, other studies have shown that HAV RNA could be detected in saliva within 5 days after the onset of symptoms [80], with a probability of detection of about 50% during the first 30 days following infection [2].

For the detection of IgM anti-HAV antibodies, analysis of urine specimens has been shown to have high diagnostic accuracy, with a sensitivity and specificity of 95.7% and 100%, respectively [55]. However, urine testing requires a large volume of fresh urine, as freezing affects the stability of the urine sample [105]. Urine samples may be preserved at −70 °C if the test cannot be performed immediately [55].

For the detection of IgM anti-HAV antibodies in saliva, the specimen may be viable for 150 days with antibodies still detectable within 30 days after infection [2]. Consequently, this alternative type of specimen may be considered for the detection of HAV during the early course of infection with the advantages of simple, inexpensive, and noninvasive specimen collection when compared with venipuncture and conventional serum sampling.

In summary, the routine clinical specimen used for HAV detection is the serum sample. In disease outbreaks, especially in children, alternative specimens, such as stool, saliva, and urine, are proposed with the advantages of noninvasive diagnostic sample collection. However, the processes of specimen collection, laboratory preparation, and RNA extraction are crucial to ensure accurate diagnostic results. The combination of molecular techniques and serology can increase the diagnostic value of HAV detection in children suspected of having infection. Figure 5.2 demonstrates the timeline for HAV detection and the clinical and laboratory findings in HAV-infected patients.

5.5 Management of HAV Infection

Following the identification of HAV infection in children, prompt reporting to the local health department and health authority is required, with the establishment of early investigation to detect the source of infection, the exposed children, and to prevent the spread of the outbreak of the infection. Post-exposure prophylaxis is encouraged for individuals exposed to HAV. If available, vaccination is recommended to provide immunoprophylaxis with the benefit of lifelong immunity.

According to the Centers for Disease Control and Prevention (CDC) in 1981 [24], up to 52% of HAV-infected patients could not identify the source of their infections. However, the recognized risk factors to exclude include injection drug use (14%), close personal contact with persons infected with HAV (12%), household or personal contact with a child who attends a childcare center (11%), international travel (4%), men who have sex with men (7%), and others, including those with household or personal contact with a newly arrived international child, recent blood transfusion, and those with exposure to a recent restaurant outbreak of HAV infection. For pediatric patients infected with HAV, daycare exposure to the virus seems to be the major source of outbreaks of HAV infection worldwide [3, 4, 13, 42, 63, 99, 107]. The following section described the management of children infected with HAV.

5.5.1 Management of Children Infected with HAV

Supportive treatment includes bedrest, adequate nutrition and hydration, and routine care to manage fever and gastrointestinal disturbances (diarrhea, nausea, and vomiting). Avoidance, or careful use, of drugs that have a hepatotoxic effect such as acetaminophen is required. About 30% of symptomatic patients require hospitalization; less than 1% will develop fulminant hepatic failure. A study in the Unites States found that 13% of patients required hospitalization, with a range from 7% for children younger than 15 years of age to 27% of adults aged 45 years old or older [10]. Approximately 100 deaths each year in the United States are attributed to fulminant hepatitis A infection [24]. There is a correlation between high viral shedding and the prognosis of the disease, as patients with underlying chronic liver disease, such as chronic viral hepatitis B or C, have an increased risk of morbidity and mortality. Because patients with HAV infection can present with mild nonspecific symptoms, pediatric cases should be admitted to the hospital if possible for close observation to prevent the development of serious complications.

The clinical clues for prediction of the severity of HAV infection that may indicate a need for patient monitoring include the following:

1. Prolonged jaundice >2 weeks, without clinical improvement, especially with symptoms of nausea and vomiting
2. Cholestatic jaundice with a total bilirubin >342 μmol/L
3. Prolonged PT or low serum albumin (<3.5 g/dL) [19]
4. Rising serum aminotransferases >3400 IU/L [19]
5. Inability to palpate the liver, despite a previously enlarged liver
6. Ascites
7. Hypoglycemia
8. Leukocytosis with a predominance of polymorphonuclear cells
9. Electroencephalogram (EEG) demonstrating bilateral frontal slow-wave activity (2–3/s)
10. Low total cholesterol <90 mg/dL [19, 74]
11. Leukopenia (<4000/L) [60]
12. Thrombocytopenia (<150,000/L) [60]
13. High serum C-reactive protein (CRP) (>8 mg/L) [60]
14. Other indices, such as high viral load [50, 104], serum LDH [74], gammaglobulin [1], or creatinine [74].

5.5.2 Identification of Individuals with HAV Infection and Their Control

5.5.2.1 The Hospital Setting

When hospitalization is necessary, contact precautions in general with standard precautions are recommended. In cases of an HAV-infected child with diapers for at least 1 week after onset of the symptoms might be enough.

5.5.2.2 Adults Who Work in Childcare or Who Work as Food Handlers

These individuals who have been infected with HAV from a child should isolate themselves from such work for at least 1 week following the onset of symptoms.

Care workers, childminders, close contacts, and household members may be identified.

Recognized symptomatic (icteric) patients can be clearly identified. However, in contrast, most infected children younger than 6 years of age are asymptomatic or have nonspecific symptoms. Therefore, HAV can spread widely outside a childcare center and for a long period. The control of outbreaks of HAV infection in children is outlined below (Fig. 5.3).

5.5.2.3 Diapered Infants and Children in Childcare Centers

Children of this age group are at risk of HAV infection if there is an infant or child who is a carrier of HAV among them, and childcare providers should be aware of direct contact. It may be difficult to determine the time of infectivity in children, as children may continue to shed HAV RNA in their stool for up to 6 months. If HAV infection has been identified in two or more families, all household members including diapered infants and children within a household should be considered for post-exposure prophylaxis [38].

There is no cost-efficacy of immune detection in non-endemic areas so immunization for non-immunized caregivers should be encouraged. Active immune protection takes 1 week. Therefore, injection of immune globulin to hepatitis A, providing passive immunity, should be provided for individuals who are at high risk following exposure to HAV, including (1) patients with chronic underlying liver disease, (2) patients who are >40 years old, or (3) infants who are contraindicated for active immunization as they are <12 months old.

Immune globulin to hepatitis A, administered within 2 weeks following exposure, can prevent symptomatic infection in between 69% and 89% of cases [90]. In case the disease persists, immune globulin decreases the severity and duration of illness of any subsequent infection and further reduces viral transmission. The recommended dose of gamma globulin is 0.02 mL/kg intramuscularly, which provides protection for about 3 months; a dose of 0.06 mL/kg provides protection for approximately 3–5 months. However, to promote lifelong immunity, vaccination is also

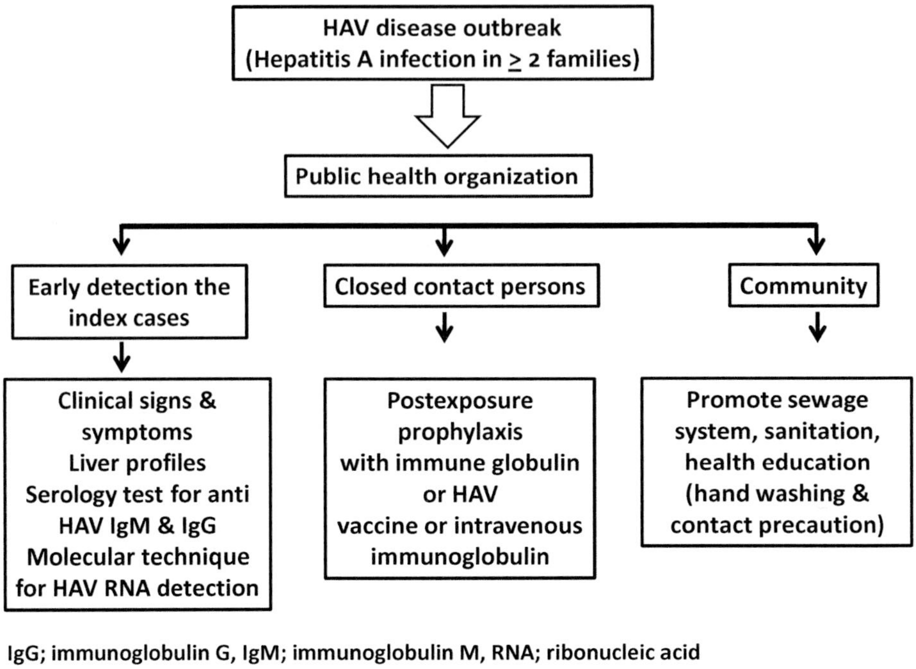

Fig. 5.3 A summary of actions required during an outbreak of hepatitis A virus (HAV) infection. *IgG* immunoglobulin G, *IgM* immunoglobulin M, *RNA* ribonucleic acid

encouraged in this group of patients if there is no contraindication (age <12 months).

Recent studies have demonstrated heterogeneity in the potency of available immune globulin preparations. Recently, Tegada-Strop et al. [119] studied nine immune globulin products with a dose of 0.02 ml/kg IM and found that only two products could raise the serum anti-HAV IgG level above the protective level (20 mIU/mL). Furthermore, these two products could maintain the anti-HAV neutralizing antibody levels above the protective level for only 18 and 35 days after injection. Consequently, the HAV vaccine is preferable as prophylaxis.

The HAV vaccine can be given if the exposure duration is less than 2 weeks. The HAV vaccine is considered to be as effective as immune globulin [128]. For the low-risk patient group, aged <40 years, without underlying chronic liver disease, active vaccination is enough. The use of immune globulin is limited, as it is available in only selected areas such as the United States, but not in Eastern countries.

However, published studies have shown that the HAV vaccine is less immunogenic in patients with chronic liver diseases (seroconversion rate 93%) [59, 73], in immunocompromised individuals (88%) [92], in transplant recipients (26%) [7], and in the elderly (65%) [133]. Alternatively, passive immunization that can be used for immunocompromised individuals consists of intravenous immunoglobulin (IVIG). Farcet and colleagues [34] have evaluated HAV antibody titers following IVIG, from human plasma pools derived from US and EU patients, and have found that, despite the low positive seroprevalence of HAV antibody in these countries, HAV antibody titers in IVIG appeared to remain adequate for antibody replacement therapy for these specific patients. A recent study [75] has also confirmed that the available IVIG from Korea, Japan, and the United States pro-

Table 5.2 Recommendations for post-exposure prophylaxis (PEP) of hepatitis A virus (HAV) infection in children

Time since exposure	Age (years)	Type of immunization	
		First-line agent	Alternative agent
≤2 weeks	≤1 year	Immune globulin 0.02–0.06[a] ml/kg IM	IVIG 400 mg/kg IV[b] if immune globulin is unavailable especially in high-risk groups (immunocompromised persons and patients with chronic liver diseases)
	1–18 year	Immune globulin 0.02–0.06[a] ml/kg IM and/or HAV vaccine 0.5 ml or pediatric dosage IM (alternate side)	
>2 weeks	No prophylaxis but HAV vaccine may be indicated for ongoing exposure		

IM intramuscular, *IVIG* intravenous immunoglobulin
[a]Preferable high dose
[b]According to study of passive immunity to HAV of IVIG in patients with primary immune deficiency [75]

vides sufficient antibodies against HAV to protect patients with primary immune deficiency (PID). In view of these findings, IVIG is recommended for administration to high-risk patients, especially those with underlying chronic liver disease, if post-exposure prophylaxis instead of immune globulin is available, or in the setting that immune globulin is not available (Table 5.2). Further studies on the role of IVIG as post-exposure prophylaxis for HAV infection are needed.

5.5.2.4 Non-diapered Childcare Center Infants and Children

Vaccination or immune globulin HAV prophylaxis is only necessary for classroom contacts or childhood index cases. Also, prophylaxis is not needed for individuals in contact with a person who has HAV infection when a single case occurs in an elementary or secondary school or an office setting, or if the source of infection is outside that setting, such as a hepatitis A patient who is admitted to hospital.

5.5.3 Environmental Sources of HAV Infection

HAV can survive in water and soil for several weeks, depending on the temperature. For example, HAV can persist in seawater at temperatures below 4 °C up to 90 days and below 25 °C for up to 60 days. Survival of HAV in cookies kept at room temperature has been demonstrated for at least a week. Moreover, a large amount of cellular material attached to the HAV surface has a protective effect, so that HAV exhibits an extremely high stability at low pH [113]. However, temperatures above 85 °C can kill HAV immediately, while temperatures of 70 °C can kill HAV over a period of 4 min [82]. Therefore, sanitation and food handling measures and handwashing especially after changing diapers and before handling food are important preventive measures for the transmission of HAV infection. Furthermore, prepared food should be cooked at a temperature of more than 85 °C (or 185 °F) for at least 1 min. Use of a 1:100 solution of household bleach, handwashing after defecation and diaper changing, and sanitary disposal of uncooked food or waste are reasonable public health preventive measures for decreasing the transmission of HAV (Table 5.3).

Disease outbreaks in children occur sporadically, mainly via food and water, causing a large public health problem. Examples of recent HAV infection outbreaks include those associated with green onions in Pennsylvania [132], with clams in Shanghai [30], with mussels and clams in Italy [79], and with ice in Thailand [100]. Early recognition and notification of the appropriate public health organizations are important, as are sanitation improvements and immunization programs. PEP for the contact persons, especially within the high-risk groups, is necessary. Molecular techniques are crucial to detecting the HAV RNA including the strain and infectious stage to plan for infection control.

Table 5.3 The stability of the hepatitis A virus (HAV) in the environment and the methods used to eradicate HAV

Environment	Survival	Environment	Survival
Freshwater, wastewater, various soil (clay, sand, and muck), 25 °C	>12 weeks	Heat >85 °C	Nearly all die immediately
Crème-filled cookies, 25 °C	>4 weeks	Heat 80 °C	5 s
Oyster, 24 °C	>5 days	Heat 75 °C	30 s
pH 1, 38 °C (gastric acid in the human body)	90 min	Heat 70 °C	4 min
pH 1, 25 °C	8 h	Heat 60 °C	12 h
Ether, alcohol, phenolics, iodine-based products, solution of acetic, peracetic, citric, and phosphoric acid	Do not die in 1 min	Chlorine component (bleach, handwashing)	10 s
		Formalin, 2% glutaraldehyde, toilet bowl cleaner, sodium hypochlorite	1 min

[31, 82, 86, 87]

5.6 Summary

Finally, for the prevention of HAV infection in children, active immunization with HAV vaccine is the best way for prevention and the best hope for eradication. The recommended age for childhood immunization is after 1 year of age, as infants will receive passive acquired maternal HAV antibody after birth, with maternal immunity protecting the infant from HAV infection and interfering with the response to the HAV vaccine [37, 96].

A full HAV vaccination course consists of two doses, between 1 and 6 months apart that generates an antibody level above the minimal protective level [138]. Humoral immunity following HAV vaccination can persist more than 12 years [124], but mathematical modeling studies of potential immune responses predict that, in some cases, immunity may last for at least 25 years [25]. Moreover, experimental studies guarantee that HAV vaccine can induce lifelong immunological memory. Therefore, a booster dose is unnecessary and not recommended at this time [123].

Immunocompromised patients with HAV infection and patients with chronic liver disease should be encouraged to be immunized. A booster dose of HAV vaccine may be needed, but further studies on its efficacy are required before this can be recommended worldwide.

Acknowledgments We would like to thank the Research Chair Grant NSTDA (P-15-50004), the Center of Excellence in Clinical Virology (GCE 58-014-30-004), MK Restaurant Company Limited, Siam Cement Group, Chulalongkorn University, and King Chulalongkorn Memorial Hospital for supporting our group and the Ratchadapiseksomphot Endowment Fund of Chulalongkorn University for a postdoctoral fellowship to Pattaratida Sa-nguanmoo.

References

1. Abdel-Ghaffar TY, Sira MM, Sira AM, Salem TA, El-Sharawy AA, El Naghi S (2015) Serological markers of autoimmunity in children with hepatitis A: relation to acute and fulminant presentation. Eur J Gastroenterol Hepatol 27(10):1161–1169
2. Amado Leon LA, de Almeida AJ, de Paula VS, Tourinho RS, Villela DA, Gaspar AM, Lewis-Ximenez LL, Pinto MA (2015) Longitudinal study of hepatitis A infection by saliva sampling: the kinetics of HAV markers in saliva revealed the application of saliva tests for hepatitis A study. PLoS One 10(12):e0145454
3. Amado LA, Villar LM, de Paula VS, Gaspar AM (2008) Comparison between serum and saliva for the detection of hepatitis A virus RNA. J Virol Methods 148(1–2):74–80
4. Amado LA, Villar LM, de Paula VS, Pinto MA, Gaspar AM (2011) Exposure to multiple subgenotypes of hepatitis A virus during an outbreak using matched serum and saliva specimens. J Med Virol 83(5):768–775
5. American Medical Association, American Nurses Association-American Nurses Foundation, Centers for Disease Control and Prevention, Center for Food Safety and Applied Nutrition, Food and Drug Administration, Food Safety and Inspection Service,

US Department of Agriculture (2004) Diagnosis and management of foodborne illnesses: a primer for physicians and other health care professionals. MMWR Recomm Rep 53:1–33
6. Anderson DA, Coulepis AG, Chenoweth MP, Gust ID (1986) Indirect immunofluorescence assay for the detection of hepatitis A virus-specific serum immunoglobulins. J Clin Microbiol 24(1):163–165
7. Arslan M, Wiesner RH, Poterucha JJ, Zein NN (2001) Safety and efficacy of hepatitis A vaccination in liver transplantation recipients. Transplantation 72(2):272–276
8. Basaranoglu M, Balci NC, Klor HU (2006) Gallbladder sludge and acute pancreatitis induced by acute hepatitis A. Pancreatology 6(1–2):141–144
9. Belalov IS, Isaeva OV, Lukashev AN (2011) Recombination in hepatitis A virus: evidence for reproductive isolation of genotypes. J Gen Virol 92(Pt 4):860–872
10. Bell BP, Shapiro CN, Alter MJ, Moyer LA, Judson FN, Mottram K, Fleenor M, Ryder PL, Margolish HS (1998) The diverse patterns of hepatitis A epidemiology in the United States-implications for vaccination strategies. J Infect Dis 178(6):1579–1584
11. Bernuau JSD, Durand F, Saliba F, Bourliere M, Adam R, Gugenheim J, Castaing D, Bismuth H, Rueff B, Erlinger S, Benhamou JP (1991) Criteria for emergency liver transplantation in patients with acute viral hepatitis and factor V below 50% of normal: a prospective study. Hepatology 14(S41–S290):49A (Abstract)
12. Blechova Z, Trojanek M, Kyncl J, Castkova J, John J, Maly M, Herrmannova K, Maresova V (2013) Clinical and laboratory features of viral hepatitis A in children. Wien Klin Wochenschr 125(3–4):83–90
13. Cabrera-Gaytan DA, Nava-Martinez ML, Ontiveros D, Niebla-Fuentes MR, Grajales-Muniz C, Rojas-Mendoza T (2014) Experience on the management of a hepatitis A outbreak in a children daycare center. Rev Med Inst Mex Seguro Soc 52(6):630–636
14. Casas N, Amarita F, de Maranon IM (2007) Evaluation of an extracting method for the detection of hepatitis A virus in shellfish by SYBR-Green real-time RT-PCR. Int J Food Microbiol 120(1–2):179–185
15. Cetinkaya B, Tezer H, Ozkaya Parlakay A, Revide Sayli T (2014) Evaluation of pediatric patients with hepatitis A. J Infect Dev Ctries 8(3):326–330
16. Chang HJ, Sinn DH, Cho SG, Oh TH, Jeon TJ, Shin WC, Choi WC (2014) Pure red-cell aplasia and autoimmune hemolytic anemia in a patient with acute hepatitis A. Clin Mol Hepatol 20(2):204–207
17. Chen CM, Chen SC, Yang HY, Yang ST, Wang CM (2016) Hospitalization and mortality due to hepatitis A in Taiwan: a 15-year nationwide cohort study. J Viral Hepat 23(11):940–945
18. Chitambar SD, Fadnis RS, Joshi MS, Habbu A, Bhatia SG (2006) Case report: hepatitis A preceding Guillain-Barre syndrome. J Med Virol 78(8):1011–1014
19. Cho SY, Choi SH, Park JH, Chung JW (2011) Initial laboratory predictors of severe hepatitis and acute kidney injury in patients with acute hepatitis A. Diagn Microbiol Infect Dis 69(4):400–404
20. Choi HK, Song YG, Han SH, Ku NS, Jeong SJ, Baek JH, Kim H, Kim SB, Kim CO, Kim JM, Choi JY (2011) Clinical features and outcomes of acute kidney injury among patients with acute hepatitis A. J Clin Virol 52(3):192–197
21. Christenson JC, Manaloor JJ (2016) Hepatitis A, B, and C. Pediatr Rev 37(10):426–438
22. Ciocca M (2000) Clinical course and consequences of hepatitis A infection. Vaccine 18(Suppl 1):S71–S74
23. Costafreda MI, Bosch A, Pinto RM (2006) Development, evaluation, and standardization of a real-time TaqMan reverse transcription-PCR assay for quantification of hepatitis A virus in clinical and shellfish samples. Appl Environ Microbiol 72(6):3846–3855
24. Craig AS, Schaffner W (2004) Prevention of hepatitis A with the hepatitis A vaccine. N Engl J Med 350(5):476–481
25. Curran D, de Ridder M, Van Effelterre T (2016) The impact of assumptions regarding vaccine-induced immunity on the public health and cost-effectiveness of hepatitis A vaccination: is one dose sufficient? Hum Vaccin Immunother 12(11):2765–2771
26. Dan M, Yaniv R (1990) Cholestatic hepatitis, cutaneous vasculitis, and vascular deposits of immunoglobulin M and complement associated with hepatitis A virus infection. Am J Med 89(1):103–104
27. De Filippis P, Divizia M, Mele A, Adamo B, Pana A (1987) Detection of hepatitis A virus in the stools of healthy people from endemic areas. Eur J Epidemiol 3(2):172–175
28. De Paula VS, Villar LM, Morais LM, Lewis-Ximenez LL, Niel C, Gaspar AM (2004) Detection of hepatitis A virus RNA in serum during the window period of infection. J Clin Virol 29(4):254–259
29. Debray D, Cullufi P, Devictor D, Fabre M, Bernard O (1997) Liver failure in children with hepatitis A. Hepatology 26(4):1018–1022
30. Desenclos JC, Klontz KC, Wilder MH, Nainan OV, Margolis HS, Gunn RA (1991) A multistate outbreak of hepatitis A caused by the consumption of raw oysters. Am J Public Health 81(10):1268–1272
31. Divizia M, Filippis D, Napoli AD, Gabrieli R, Santi AL, Pana A (1988) Recovery of hepatitis A virus from seeded tap water. In: Zuckerman AJ (ed) Viral hepatitis and liver diseases. Alan R Liss, Inc, New York, pp 125–130
32. Eisenbach C, Longerich T, Fickenscher H, Schalasta G, Stremmel W, Encke J (2006) Recurrence of clinically significant hepatitis A following liver trans-

plantation for fulminant hepatitis A. J Clin Virol 35(1):109–112
33. Fagan E, Yousef G, Brahm J, Garelick H, Mann G, Wolstenholme A, Portmann B, Harrison T, Mowbray JF, Mowat A (1990) Persistence of hepatitis A virus in fulminant hepatitis and after liver transplantation. J Med Virol 30(2):131–136
34. Farcet MR, Planitzer CB, Stein O, Modrof J, Kreil TR (2010) Hepatitis A virus antibodies in immunoglobulin preparations. J Allergy Clin Immunol 125(1):198–202
35. Feigelstock DA, Thompson P, Kaplan GG (2005) Growth of hepatitis A virus in a mouse liver cell line. J Virol 79(5):2950–2955
36. Fiore AE (2004) Hepatitis A transmitted by food. Clin Infect Dis 38(5):705–715
37. Fiore AE, Shapiro CN, Sabin K, Labonte K, Darling K, Culver D, Bell BP, Margolis HS (2003) Hepatitis A vaccination of infants: effect of maternal antibody status on antibody persistence and response to a booster dose. Pediatr Infect Dis J 22(4):354–359
38. Flehmig B, Normann A, Bohnen D (2000) Transmission of hepatitis A virus infection despite vaccination. N Engl J Med 343(4):30130–30132
39. Gane E, Sallie R, Saleh M, Portmann B, Williams R (1995) Clinical recurrence of hepatitis A following liver transplantation for acute liver failure. J Med Virol 45(1):35–39
40. Gargouri S, Fki Berrajah L, Ayadi I, Messedi E, Jallouli H, Hammami A, Karray-Hakim H (2016) Epidemiological and clinical analysis of hepatitis virus A infections during three successive outbreaks in Sfax (Tunisia) between 2007 and 2010. Med Sante Trop 26(2):159–164
41. Gauss-Muller V, Frosner GG, Deinhardt F (1981) Propagation of hepatitis A virus in human embryo fibroblasts. J Med Virol 7(3):233–239
42. Gharbi-Khelifi H, Ben Salem Abid N, Sdiri K, Harrath R, Beji A, Bhiri L, Billauel S, Ferre V, Aouni M (2011) Characterization of outbreak hepatitis a isolates in five Tunisian childcare centers. Braz J Microbiol 42(3):1204–1212
43. Gimson AE, White YS, Eddleston AL, Williams R (1983) Clinical and prognostic differences in fulminant hepatitis type A, B and non-A non-B. Gut 24(12):1194–1198
44. Gingrich GA, Hadler SC, Elder HA, Ash KO (1983) Serologic investigation of an outbreak of hepatitis A in a rural day-care center. Am J Public Health 73(10):1190–1193
45. Glikson M, Galun E, Oren R, Tur-Kaspa R, Shouval D (1992) Relapsing hepatitis A. Review of 14 cases and literature survey. Medicine (Baltimore) 71(1):14–23
46. Hadler SC, Webster HM, Erben JJ, Swanson JE, Maynard JE (1980) Hepatitis A in day-care centers. A community-wide assessment. N Engl J Med 302(22):1222–1227
47. Hegazi MA, Mansor I, Rahman FA, El-Sayed M (2011) Hepatitis A virus presenting as fatal encephalitis in a child. Pediatr Infect Dis J 30(11):1012
48. Hilzenrat N, Zilberman D, Klein T, Zur B, Sikuler E (1999) Autoimmune hepatitis in a genetically susceptible patient: is it triggered by acute viral hepatitis A? Dig Dis Sci 44(10):1950–1952
49. Huppertz HI, Treichel U, Gassel AM, Jeschke R, Meyer zum Buschenfelde KH (1995) Autoimmune hepatitis following hepatitis A virus infection. J Hepatol 23(2):204–208
50. Hussain Z, Husain SA, Almajhdi FN, Kar P (2011) Immunological and molecular epidemiological characteristics of acute and fulminant viral hepatitis A. Virol J 8:254
51. Ilan Y, Hillman M, Oren R, Zlotogorski A, Shouval D (1990) Vasculitis and cryoglobulinemia associated with persisting cholestatic hepatitis A virus infection. Am J Gastroenterol 85(5):586–587
52. Inman RD, Hodge M, Johnston ME, Wright J, Heathcote J (1986) Arthritis, vasculitis, and cryoglobulinemia associated with relapsing hepatitis A virus infection. Ann Intern Med 105(5):700–703
53. Innis BL, Snitbhan R, Kunasol P, Laorakpongse T, Poopatanakool W, Kozik CA, Suntayakorn S, Sukuntapong T, Safary A, Tang DB (1994) Protection against hepatitis A by an inactivated vaccine. JAMA 271(17):1328–1334
54. Johnston DE (1999) Special considerations in interpreting liver function tests. Am Fam Physician 59(8):2223–2230
55. Joshi MS, Chitambar SD, Arankalle VA, Chadha MS (2002) Evaluation of urine as a clinical specimen for diagnosis of hepatitis a. Clin Diagn Lab Immunol 9(4):840–845
56. Joshi MS, Bhalla S, Kalrao VR, Dhongade RK, Chitambar SD (2014) Exploring the concurrent presence of hepatitis A virus genome in serum, stool, saliva, and urine samples of hepatitis A patients. Diagn Microbiol Infect Dis 78(4):379–382
57. Jung YJ, Kim W, Jeong JB, Kim BG, Lee KL, Oh KH, Yoon JH, Lee HS, Kim YJ (2010) Clinical features of acute renal failure associated with hepatitis A virus infection. J Viral Hepat 17(9):611–617
58. Kamath SR, Sathiyasekaran M, Raja TE, Sudha L (2009) Profile of viral hepatitis A in Chennai. Indian Pediatr 46(7):642–643
59. Keeffe EB, Iwarson S, McMahon BJ, Lindsay KL, Koff RS, Manns M, Baumgarten R, Wiese M, Fourneau M, Safary A, Clemens R, Krause DS (1998) Safety and immunogenicity of hepatitis A vaccine in patients with chronic liver disease. Hepatology 27(3):881–886
60. Kim SY, Kim MG, Choi WC (2008a) Acute transverse myelitis after acute hepatitis a: findings on magnetic resonance imaging. Clin Gastroenterol Hepatol 6(9):xxviii–xxvie1
61. Kim HS, Kim HS, Lee JY, Jang JS, Shin WG, Kim KH, Park JY, Lee JH, Kim HY, Jang MK (2008b)

Initial thrombocytopenia as a simple, valuable predictor for clinical manifestation in acute hepatitis A. Scand J Gastroenterol 43(1):81–88
62. Kim YD, Kim KA, Rou WS, Lee JS, Song TJ, Bae WK, Kim NH (2011) A case of autoimmune hepatitis following acute hepatitis A. Korean J Gastroenterol 57(5):315–318
63. Klevens RM, Miller JT, Iqbal K, Thomas A, Rizzo EM, Hanson H, Sweet K, Phan Q, Cronquist A, Khudyakov Y, Xia GL, Sprading P (2010) The evolving epidemiology of hepatitis a in the United States: incidence and molecular epidemiology from population-based surveillance, 2005-2007. Arch Intern Med 170(20):1811–1818
64. Koff RS (1992) Clinical manifestations and diagnosis of hepatitis A virus infection. Vaccine 10(Suppl 1):S15–S17
65. Koff RS, Feinstone SM, Kapikian AZ, Purcell RH (2002) Hepatitis A: detection by immune electron microscopy of a virus like antigen associated with acute illness [Science 1973;182:1026-1028]. J Hepatol 37(1):2–6
66. Kojaoghlanian T (2010) Hepatitis A. Pediatr Rev 31(8):348–350
67. Krawczyk M, Grunhage F, Langhirt M, Bohle RM, Lammert F (2012) Prolonged cholestasis triggered by hepatitis A virus infection and variants of the hepatocanalicular phospholipid and bile salt transporters. Ann Hepatol 11(5):710–714
68. Kumar P, Bhatia V (2011) Prolonged cholestasis due to hepatitis A virus infection. Indian Pediatr 48(6):485–486
69. Kumar KJ, Kumar HC, Manjunath VG, Anitha C, Mamatha S (2014) Hepatitis A in children- clinical course, complications and laboratory profile. Indian J Pediatr 81(1):15–19
70. La Rosa G, Libera SD, Iaconelli M, Ciccaglione AR, Bruni R, Taffon S, Equestre M, Alfonsi V, Rizzo C, Tosti ME, Chironna M, Romano L, Zanett AR, Muscillo M (2014) Surveillance of hepatitis A virus in urban sewages and comparison with cases notified in the course of an outbreak, Italy 2013. BMC Infect Dis 14:419
71. Lapp RT, Rochling F (2013) Acute cholestatic hepatitis a virus infection presenting with hemolytic anemia and renal failure: a case report. Case Rep Hepatol 2013:438375
72. Leblebisatan G, Tumgor G, Sasmaz I, Ozgur O, Antmen B (2012) Hepatitis A-associated immune thrombocytopenia. Tur J Gastroenterol 23(2):195–197
73. Lee SD, Chan CY, Yu MI, Wang YJ, Chang FY, Lo KJ, Safary A (1997) Safety and immunogenicity of inactivated hepatitis A vaccine in patients with chronic liver disease. J Med Virol 52(2):215–218
74. Lee HW, Chang DY, Moon HJ, Chang HY, Shin EC, Lee JS, Kim KA, Kim HJ (2015) Clinical factors and viral load influencing severity of acute hepatitis A. PLoS One 10(6):e0130728
75. Lee S, Kim HW, Kim KH (2016) Antibodies against hepatitis A and hepatitis B virus in intravenous immunoglobulin products. J Korean Med Sci 31(12):1937–1942
76. Lemon SM, Murphy PC, Provost PJ, Chalikonda I, Davide JP, Schofield TL, Dr N, Lewis JA (1997) Immunoprecipitation and virus neutralization assays demonstrate qualitative differences between protective antibody responses to inactivated hepatitis A vaccine and passive immunization with immune globulin. J Infect Dis 176(1):9–19
77. Lim PS, Kim IH, Kim SH, Lee SO, Kim SW (2012) A case of severe acute hepatitis a complicated with pure red cell aplasia. Korean J Gastroenterol 60(3):177–181
78. Liu CC, Wang JY, Yao WJ (1994) Seroepidemiology of hepatitis A virus infection in southern Taiwan. Zhonghua Min Guo Xiao Er Ke Yi Xue Hui Za Zhi 35(5):391–396
79. Lucioni C, Cipriani V, Mazzi S, Panunzio M (1998) Cost of an outbreak of hepatitis A in Puglia, Italy. PharmacoEconomics 13(2):257–266
80. Mackiewicz V, Dussaix E, Le Petitcorps MF, Roque-Afonso AM (2004) Detection of hepatitis A virus RNA in saliva. J Clin Microbiol 42(9):4329–4331
81. Margolis HS, Nainan OV, Krawczynski K, Bradley DW, Ebert JW, Spelbring J et al (1988) Appearance of immune complexes during experimental hepatitis A infection in chimpanzees. J Med Virol 26(3):315–326
82. Mark D, Sobsey PAS, Fred S, Hauchman ALD, Rullman VA, Bosch A (1988) Survival and persistence of hepatitis A virus in environmental samples. In: Zuckerman AJ (ed) Viral hepatitis and liver disease. Alan R Liss, INC, New York, pp 121–124
83. Martin A, Lemon SM (2006) Hepatitis A virus: from discovery to vaccines. Hepatology 43(2 Suppl 1):S164–S172
84. Matheny SC, Kingery JE (2012) Hepatitis A. Am Fam Physician 86(11):1027–1034 quiz 10-12
85. Mathiesen LR, Feinstone SM, Purcell RH, Wagner JA (1977) Detection of hepatitis A antigen by immunofluorescence. Infect Immun 18(2):524–530
86. Mbithi JN, Springthorpe VS, Sattar SA (1990) Chemical disinfection of hepatitis A virus on environmental surfaces. Appl Environ Microbiol 56(11):3601–3604
87. Mbithi JN, Springthorpe VS, Sattar SA (1993) Comparative in vivo efficiencies of hand-washing agents against hepatitis A virus (HM-175) and poliovirus type 1 (Sabin). Appl Environ Microbiol 59(10):3463–3349
88. Mesquita JR, Vaz L, Cerqueira S, Castilho F, Santos R, Monteiro S, Manso CF, Romalde JL, Nascimento MS (2011) Norovirus, hepatitis A virus and enterovirus presence in shellfish from high quality harvesting areas in Portugal. Food Microbiol 28(5):936–941
89. Moratorio G, Costa-Mattioli M, Piovani R, Romero H, Musto H, Cristina J (2007) Bayesian coalescent inference of hepatitis A virus populations: evolutionary rates and patterns. J Gen Virol 88(Pt 11):3039–3042

90. Mosley JW, Reisler DM, Brachott D, Roth D, Weiser J (1968) Comparison of two lots of immune serum globulin for prophylaxis of infectious hepatitis. Am J Epidemiol 87(3):539–550
91. Nainan OV, Xia G, Vaughan G, Margolis HS (2006) Diagnosis of hepatitis a virus infection: a molecular approach. Clin Microbiol Rev 19(1):63–79
92. Neilsen GA, Bodsworth NJ, Watts N (1997) Response to hepatitis A vaccination in human immunodeficiency virus-infected and -uninfected homosexual men. J Infect Dis 176(4):1064–1067
93. O'Grady JG, Alexander GJ, Hayllar KM, Williams R (1989) Early indicators of prognosis in fulminant hepatic failure. Gastroenterology 97(2):439–445
94. Ozaras R, Tahan V, Tabak F (2016) More on autoimmune hepatitis and acute hepatitis A. Eur J Gastroenterol Hepatol 28(3):360
95. Park GC, Hwang S, Yu YD, Park PJ, Choi YI, Song GW, Jung DH, Ahn CS, Kim KH, Moon DB, Ha TY, Lee SG (2010) Intractable recurrent hepatitis A virus infection requiring repeated liver transplantation: a case report. Transplant Proc 42(10):4658–4660
96. Piazza M, Safary A, Vegnente A, Soncini R, Pensati P, Sardo M, Orlando R, Tosone G, Picciotto L (1999) Safety and immunogenicity of hepatitis A vaccine in infants: a candidate for inclusion in the childhood vaccination programme. Vaccine 17(6):585–588
97. Pinto MA, Marchevsky RS, Baptista ML, de Lima MA, Pelajo-Machado M, Vitral CL, Kubelka CF, Pissurno JW, Franca MS, Schatzmayr HG, Gaspar AM (2002) Experimental hepatitis A virus (HAV) infection in Callithrix jacchus: early detection of HAV antigen and viral fate. Exp Toxicol Pathol 53(6):413–420
98. Poddar U, Thapa BR, Prasad A, Singh K (2002) Changing spectrum of sporadic acute viral hepatitis in Indian children. J Trop Pediatr 48(4):210–213
99. Poovorawan Y, Theamboonlers A, Chongsrisawat V, Jantaradsamee P, Chutsirimongkol S, Tangkijvanich P (2005) Clinical features and molecular characterization of hepatitis A virus outbreak in a child care center in Thailand. J Clin Virol 32(1):24–28
100. Poovorawan K, Chattakul P, Chattakul S, Thongmee T, Theamboonlers A, Komolmit P, Poovorawan Y (2013) The important role of early diagnosis and preventive management during a large-scale outbreak of hepatitis A in Thailand. Pathogens Glob Health 107(7):367–372
101. Pramoolsinsap C (2000) Acute hepatitis A and acquired immunity to hepatitis A virus in hepatitis B virus (HBV) carriers and in HBV- or hepatitis C virus-related chronic liver diseases in Thailand. J Viral Hepat 7(Suppl 1):11–12
102. Provost PJ, Wolanski BS, Miller WJ, Ittensohn OL, McAleer WJ, Hilleman MR (1975) Physical, chemical and morphologic dimensions of human hepatitis A virus strain CR326 (38578). Proc Soc Exp Biol Med 148(2):532–539
103. Rachima CM, Cohen E, Garty M (2000) Acute hepatitis A: combination of the relapsing and the cholestatic forms, two rare variants. Am J Med Sci 319(6):417–419
104. Rezende G, Roque-Afonso AM, Samuel D, Gigou M, Nicand E, Ferre V, Dussaix E, Bismuth H, Feray C (2003) Viral and clinical factors associated with the fulminant course of hepatitis A infection. Hepatology 38(3):613–618
105. Rodriguez Lay Lde L, Larralde Diaz O, Martinez Casanueva R, Gutierrez Moreno A (2003) Anti-hepatitis A virus immunoglobulin M antibodies in urine samples for rapid diagnosis of outbreaks. Clin Diagn Lab Immunol 10(3):492–494
106. Ruddy SJ, Johnson RF, Mosley JW, Atwater JB, Rossetti MA, Hart JC (1969) An epidemic of clam-associated hepatitis. JAMA 208(4):649–655
107. Rump BO, Visser O, Te Wierik MJ, Vennema H, Fanoy EB (2013) Use of PCR for detection of faecal HAV as a screening tool in an outbreak of hepatitis A in daycare centres. Epidemiol Infect 141(3):549–555
108. Sagnelli E, Coppola N, Marrocco C, Onofrio M, Scarano F, Marotta A, Scoilastico C, Catuogno A, Salzillo A, Sagnelli C, Piccinino F, Filippini P (2003) HAV replication in acute hepatitis with typical and atypical clinical course. J Med Virol 71(1):1–6
109. Sanchez G, Bosch A, Pinto RM (2007) Hepatitis A virus detection in food: current and future prospects. Lett Appl Microbiol 45(1):1–5
110. Sata M, Nakano H, Tanaka E, Kumashiro R, Suzuki H, Tanikawa K (1996) Analysis of serum hepatitis A virus antibody response in different courses of hepatitis A virus infection. J Gastroenterol 31(6):812–817
111. Saxena P, Bihari C, Rastogi A, Sood V, Khanna R, Alam S, Sarin SK (2014) Hepatitis A induced hemophagocytic syndrome. Trop Gastroenterol 35(2):122–124
112. Schiff ER (1992) Atypical clinical manifestations of hepatitis A. Vaccine 10(Suppl 1):S18–S20
113. Scholz E, Heinricy U, Flehmig B (1989) Acid stability of hepatitis A virus. J Gen Virol 70(Pt 9):2481–2485
114. Segev A, Hadari R, Zehavi T, Schneider M, Hershkoviz R, Mekori YA (2001) Lupus-like syndrome with submassive hepatic necrosis associated with hepatitis A. J Gastroenterol Hepatol 16(1):112–114
115. Sinlaparatsamee S, Nuniem J, Kankao J, Theamboonlers A, Chumdermpadetsuk S, Poovorawan Y (1995) An outbreak of hepatitis A in school children at Nakhon Si Thammarat, southern Thailand. Southeast Asian J Trop Med Public Health 26(1):104–108
116. Stapleton JT (1995) Host immune response to hepatitis A virus. J Infect Dis 171(Suppl 1):S9–S14
117. Stone JH, Murali MR (2013) Case records of the Massachusetts General Hospital. Case 10-2013. A

30-year-old man with fever, myalgias, arthritis, and rash. N Engl J Med 368(13):1239–1245
118. Tabak F, Ozdemir F, Tabak O, Erer B, Tahan V, Ozaras R (2008) Autoimmune hepatitis induced by the prolonged hepatitis A virus infection. Ann Hepatol 7(2):177–179
119. Teijada-Strop ACM, Dimitriva Z, Kaplan GG, Teo C-G (2017) Evaluation of potencies of immune globulin products against hepatitis A [published online January 9, 2017]. JAMA Intern Med
120. Tong MJ, Thursby M, Rakela J, McPeak C, Edwards VM, Mosley JW (1981) Studies on the maternal-infant transmission of the viruses which cause acute hepatitis. Gastroenterology 80(5 pt 1):999–1004
121. Tong MJ, El-Farra NS, Grew MI (1995) Clinical manifestations of hepatitis A: recent experience in a community teaching hospital. J Infect Dis 171(Suppl 1):S15–S158
122. Tsatsralt-Od B, Baasanjav N, Nyamkhuu D, Ohnishi H, Takahashi M, Kobayashi T, Nagashima S, Nishizawa T, Okamoto H (2016) Molecular analysis of hepatitis A virus strains obtained from patients with acute hepatitis A in Mongolia, 2004-2013. J Med Virol 88(4):622–630
123. Van Damme P, Van Herck K (2007) A review of the long-term protection after hepatitis A and B vaccination. Travel Med Infect Dis 5(2):79–84
124. Van Damme P, Banatvala J, Fay O, Iwarson S, McMahon B, Van Herck K, Shouval D, Bonanni P, Connor B, Cooksley G, Leroux-Roels G, Von Sonnenburg F, International Consensus Group on Hepatitis A Virus Immunity (2003) Hepatitis A booster vaccination: is there a need? Lancet 362(9389):1065–1071
125. Vento S (2000) Fulminant hepatitis associated with hepatitis A virus superinfection in patients with chronic hepatitis C. J Viral Hepat 7(Suppl 1):7–8
126. Vento S, Garofano T, Di Perri G, Dolci L, Concia E, Bassetti D (1991) Identification of hepatitis A virus as a trigger for autoimmune chronic hepatitis type 1 in susceptible individuals. Lancet 337(8751):1183–1187
127. Verucchi G, Calza L, Chiodo F (1999) Viral hepatitis A with atypical course. Clinical, biochemical, and virologic study of 7 cases. Ann Ital Med Int 14(4):239–245
128. Victor JC, Monto AS, Surdina TY, Suleimenova SZ, Vaughan G, Nainan OV et al (2007) Hepatitis A vaccine versus immune globulin for postexposure prophylaxis. N Engl J Med 357(17):1685–1694
129. Wands JR, Mann E, Alpert E, Isselbacher KJ (1975) The pathogenesis of arthritis associated with acute hepatitis-B surface antigen-positive hepatitis. Complement activation and characterization of circulating immune complexes. J Clin Invest 55(5):930–936
130. Wasley A, Samandari T, Bell BP (2005) Incidence of hepatitis A in the United States in the era of vaccination. JAMA 294(2):194–201
131. Werzberger A, Mensch B, Kuter B, Brown L, Lewis J, Sitrin R et al (1992) A controlled trial of a formalin-inactivated hepatitis A vaccine in healthy children. N Engl J Med 327(7):453–457
132. Wheeler C, Vogt TM, Armstrong GL, Vaughan G, Weltman A, Nainan OV, Dato V, Xia G, Waller K, Amon J, Lee TM, Highbaugh-Battle A, Hembree C, Evenson S, Ruta MA, Williams IT, Fiore AE, Bell BP (2005) An outbreak of hepatitis A associated with green onions. N Engl J Med 353(9):890–897
133. Wolters B, Junge U, Dziuba S, Roggendorf M (2003) Immunogenicity of combined hepatitis A and B vaccine in elderly persons. Vaccine 21(25–26):3623–3628
134. Yeh HY, Hwang YC, Yates MV, Mulchandani A, Chen W (2008) Detection of hepatitis a virus by using a combined cell culture-molecular beacon assay. Appl Environ Microbiol 74(7):2239–2243
135. Yilmaz-Ciftdogan D, Kose E, Aslan S, Gayyurhan E (2015) Atypical clinical manifestations of hepatitis a among children aged 1-16 years in South-Eastern Region of Turkey. Turk J Pediatr 57(4):339–344
136. Yoon EL, Yim HJ, Kim SY, Kim JH, Lee JH, Lee YS, Lee HJ, Jung SW, Lee SW, Choi JH (2010) Clinical courses after administration of oral corticosteroids in patients with severely cholestatic acute hepatitis A; three cases. Korean J Hepatol 16(3):329–333
137. Yu JH, Kim JK, Park JY, Paik YH, Kim DY, Ahn SH, Han KH, Chon CY, Lee KS (2012) Clinical characteristics of acute hepatitis A complicated by acute kidney injury. Scand J Infect Dis 44(2):144–148
138. Zaaijer HL, Leentvaar-Kuijpers A, Rotman H, Lelie PN (1993) Hepatitis A antibody titres after infection and immunization: implications for passive and active immunization. J Med Virol 40(1):22–27

Prevention of Hepatitis A

6

Daniel Shouval

Abstract

Hepatitis A virus (HAV) infection is a preventable, acute inflammatory disease of the liver caused by a member of the Picornavirus family. The HAV is a non-cytopatic, hepatotrophic RNA virus which replicates in hepatocytes and generates immune-mediated liver injury. Infection is mainly transmitted through fecal-oral route, close person-to-person contact, and intake of contaminated water or food. HAV endemicity is classified as high, intermediate, low, and very low, depending on age-adjusted prevalence of anti-HAV(IgG) antibodies in the population. The epidemiology and susceptibility to infection are driven by a number of factors including sanitary and socioeconomic conditions, age at exposure, and herd immunity. Improvement in socioeconomic conditions and in the level of hygienic standards in many countries with intermediate endemicity in transition has led to a shift in susceptibility to infection in adolescents and young adults. Major progress has been made in the past decades in prevention of hepatitis A. Pre- and postexposure prophylaxis using formaldehyde-inactivated HAV vaccines has gradually replaced the use of immune serum globulin for protection of subjects at risk. Live attenuated HAV vaccines have been developed in China for preexposure prophylaxis. Several attenuated HAV strains have been used for over 20 years in the United States, Europe, and China for manufacturing of formalin-inactivated vaccines. Administration of such highly immunogenic vaccines, given at two doses, separated by a flexible interval of 6–12 months, has had an excellent record of safety and tolerability. While most countries still employ a two-dose immunization strategy, Argentina and China chose to use a single-dose immunization strategy for UMV, using a formaldehyde-inactivated and live attenuated vaccine, respectively. Immunization strategies include universal mass vaccination (UMV) of toddlers, regional mass vaccination (RMV), and immunization of distinct risk groups. Introduction of UMV and RMV programs in the United States, Israel, several European countries, and in Australia has led to an unprecedented decline in the incidence of HAV infection and a rise in herd immunity in these regions.

D. Shouval (✉)
Liver Unit, Institute of Gastroenterology and Hepatology, Jerusalem, Israel

Division of Medicine, Hadassah-Hebrew University Hospital, Jerusalem, Israel
e-mail: Shouval@hadssah.org.il

M.-H. Chang, K. B. Schwarz (eds.), *Viral Hepatitis in Children*,
https://doi.org/10.1007/978-981-13-0050-9_6

Abbreviations

ACIP	Advisory Committee on Immunization Practices
AE	Adverse event
Anti-HAV	Antibodies to the hepatitis A virus
CDC	Centers for Disease Control
EPI	Expanded program of immunization
HAV	Hepatitis A virus
IG	Immune globulin
IgA	Immune globulin A
IgG	Immune globulin G
IgM	Immune globulin M
MMR	Mumps, measles, and rubella vaccine
MSM	Men who have sex with men
PEP	Postexposure prophylaxis
RMV	Regional mass vaccination
SAE	Serious adverse event
UMV	Universal mass vaccination
WHO	World Health Organization

6.1 Introduction

There are several measures for protection against hepatitis A virus (HAV) infection: (1) general actions including maintenance of personal hygiene, adequate sanitation, and improvement of socioeconomic status, (2) pre- or postexposure passive prophylaxis with immune globulin (IG), and (3) pre- or postexposure active immunization with formaldehyde-inactivated vaccines. Live attenuated vaccines are only used for preexposure prophylaxis.

6.2 Personal Hygiene and Sanitation

HAV is a robust virus which is resistant to low pH and may persist in feces, in sewage, and in soil for a prolonged period [1]. Personal hygiene and environmental sanitation to prevent transmission through fecal contamination of food and water or by personal contact are primary means to control hepatitis A in any setting.

6.3 Passive Pre- and Postexposure Prophylaxis Against Hepatitis A with Immune Globulin (IG)

Administration of human immune globulin (IG) prepared from pooled human plasma through ethanol fractionation and containing high concentration of anti-HAV (IgG) antibodies has been used historically since 1942 as an efficient and rapid means for pre- and postexposure prophylaxis (PEP) against HAV infection [2, 3]. The protective efficacy of IG is dose dependent and limited to 12–20 weeks following intramuscular (i.m.) injection of 0.02 and 0.06 ml/kg weight, respectively. In view of the declining incidence of HAV infection in some countries in the Western Hemisphere, pooled plasma used for preparation of IG contains lower concentration of neutralizing anti-HAV(IgG) antibodies, raising doubt regarding the potential protective efficacy of IG against HAV [4]. Preexposure prophylaxis with IG is achieved rapidly. The putative mechanism of protection against hepatitis A conferred by IG involves neutralization of circulating virus and possibly prevention of uptake of virus through the gut mucosa and/or hepatocytes.

Little information is available regarding the safety of IG in the pediatric population [5]. Reports on serious systemic adverse events (AEs) in children receiving IG are rare, and the cumulative clinical experience, mainly collected during the pre-HAV vaccine era, suggests that administration of IG to adults and most probably to children is very safe [2, 6], except in patients with IgA deficiency. However, IG administration may interfere with live attenuated vaccines such as measles, mumps, rubella (MMR) and varicella. Co-administration of IG with an active hepatitis A vaccine may blunt the initial quantitative anti-HAV (IgG) antibody response after the first vaccine dose [7]. This effect, which is similar to the effect of passively transferred maternal anti-HAV

(IgG) antibodies, is of minor significance, and such vaccinees respond well to a booster dose given 6 months after the primary immunization. Finally, the use of immune globulin worldwide is now declining for a number of reasons: (a) nonspecific IG preparations increasingly fail to contain adequate amounts of anti-HAV (IgG), (b) cost of specific HAV IG preparations is high, (c) duration of IG-mediated protection against HAV infection lasts only several months as compared to hepatitis A vaccines, and (d) hepatitis A vaccines have already been shown to induce rapid and efficient pre- as well as postexposure protection against HAV following the first of two recommended doses [3].

6.4 Active Pre- and Postexposure Prophylaxis Against Hepatitis A

6.4.1 Immunization with Inactivated Hepatitis A Vaccines

All HAV vaccines contain cell culture-derived HAV antigen containing attenuated HAV strains adapted to grow in human and nonhuman mammalian cells through serial passage of originally wild-type HAV. Viral attenuation is associated with a small number of HAV mutations, distributed throughout the genome [8]. Cell culture-derived HAV antigen is purified, inactivated by formaldehyde, and adsorbed to aluminum hydroxide for the following vaccines: HAVRIX®, VAQTA®, and AVAXIM®. The HAV antigen in EPAXAL® is formulated in influenza-reconstituted virosomes. VAQTA®, HAVRIX®, EPAXAL®, HEALIVE®, and the Chinese Lv-8 inactivated HAV vaccine are at present preservative free (Table 6.1). The WHO has released recommendations for production and quality control of HAV vaccines [9]. The biological activity of inactivated hepatitis A vaccines is measured either by an in vivo relative potency assay or by an immunochemical determination of antigen.

For children, several manufacturers provide a half-volume presentation of the vaccine with the same antigen concentration as the adult formulation. Inactivated hepatitis A vaccines should be refrigerated at 2–8 °C; the vaccines should not be frozen. When stored at the recommended temperature, the shelf-life for inactivated hepatitis A vaccines ranges between 24 and 36 months, as specified by the manufacturers [9].

In addition to monovalent HAV vaccines, formaldehyde-inactivated combination vaccines have been developed in Europe against HAV and HBV or HAV and typhoid [3, 10].

Formaldehyde-inactivated hepatitis A vaccines are highly immunogenic and safe, providing rapid, protective immunity to hepatitis A within 2–4 weeks after primary immunization. A second dose is usually administered within 6–12 months after the priming injection, but the interval may be extended to 18–36 months depending on vaccine type.

Table 6.1 Monovalent HAV vaccines[a]

Attenuated HAV strain	Trade name	Adjuvant	HAV antigen dose/injection		Manufactures
			Pediatric	Adult	
HM-175	HAVRIX®	Alum hydroxide	720 EU	1440 EU	GSK [34]
CR-326	VAQTA®	Alum hydroxide	25 U	50 U	MSD [33]
GBM	AVAXIM®	Alum hydroxide	80 U	160 U	Aventis Pasteur [11]
TZ84	HEALIVE®	Alum hydroxide	250 U	500 U	Sinovac [15]
RG-SB	EPAXAL®	Virosome	24 U	24 U	Crucell/Berna Biotech [35]

[a]Reproduced with permission from Ref. [3]

6.4.2 Immunization with Live Attenuated Hepatitis A Vaccines

Two live attenuated hepatitis A vaccines were developed in China containing the H2 and LA-1 strains [12–15] . Both these vaccines as well as two formaldehyde-inactivated vaccines, administered in two doses, were tested in clinical trials in China using one or two doses and integrated into the Chinese EPI in 2008 (http://www.who.int/wer/2010/wer8530/en/index.html). A recent review summarizes the immunogenicity of six controlled clinical trials with the live attenuated HAV vaccine conducted in children in China, reporting 72–97.9% seroconversion rates and a good safety record [16]. Currently, the live attenuated vaccine is usually administered as a single subcutaneous dose.

6.4.3 Serologic Measurement of Protection

A positive (qualitative) test for anti-HAV (IgG) antibodies signifies immunity to hepatitis A. Although the lowest protective level against challenge with HAV is unknown, the reported minimal serum levels of anti-HAV (IgG) antibodies required for protection against HAV in humans varies between 10 and 33 mIU/ml depending on the immunoassay used for detections. Clinical experience suggests that protection against hepatitis A following passive immunization with IG or active vaccination may still be present even in the absence of detectable anti-HAV antibodies using standard immunoassays [17]. Low levels of anti-HAV (IgM) antibodies may be detectable by a conventional assay for a few weeks in ~20% of recipients of HAV vaccines. Therefore, anti-HAV (IgM) antibody assays cannot be used for reliable distinction between acute hepatitis A and anti-HAV response to vaccination.

6.4.4 Vaccine-Mediated Immune Response Against Hepatitis A Virus

Following infection with live, wild-type HAV, the virus penetrates the gut mucosa and is transported to the liver. Passage of the virus through the gut wall and virus replication in liver cells is associated with an active cellular and humoral immune response against the virus which induces hepatocellular injury [18–25]. In contrast, viral replication does not occur after immunization with a killed HAV vaccine, and protection against HAV is primarily antibody based. Evidence has now been obtained to suggest that immunization against HAV with a killed vaccine also leads to a measurable cellular protective immune response which is long-lasting for at least 6 years and may be boosted to revive the immune memory [3].

6.4.5 Duration of HAV Vaccine-Mediated Protection

Immune memory-mediated long-term protection against HAV infection, following a complete two-dose inactivated vaccine administration in children born to anti-HAV(IgG) negative mothers, has been predicted by modeling in 97% of vaccinees for at least 40 years and already documented through sero-surveillance for 20 years [26]. Similar data have been reported for a virosomal formulated HAV vaccine [27]. Consequently, booster doses are not recommended in vaccinees who completed a two-dose vaccination schedule.

Argentina and several countries in South America as well as China are pioneering a different immunization strategy, using single-vaccine dose immunization instead of the two-dose schedule licensed in most countries. Limited data on persistence of immune memory following one dose of a killed inactivated or live attenuated vaccine suggest persistence of protection for at least 7.5–9 and 5 years, respectively [28–30].

The immunogenicity of formaldehyde-inactivated hepatitis A vaccines is blunted somewhat by preexisting anti-HAV(IgG) antibodies, such as that which occurs when vaccine is co-administered with IG or when given to infants of previously infected HAV immune mothers [31, 32]. Yet, the practical consequences of this phenomenon are most likely negligible.

6.5 Strategies of Preexposure Prophylaxis Through Active Immunization

Inactivated hepatitis A vaccines have been licensed in Europe, Asia, Australia, and the Americas. The high efficacy of these vaccines in preventing hepatitis A in children has been shown in two pivotal placebo-controlled clinical trials conducted in Thailand and the United States demonstrating a 99% efficacy after three doses and 100% after two doses of aluminum hydroxide-formulated vaccines, respectively [33, 34].

In a third study, a single dose of an inactivated vaccine formulated in virosomes was shown to provide complete protection against disease [35]. Several factors had a marginal impact on blunting of anti-HAV (IgG) antibody levels following immunization. These include overweight, older age, smoking, as well as passively transferred anti-HAV (IgG) antibodies from pregnant mothers to their newborns. Lower sero-protection rates following vaccination have been reported in human immunodeficiency virus-infected patients as well as solid organ and stem-cell transplant recipients. As observed with other vaccines, anti-HAV (IgG) levels were reported to be higher in female vaccinees as compared to males, following a priming and booster dose of the vaccine [3].

As more information has become available on the extra-ordinary immunogenicity, effectiveness, and safety of hepatitis A vaccines, immunization strategies have shifted from vaccination of individuals belonging to specific risk groups to mass vaccination campaigns and then to universal mass vaccination (UMV), which is however still restricted to a limited number of countries [3, 29].

Following the licensure of HAV vaccines, four immunization strategies have been evaluated for preexposure prophylaxis. *First* is the early efforts at immunization of individuals at increased risk including international travelers to areas of HAV endemicity, men who have sex with men (MSM), intravenous drug users, patients with chronic liver disease, food handlers, day-care center staff, caretakers of nonhuman primates, and patients with blood-clotting disorders. This policy is still valid but has no or little public health impact on herd immunity at large.

The second strategy included regional mass vaccination (RMV) of pediatric populations at risk. Three demonstration projects conducted in the United States in Native Americans in Alaska, in Native American Indians, and in Butte County, California, documented a 94–97% reduction in incidence of symptomatic acute hepatitis A [36]. Consequently, in 1999, the US Advisory Committee on Immunization Practices (ACIP) issued a recommendation to introduce universal hepatitis A vaccination into routine childhood vaccination (2 doses in children >2 years old and catch-up at the age of 10–12 years) in 17 states in the United States with an annual incidence of >20 cases/100,000. Postimmunization surveillance revealed that, despite variable first vaccine coverage of 50–80%, a progressive decline in reported incidence of hepatitis A was observed from 21.1 cases/100000 to 2.5 cases/100000, which represents an 88% drop [36]. Similar projects were introduced in Puglia, Italy, in 1997 [37]; in Catalonia, Spain, in 1998 [38]; and in North Queensland, Australia, in 1999 [, leading to a 90–97% decline in the reported incidence in these regions. The results of these highly successful vaccination projects in selected geographic regions worldwide suggested that mass vaccination of children in communities at risk is effective and will lead to herd immunity even under moderate coverage.

These early projects paved the way for the introduction of *the third immunization strategy*, namely, universal mass vaccination (UMV) against HAV in selected countries with intermediate endemicity in transition. By 2010, 11 countries have embarked on the road toward universal HAV vaccination in babies. In 1999, Israel, a

areas, with all reported cost-effectiveness ratios falling below ~US$ 35,000 per QALY. For targeted vaccination, cost-effectiveness was highly dependent on the risk of infection in the targeted groups" [9].

6.6 Postexposure Prophylaxis (PEP)

The incubation of hepatitis A varies between 15 and 50 days (average 20–30 days). Evidence obtained in a number of clinical trials suggested that postexposure immunization against hepatitis A may also have similar effectiveness as IG, provided that immunization is started within 2 weeks of exposure. Support for this conclusion was initially obtained from the hepatitis A efficacy trial conducted in the United States, where the HAV vaccine was administered during an HAV outbreak. In this pivotal clinical trial, no new cases of acute hepatitis were identified from day 17 onwards after vaccination [33]. A similar experience was obtained, in Slovakia [47], in Israel [48], and in Italy [49], where a 79% protective efficacy of postexposure immunization was documented in Italian household contacts of acute hepatitis A cases. In Israel, as in Slovakia, prompt intervention with an active vaccine in a community outbreak of hepatitis A led to effective control of an epidemic within 2 weeks of starting the intervention. Final proof for the use of inactivated HAV vaccines for postexposure prophylaxis was obtained in a study conducted in Kazakhstan [50]. In this controlled clinical trial, 1090 household and day-care contacts (2–40 years old) of index cases with acute hepatitis were randomized to receive hepatitis A vaccine or IG. Transmission of HAV, confirmed by anti-HAV (IgM) testing, occurred in 4.4% and 3.3% of the study groups, respectively (RR 1.35; 95% CI = 0.70–2.67). Consequently, the US ACIP is now recommending postexposure immunization with an active HAV vaccine in 2–40-year-old individuals at risk. The field effectiveness of PEP using an active HAV vaccine administered within 14 days of exposure was later also confirmed in Australia in a retrospective survey of susceptible contacts of patients with acute HAV infection [51]. Altogether, the use of hepatitis A vaccines instead of IG for PEP has a number of advantages, including induction of long-term protection against HAV, ease of administration, and acceptance at a similar cost per dose.

6.7 Co-administration of Hepatitis A Vaccines with Other Childhood or Traveler Vaccines

Concurrent administration of a number of routine childhood and traveler monovalent and trivalent vaccines with an HAV vaccine does not lead to significant interference in immunogenicity, reactogenicity, or safety of the individual vaccines. As demonstrated in a number of controlled studies conducted among 12–15-month-old infants, in children <18 years, and in adults, inactivated HAV vaccines can be administered simultaneously with diphtheria, tetanus, acellular pertussis (DTaP), polio (oral and inactivated), *Haemophilus influenzae* (Hib), MMR typhoid (oral and intramuscular), hepatitis B, cholera, Japanese encephalitis, rabies, and yellow fever vaccines. It is recommended that injections should be given at different sites [3].

6.7.1 Safety of Hepatitis A Vaccines

Inactivated HAV vaccines have an excellent safety and tolerability record in children and adults alike and are interchangeable [3]. Almost 200 million doses of inactivated hepatitis A vaccines were sold worldwide between 1995 and early 2006 and many more afterwards. Based on the cumulative experience gained until 2006, the overall safety profile of all formaldehyde-inactivated hepatitis A vaccines administered to children and adults has been excellent, irrespective of manufacturer [3]. The following information is quoted from a US Centers for Disease Control (CDC) review [52]:

"*Reactogenicity*: Local reactions, including soreness or tenderness at injection site, were reported in pre-licensure clinical trials in 56% (N = 50,000) and 53% (N = 10,000) of adult recipients of HAVRIX® and VAQTA® respectively, while in children these figures were at a range of 15% and 17%. Headaches were reported in 14–16% of adults for both vaccines respectively, and in 4% of children receiving HAVRIX® in whom ~8% had feeding problems". A recent retrospective evaluation was conducted in 1.4 million children, age 1–6 years, who received 6.0 million intramuscular injections of various vaccines including HAV vaccines. Results confirmed the low incidence of local site reactions in recipient of such vaccines [53].

Serious Adverse Events (SAE): An estimated 1.3 million persons in Asia and Europe were vaccinated with HAVRIX® before the vaccine's licensure in the United States in 1995. Reports of serious adverse events, without regard to causality, received by the vaccine manufacturer, included anaphylaxis, Guillain-Barré syndrome, brachial plexus neuropathy, transverse myelitis, multiple sclerosis, encephalopathy and erythema multiform. The majority of these events occurred among adults, and approximately one third occurred among persons concurrently receiving other vaccines. For serious adverse events for which background incidence data can be estimated (e.g. Guillain-Barré syndrome and brachial plexus neuropathy), rates for vaccine recipients were no higher than would be expected for an unvaccinated population.

No vaccine-related serious adverse events were reported for approximately 40,000 children who were administered the 360 EL.U. dose of HAVRIX® in the protective efficacy study. In a post-licensure study of 11,417 children and 25,023 adults who were administered VAQTA®, no serious adverse events occurred that were considered to be associated with administration of vaccine. A published post-licensure evaluation of safety among 2000 child and adult recipients identified no serious adverse events associated with VAQTA®.

According to information received from the China Centers for Disease Control, between 1992 and 2007, 60 million doses of mainly live attenuated HAV vaccines were administered in China. Since 2005, 8 million doses are distributed annually to 18-month-old toddlers and older children. With respect to the Chinese inactivated and live attenuated hepatitis A vaccines, experience during clinical trials and through passive surveillance did not identify any substantial safety issues. Further up-to-date information on the immunogenicity and safety of live attenuated vaccines used in China has recently been released [16]. However, post-marketing surveillance in selected communities to measure and monitor safety and adverse reactions is still desirable [54]. Studies of children vaccinated with live attenuated vaccines have shown shedding of the vaccine virus and possibly secondary infection among contacts, so post-marketing surveillance may provide a context in which to conduct specific studies to examine the outcome of secondary infection and virus circulation if it occurs. Data of particular interest include molecular markers of attenuation and the genetic stability of attenuation markers after human passage. (http://www.who.int/wer/2010/wer8530/en/index.html)

6.8 Summary

Despite the availability of efficacious and safe hepatitis A vaccines for more than 20 years, hepatitis A still remains a frequent and debilitating disease affecting millions of individuals worldwide annually. The continuous improvement in sanitary and socioeconomic conditions has led to a shift in prevalence of HAV infection from high to intermediate and even low endemicity. Consequently a growing population of adolescents and young adults becomes susceptible to HAV infection.

The following recommendations were released through the WHO 2012 position paper [9]*:*

- Both inactivated and live attenuated hepatitis A vaccines are highly immunogenic, and immunization will generate long-lasting, possibly lifelong, protection against hepatitis A in children as well as in adults.
- Evidence testifies to the excellent safety profile of inactivated vaccines. Although considered safe, internationally published evidence on the safety and tolerability of the live attenuated hepatitis A vaccines is more limited.
- WHO recommends that vaccination against HAV be integrated into the national immunization schedule for children aged ≥1 year if indicated on the basis of incidence of acute hepatitis A, change in the endemicity from high to intermediate, and consideration of cost-effectiveness.
- Vaccination against hepatitis A should be part of a comprehensive plan for the prevention and control of viral hepatitis, including measures to improve hygiene and sanitation and measures for outbreak control.
- Targeted vaccination of high-risk groups should be considered in low and very low endemicity settings to provide individual health benefits.
- The use of hepatitis A vaccine rather than passive prophylaxis with immune globulin should be considered for preexposure prophylaxis (e.g., for travelers to areas of higher hepatitis A endemicity) and postexposure prophylaxis (e.g., for close contacts of acute cases of hepatitis A).
- The use of a single-dose regimen of hepatitis A vaccine to control community-wide outbreaks has been most successful in small self-contained communities, when vaccination was started early in the course of the outbreak and when high coverage of multiple age cohorts was achieved.
- National immunization programs may consider inclusion of single-dose inactivated hepatitis A vaccines in immunization schedules. This option seems to be comparable in terms of effectiveness and is less expensive. However, until further experience has been obtained with a single-dose schedule, in individuals at substantial risk of contracting hepatitis A, and in immunocompromised individuals, a two-dose schedule is preferred.
- Inactivated hepatitis A vaccines produced by different manufacturers, including combined hepatitis A vaccines, are interchangeable

References

1. Siegl G, Weitz M, Kronauer G (1984) Stability of hepatitis A virus. Intervirology 22(4):218–226
2. Liu JP, Nikolova D, Fei Y (2009) Immunoglobulins for preventing hepatitis A. Cochrane Database Syst Rev 2:CD004181
3. Shouval D (2010) Hepatitis A. The immunological basis for immunization series. Module 18,World Health Organization. http://whqlibdoc.who.int/publications/2011/9789241501422_eng.pdf
4. Tejada-Strop A, Costafreda MI, Dimitrova Z, Kaplan GG, Teo CG (2017) Evaluation of potencies of immune globulin products against hepatitis A. JAMA Intern Med 177(3):430–432
5. Zhang RL, Zeng JS, Zhang HZ (1990) Survey of 34 pregnant women with hepatitis A and their neonates. Chin Med J 103(7):552–555
6. Ashur Y, Adler R, Rowe M, Shouval D (1999) Comparison of immunogenicity of two hepatitis A vaccines--VAQTA and HAVRIX--in young adults. Vaccine 17(18):2290–2296
7. Wagner G, Lavanchy D, Darioli R et al (1993) Simultaneous active and passive immunization against hepatitis A studied in a population of travellers. Vaccine 11(10):1027–1032
8. Martin A, Lemon SM (2006) Hepatitis A virus: from discovery to vaccines. Hepatology 43(2 Suppl 1):S164–S172
9. WHO position paper on hepatitis A vaccines (2012) Wkly Epidemiol Rec 87(28/29):261–276
10. Van Damme P, Van Herck K (2004) A review of the efficacy, immunogenicity and tolerability of a combined hepatitis A and B vaccine. Expert Rev Vaccines 3(3):249–267
11. Vidor E, Dumas R, Porteret V, Bailleux F, Veitch K (2004) Aventis Pasteur vaccines containing inactivated hepatitis A virus: a compilation of immunogenicity data. Eur J Clin Microbiol Infect Dis 23(4):300–309
12. Wu JY, Liu Y, Chen JT, Xia M, Zhang XM (2012) Review of 10 years of marketing experience with Chinese domestic inactivated hepatitis A vaccine Healive(R). Hum Vaccin Immunother 8(12):1836–1844
13. Zhang X, An J, Tu A et al (2016) Comparison of immune persistence among inactivated and live attenuated hepatitis a vaccines 2 years after a single dose. Hum Vaccin Immunother 12(9):2322–2326

14. Liu XE, Wushouer F, Gou A et al (2013) Comparison of immunogenicity between inactivated and live attenuated hepatitis A vaccines: a single-blind, randomized, parallel-group clinical trial among children in Xinjiang Uighur Autonomous Region. China Hum Vaccin Immunother 9(7):1460–1465
15. Cui F, Liang X, Wang F, Zheng H, Hutin YJ, Yang W (2014) Development, production, and postmarketing surveillance of hepatitis A vaccines in China. J Epidemiol 24(3):169–177
16. Rao S, Mao JS, Motlekar S, Fangcheng Z, Kadhe G (2016) A review of immunogenicity and tolerability of live attenuated Hepatitis A vaccine in children. Hum Vaccin Immunother 12(12):3160–3165
17. Shouval D, Ashur Y, Adler R et al (1993) Single and booster dose responses to an inactivated hepatitis A virus vaccine: comparison with immune serum globulin prophylaxis. Vaccine 11(Suppl 1):9–14
18. Lemon SM (1993) Immunologic approaches to assessing the response to inactivated hepatitis A vaccine. J Hepatol 18(Suppl 2):S15–S19
19. Vallbracht A, Maier K, Stierhof YD, Wiedmann KH, Flehmig B, Fleischer B (1989) Liver-derived cytotoxic T cells in hepatitis A virus infection. J Infect Dis 160(2):209–217
20. Hashimoti E, Kojimahara N, Noguchi S, Taniai M, Ishiguro N, Hayashi N (1996) Immunohistochemical characterization of hepatic lymphocytes in acute hepatitis A, B, and C. J Clin Gastroenterol 23(3):199–202
21. Sanchez G, Pinto RM, Bosch A (2004) A novel CD4+ T-helper lymphocyte epitope in the VP3 protein of hepatitis A virus. J Med Virol 72(4):525–532
22. Baba M, Fukai K, Hasegawa H, Nakayabu M, Suzuki S (1992) The role of natural killer cells and lymphokine activated killer cells in the pathogenesis of hepatic injury in hepatitis A [corrected]. J Clin Lab Immunol 38(1):1–14
23. Vallbracht A, Gabriel P, Maier K et al (1986) Cell-mediated cytotoxicity in hepatitis A virus infection. Hepatology 6(6):1308–1314
24. Kurane I, Binn LN, Bancroft WH, Ennis FA (1985) Human lymphocyte responses to hepatitis A virus-infected cells: interferon production and lysis of infected cells. J Immunol 135(3):2140–2144
25. Perrella A, Vitiello L, Atripaldi L et al (2008) Impaired function of CD4+/CD25+ T regulatory lymphocytes characterizes the self-limited hepatitis A virus infection. J Gastroenterol Hepatol 23(7 Pt 2):e105–e110
26. Van Damme P, Leroux-Roels G, Suryakiran P, Folschweiller N, Van Der Meeren O (2017) Persistence of antibodies 20 y after vaccination with a combined hepatitis A and B vaccine. Hum Vaccin Immunother 10:1–9
27. Chappuis F, Farinelli T, Deckx H et al (2017) Immunogenicity and estimation of antibody persistence following vaccination with an inactivated virosomal hepatitis A vaccine in adults: a 20-year follow-up study. Vaccine 35(10):1448–1454
28. Mayorga O, Buhler S, Jaeger VK et al (2016) Single-dose hepatitis A immunization: 7.5-year observational pilot study in Nicaraguan children to assess protective effectiveness and humoral immune memory response. J Infect Dis 214(10):1498–1506
29. Uruena A, Gonzalez JE, Rearte A et al (2016) Single-dose universal hepatitis A immunization in one-year-old children in Argentina: high prevalence of protective antibodies up to 9 years after vaccination. Pediatr Infect Dis J 35(12):1339–1342
30. Zhang Z, Zhu X, Hu Y et al (2017) Five-year antibody persistence in children after one dose of inactivated or live attenuated hepatitis A vaccine. Hum Vaccin Immunother 14:1–6
31. Leentvaar-Kuijpers A, Coutinho RA, Brulein V, Safary A (1992) Simultaneous passive and active immunization against hepatitis A. Vaccine 10(Suppl 1):S138–S141
32. Spradling PR, Bulkow LR, Negus SE, Homan C, Bruce MG, McMahon BJ (Mar 2016) Persistence of seropositivity among persons vaccinated for hepatitis A during infancy by maternal antibody status: 15-year follow-up. Hepatology 63(3):703–711
33. Werzberger A, Mensch B, Kuter B et al (1992) A controlled trial of a formalin-inactivated hepatitis A vaccine in healthy children. N Engl J Med 327(7):453–457
34. Innis BLSR, Kunasol P et al (1994) Protection against hepatitis A by an inactivated vaccine. JAMA 271:1328–1334
35. Mayorga Perez O, Herzog C, Zellmeyer M, Loaisiga A, Frosner G, Egger M (2003) Efficacy of virosome hepatitis A vaccine in young children in Nicaragua: randomized placebo-controlled trial. J Infect Dis 188(5):671–677
36. Klevens RM, Kruszon-Moran D, Wasley A et al (2011) Seroprevalence of hepatitis A virus antibodies in the U.S.: results from the national health and nutrition examination survey. Public Health Rep 126(4):522–532
37. Dominguez A, Salleras L, Carmona G, Batalla J (2003) Effectiveness of a mass hepatitis A vaccination program in preadolescents. Vaccine 21(7–8):698–701
38. Hanna JN, Hills SL, Humphreys JL (2004) Impact of hepatitis A vaccination of Indigenous children on notifications of hepatitis A in north Queensland. Med J Aust 181(9):482–485
39. Dagan R, Leventhal A, Anis E, Slater P, Ashur Y, Shouval D (2005) Incidence of hepatitis A in Israel following universal immunization of toddlers. JAMA 294(2):202–210
40. Chodick G, Heymann AD, Ashkenazi S, Kokia E, Shalev V (2008) Long-term trends in hepatitis A incidence following the inclusion of hepatitis A vaccine in the routine nationwide immunization program. J Viral Hepat 15(Suppl 2):62–65
41. Barkai G, Belmaker I, Givon-Lavi N, Dagan R (2009) The effect of universal toddlers-only hepatitis A virus vaccination program on seropositivity rate in unvaccinated toddlers: evidence for reduced virus circulation in the community. Pediatr Infect Dis J 28(5):391–393

42. Manor Y, Lewis M, Ram D, et al (2017) Evidence for hepatitis A virus endemic circulation in Israel despite universal toddler vaccination since 1999 and low clinical incidence in all age groups. J Infect Dis 215(4) 574–580
43. Stuurman AL, Marano C, Bunge EM, De Moerlooze L, Shouval D (2017) Impact of universal mass vaccination with monovalent inactivated hepatitis A vaccines – a systematic review. Hum Vaccin Immunother 13(3):724–736
44. Van Damme P, Mathei C, Thoelen S, Meheus A, Safary A, Andre FE (1994) Single dose inactivated hepatitis A vaccine: rationale and clinical assessment of the safety and immunogenicity. J Med Virol 44(4):435–441
45. Vacchino MN (2008) Incidence of hepatitis A in Argentina after vaccination. J Viral Hepat 15(Suppl 2):47–50
46. Vizzotti C, Gonzalez J, Gentile A et al (2014) Impact of the single-dose immunization strategy against hepatitis A in Argentina. Pediatr Infect Dis J 33(1):84–88
47. Prikazsky V, Olear V, Cernoch A, Safary A, Andre FE (1994) Interruption of an outbreak of hepatitis A in two villages by vaccination. J Med Virol 44(4):457–459
48. Zamir C, Rishpon S, Zamir D, Leventhal A, Rimon N, Ben-Porath E (2001) Control of a community-wide outbreak of hepatitis A by mass vaccination with inactivated hepatitis A vaccine. Eur J Clin Microbiol Infect Dis 20(3):185–187
49. Sagliocca L, Amoroso P, Stroffolini T et al (1999) Efficacy of hepatitis A vaccine in prevention of secondary hepatitis A infection: a randomised trial. Lancet 353(9159):1136–1139
50. Victor JC, Monto AS, Surdina TY et al (2007) Hepatitis A vaccine versus immune globulin for postexposure prophylaxis. N Engl J Med 357(17):1685–1694
51. Freeman E, Lawrence G, McAnulty J, Tobin S, MacIntyre CR, Torvaldsen S (2014) Field effectiveness of hepatitis A vaccine and uptake of post exposure prophylaxis following a change to the Australian guidelines. Vaccine 32(42):5509–5513
52. Fiore AE, Wasley A, Bell BP (2006) Prevention of hepatitis A through active or passive immunization: recommendations of the Advisory Committee on Immunization Practices (ACIP). MMWR Recomm Rep 55(RR-7):1–23
53. Jackson LA, Peterson D, Nelson JC et al (2013) Vaccination site and risk of local reactions in children 1 through 6 years of age. Pediatrics 131(2):283–289
54. Irving GJ, Holden J, Yang R, Pope D (2012) Hepatitis A immunisation in persons not previously exposed to hepatitis A. Cochrane Database Syst Rev 7:CD009051

7 Natural History of Hepatitis B Virus Infection: From Infancy to Adult Life

Jia-Feng Wu and Yen-Hsuan Ni

Abstract

Hepatitis B virus (HBV) infection in endemic areas usually starts in infancy and persists until adulthood. The clinical course of chronic HBV infection varies among different individuals, HBV viral strains, and the interactions between humans and HBV. Children with chronic HBV infection usually present with immune-tolerant status initially, break through the immune tolerance and experience the inflammatory phase beyond puberty, and enter the inactive phase after hepatitis B e antigen (HBeAg) seroconversion. HBeAg-negative hepatitis flares occur in 5–25% of chronic HBV-infected subjects after HBeAg seroconversion.

The diverse course of chronic HBV infection is associated with the age of HBV infection, route of HBV acquisition, host factors (host immune system, endocrine system, and hepatocyte receptor), viral factors (viral load, HBV genotypes, and mutant strains), and host-viral interactions. The breakthrough of immune tolerance is correlated with the start of adrenarche and puberty in children with chronic HBV infection. Human cytokines, innate immunity, and human leukocyte antigens are also reported to modulate the disease course of immune clearance, inflammation, and long-term outcomes. Different immune escape HBV mutant strains, causing different impacts on viral biosynthesis, which emerge under host immune selection are noted to result in different long-term outcomes of chronic HBV infection. Early chronic HBV infection events during childhood are key predictors of late outcomes in adulthood. Realization of the mechanisms of immune-tolerant breakthrough, triggering inflammation, and their long-term impact may enhance the development of better strategies for children with chronic HBV infection.

Keywords

Hepatitis B virus · Immune-tolerant · Host viral interaction · Endocrine system

J.-F. Wu
Department of Pediatrics, National Taiwan University Children's Hospital, Taipei, Taiwan

Y.-H. Ni (✉)
Department of Pediatrics, National Taiwan University Children's Hospital, Taipei, Taiwan

Hepatitis Research Center, National Taiwan University Hospital, Taipei, Taiwan
e-mail: yhni@ntu.edu.tw

M.-H. Chang, K. B. Schwarz (eds.), *Viral Hepatitis in Children*,
https://doi.org/10.1007/978-981-13-0050-9_7

7.1 Natural Course of Chronic Hepatitis B Virus Infection

Chronic hepatitis B virus (HBV) infection remains an important disease burden globally. The clinical course of chronic HBV infection is closely related to the age of acquisition, route of transmission, host immune and endocrine factors, viral factors, and various host-viral interactions. The transmission route of HBV may be either maternal/perinatal or horizontal. Maternal/perinatal transmission and early childhood HBV acquisition are associated with a high likelihood of lifelong infection [1–3]. In endemic areas, such as Taiwan, maternal/perinatal transmission accounts for approximately half of the routes of chronic HBV infection before universal HBV vaccination program implementation, while this route accounts for 90% after the initiation of this program [4]. The natural course of chronic HBV infection is generally divided into the immune-tolerant phase, immune clearance/inflammatory phase, and post-HBeAg seroconversion phases (Table 7.1).

The immune-tolerant phase is indicated by normal alanine aminotransferase (ALT) levels, high viral load, and the presence of HBeAg. In the majority of the patients during or after adolescence, the flare-up of ALT and the HBeAg seroconversion to its antibody (anti-HBe) indicate the breakthrough of immune tolerance and the start of immune clearance/inflammatory phase. HBeAg seroconversion generally indicates the decrement of active viral replication and hepatitis activity, while delayed HBeAg seroconversion with persistently high viremia after the third–fourth decade of life indicates a high risk of liver cirrhosis and hepatocellular carcinoma (HCC) [5–9]. Due to the lack of proofreading ability of HBV polymerase, HBV is prone to development of mutant strains during the disease course of chronic infection. Various HBV mutants, such as basal core promoter (BCP) and precore/core gene mutation, are associated with different viral replication ability and clinical outcomes [10, 11].

Some infected subjects may enter the HBeAg-negative hepatitis reactivation phase and develop liver cirrhosis or HCC [12, 13]. The majority of children with chronic HBV infection present with immune-tolerant status initially, enter the immune clearance phase with various degrees of liver injury in puberty or beyond, and then settle at the inactive phase after HBeAg seroconversion [14]. Some of them may exhibit elevation of viral load with hepatitis flare-up after HBeAg seroconversion, the so-called HBeAg- negative hepatitis. In an adult study from Taiwan, the estimated incidence rates of HBeAg-negative hepatitis were 2.9%, 3.8%, and 8.5% in subjects with spontaneous HBeAg seroconversion at 16–30, 30–40, and > 40 years of age, respectively [5, 6, 9]. The annual incidence of HBeAg-negative hepatitis was estimated to be 0.26–0.41% in children with chronic HBV infection after HBeAg seroconversion [15]. Liver cirrhosis and even hepatocellular carcinoma may develop afterward [12, 13]. The HBsAg titers decreased with age, with an average annual clearance rate of 0.58% [16]. Few chronically HBV-infected subjects develop HBsAg seroclearance with

Table 7.1 Summary of the clinical course of chronic hepatitis B virus infection

	HBsAg/ anti-HBs	HBeAg/ anti-HBs	HBV viral load [107]	ALT levels	HBV mutants	HBcAg location in hepatocyte [108]
Immune-tolerant phase	(+)/(−)	(+)/(−)	>20,000 IU/mL	Normal	−	Nuclear
Immune clearance/ inflammatory phase	(+)/(−)	(+)/(−)	>20,000 IU/mL	Elevated	+	Nuclear and cytoplasmic
Post-HBeAg seroconversion phase						
HBeAg-negative inactive phase	(+)/(−)	(−)/(+)	<2000 IU/mL	Normal	+	Absent
HBeAg-negative hepatitis phase	(+)/(−)	(−)/(+)	>2000 IU/mL	Elevated	+	Cytoplasmic

positive anti-HBs (HBsAg seroconversion) [16, 17]. The overall cumulative incidence of spontaneous HBsAg seroconversion was 5.40%, whereas the annual HBsAg seroconversion rate was 0.25% in a Taiwanese cohort chronically infected with genotypes B or C [17].

Different individuals have different responses to HBV during the chronic course of infection. For example, the onset of adrenarche and puberty modulates the start of immune breakthrough and the severity of liver inflammation in chronic HBV-infected children. The genotype and phenotype of human cytokines, innate immunity, and human leukocyte antigens (HLA) are also associated with the onset of immune clearance of chronic HBV infection and severity of inflammation [18].

Both host and viral factors trigger the immune clearance/inflammatory phase, HBeAg seroclearance/seroconversion, HBsAg seroclearance/seroconversion, and even the occurrence of HBeAg-negative hepatitis flare. Several of these factors are key determinants of liver injury, chronic liver failure, liver cirrhosis, and even HCC.

7.2 Host Factors Affecting the Natural Course of Hepatitis B Virus Infection: From Hepatocyte, Human Endocrine to Immune Systems

7.2.1 Host Hepatocyte: Sodium Taurocholate Co-transporting Polypeptide (NTCP) Receptor

A liver-specific bile acid transporter, which is encoded by *SLC10A1*, has been identified as the cellular receptor for HBV [19, 20]. The NTCP-binding lipopeptide that originates from the first 47 amino acids of the pre-S1 domain of the HBV large protein blocks taurocholate transport [19, 20]. Identification of NTCP as an HBV receptor facilitates understanding of the HBV life cycle and biology, including the identification of host restriction and dependency factors. The impact of NCTP gene polymorphisms on the clinical course of chronically HBV-infected children has not been well elucidated yet. The *SLC10A1* (NTCP) S267F variant accounts for about 9% of the East Asian population and is independently associated with a decreased risk of liver cirrhosis and HCC occurrence and resistance to chronic HBV infection [21]. NTCP may also serve as a new therapeutic target in the development of new anti-HBV agents.

7.2.2 Human Endocrine Systems

In pediatric chronic HBV infection, the spontaneous HBeAg seroconversion rate was estimated to be low before 10 years of age and accelerated later after the adrenarche and puberty [14, 22–24]. The annual spontaneous HBeAg seroconversion rate was 1.70% ± 1.78% (95% CI 0.43%–2.97%) in the first decade of life, 3.78% ± 1.63% (95% CI 2.61%–4.94%) in the second decade of life, and 4.02% ± 2.29% (95% CI 1.61%–6.23%) in the third decade of life in a genotype B and C cohort with chronic HB-infection [14].

Earlier puberty onset is associated with earlier HBeAg seroconversion in boys with chronic HBV infection [23]. Earlier menarche in girls, indicating earlier puberty onset, is also associated with earlier HBeAg seroconversion [24]. The clinical course of various infections differs greatly between males and females, probably because of the interaction between sex hormones and immune systems [25, 26]. Previous animal studies showed the androgen pathway can enhance the transcription of HBV and block the tumor suppressor gene in early hepatocarcinogenesis, while the estrogen pathway can suppress the transcription of HBV gene [27–29].

Dehydroepiandrosterone sulfate (DHEAS) is known as a serum marker of adrenarche in humans. The serum DHEAS levels are usually elevated around 2 years before puberty and are significantly associated with the age of HBeAg seroconversion in chronic HBV-infected boys and girls [30]. The serum DHEAS level is usually elevated around 6–8 years of age in both genders, is persistently elevated during the second decade of life, and peaks at the third decade of life [31, 32]. DHEAS is reported as a potent immune modulator to various infectious pathogens, including parasites, *mycobacterium tuberculosis*, and even human immunodeficiency virus [31–35]. DHEAS exhibits an immune stimulatory effect and mediates the cross talk between the hypothalamic-pituitary-adrenocortical axis hormones and the systemic immune system. A high serum DHEAS level at mid-puberty has been proven to be associated with a decreased HBV viral load and HBsAg titer in adolescents and adults [30]. Endocrine factors, particularly DHEAS, may be partially responsible for the initiation of the breakthrough of the immune-tolerant phase in patients with chronic HBV infection.

7.2.3 Adaptive and Innate Immunity

Both adaptive and innate immune systems in humans are critical in terms of the clinical outcomes. Human cytokines play important roles in the adaptive immunity to defend against pathogens either by direct inhibition of viral replication or indirectly by determining the predominant pattern of host immune response, which is regulated by the human genetic background and modulates the clinical outcomes of viral infection. Previous studies showed interferon-γ and tumor necrosis factor-α (TNF-α) may contribute to the cell-mediated anti-HBV response in children with chronic HBV infection entering the immune clearance/inflammatory phase [36, 37].

A cohort study with candidate gene approach demonstrated that interleukin (IL)-10 and IL-12 correlate with the HBeAg seroconversion age and severity of inflammation during the immune clearance/inflammatory phase [38]. The *IL-10-1082 G/G* genotype is associated with higher serum IL-10 levels, while the *IL-12β – 10,993 C/G* genotype is associated with higher HBcAg-inducible IL-12 secretion of peripheral blood mononuclear cells in vitro [38]. Both are associated with earlier initiation of clearance/inflammatory phase and spontaneous HBeAg seroconversion in patients with chronic HBV infection [38]. IL-12 is a pro-inflammatory cytokine that promotes Th1 cell differentiation and suppresses Th2 cells and enhances the production of antiviral cytokines, such as INF-γ and IL-2, by mononuclear cells, and amplifies the cytotoxicity of cytotoxic T lymphocyte (CTL) and natural killer cells [39]. Although IL-10 is generally considered to be immunosuppressive during chronic viral infection, it also reportedly activates CTL in the presence of IL-2, the downstream signal of IL-12 [40].

The *A*-allele of *IL-10* single-nucleotide polymorphism (SNP) *rs1800872* and the *G*-allele of *IL-12β SNP rs3212217* were predictors of spontaneous HBsAg seroconversion and recovery from HBV infection [41]. During the immune clearance/inflammatory phase in human liver tissues, the IL-10 and IL-12β mRNA abundances were positively correlated with interferon-γ mRNA expression levels [42]. The interferon-γ mRNA abundance in human liver tissues was correlated with low furin, high program death 1 (PD-1), and high program death ligand-1 (PD-L1) mRNA levels in liver tissue from HBeAg-positive patients during the immune clearance/inflammatory phase [41, 42]. The intrahepatic interferon-γ may modulate the inflammatory response to avoid excessive hepatocyte damage through the enhancement of PD-1/PD-L1 pathway activation, whereas interferon-γ-mediated furin suppression may contribute to a suppression of HBV protein (HBeAg and HBsAg) biosynthesis [41–44].

Furin, a human proprotein peptidase, located at the endoplasmic reticulum membrane in hepatocytes, is used by HBV to facilitate the biosynthesis and maturation of HBeAg from the 25-kDa proprotein to the 17-kDa mature HBeAg [45]. The inhibition of furin either by interferon-γ, small molecular weight antagonists, or even knockdown experiments, all inhibited the biosynthesis of mature HBeAg in both in vivo and in vitro studies [41, 46].

The activation of PD-1/PD-L1 pathway is considered to be a marker of immunologic tolerance and T-cell dysfunction in the presence of various kinds of infectious pathogens, including HBV [47, 48]. The blockage of PD-1 and PD-L1 is demonstrated to enhance the reactivation of HBV-specific CTLs and secretion of interferon-γ by circulating intrahepatic lymphocytes in subjects with chronic HBV infection after their HBeAg seroconversion [49]. The non-expression of the PD-1/PD-L1 pathway was reported to be associated with the occurrence of fulminant hepatic failure in acute HBV-infected patients [50]. Hence, upregulation of the PD-1/PD-L1 pathway may efficiently mitigate pathogenic T-cell responses, limit liver inflammation, and avoid excessive liver damage and fulminant hepatic failure in patients with HBV infection [49, 50]. The PD-1/PD-L1 pathway is thus considered to play a key regulatory role in avoiding excessive liver damage when the inflammatory response is programmed to turn off or the immune response fails to clear the pathogen [41, 50–52]. Most patients with chronic HBV infection may break through the immune-tolerant status and experience a flare of hepatitis at the immune clearance/inflammatory phase, followed by an inactive phase after HBeAg seroconversion, with a decline in viral load and normalization of ALT. The interferon-γ-mediated pathway to suppress HBV during the immune clearance/inflammatory phase, including the upregulation of PD-1/PD-L1 pathway and downregulation of furin, may serve as important regulators of the transition from the cytolytic to the non-cytolytic HBV suppression pathway inside the liver. Activation of this pathway avoids excessive liver damage and occurrence of fulminant hepatic failure during the immune clearance/inflammatory phase [41].

Human T lymphocytes may identify HBV viral peptides presented by HLA on antigen- presenting cells. Variations in immune responses to various infectious pathogens are often associated with HLA gene polymorphisms in humans [53]. A previous cross-sectional study demonstrated the major histocompatibility complex (MHC) class II alleles *HLA-DRB1*1301–02* are associated with protection against persistent HBV infection in Gambia, and the findings were further confirmed by two other independent studies in Germany and Korea [54–56]. Other studies suggested a protective role of *HLA-DR2*, *HLA-DR*0406*, *HLA-B*4001*, and *HLA-DR7* against acute HBV infection in human [57, 58]. A recent genome-wide association cross-sectional study showed the association of *HLA-DP* with protection against chronic HBV and with the clinical course of HBV clearance in Korean and Japanese [59]. Our previous cohort showed the *HLA-B61* and *HLA-DQB1*0503* are associated with earlier breakthrough of immune-tolerant phase and earlier HBeAg seroconversion age in Taiwanese children with genotype B and C chronic HBV infection [60].

Mounting evidence indicates that innate immune responses play roles in human infectious diseases, especially the toll-like receptor (TLR) signaling pathway. TLR signaling pathways are essential to the defense mechanism against various pathogens by activating downstream inflammatory cascades like nuclear factor κB, interferon regulatory factor, mitogen-activated protein kinases, and pro-inflammatory cytokines to modulate the clinical course of infectious diseases in human [61, 62]. Chronically HBV-infected patients with *TLR5 rs5744174* (p.Phe616Leu) and *C*-allele at *TLR9 rs5743836* promoter region polymorphism might experience an early spontaneous HBeAg seroconversion [61]. *TLR5 rs5744174* (p.Phe616Leu) is associated with higher interferon-γ production in patients with chronic HBV infection, and the *C*-allele at the *TLR9 rs5743836* promoter polymorphism site was reported to increase TLR9 receptor expression levels, which may mediate signals from thymosin alpha-1 to suppress the replication of HBV through downstream cytokine signal cascades [61].

The *G*-allele carriers at *TLR4 SNP rs4986790* (p.Asp299Gly) in a cohort of patients with chronic HBV infection experienced spontaneous HBsAg seroconversion [61]. A recent animal study showed that gut microbiota may stimulate liver immune responses through the TLR4-dependent pathway, resulting in rapid HBV clearance in the mouse model [42, 61, 62].

These data suggest that both the adaptive immune (IL-10 and IL-12) and innate immune factors (TLR-5 and TLR-9) may modulate the interferon-γ-mediated HBV suppression pathway to promote breakthrough of the immune-tolerant phase, early HBeAg seroconversion, and clearance of HBV in humans. In the meantime, interferon-γ may fine-tune the PD-1 and PD-L1 pathway to avoid excessive liver damage in the immune clearance/inflammation phase.

7.3 Viral Factors Affecting the Natural Course of HBV Infection

7.3.1 HBV Genotypes

Eight genotypes (A–H) of HBV have been defined in the world. Different HBV genotypes are recognized to be important predictors of clinical outcomes of chronic HBV infection in humans. In India, genotype D HBV was reported to induce more severe liver damage than genotype A HBV and is associated with a higher incidence of HCC [63]. In Eastern Asian countries, genotypes B and C are the predominant HBV strains, while genotype C is noted to associate with severe liver disease, delayed spontaneous HBeAg seroconversion, and higher incidence of HBeAg-negative hepatitis than genotype B HBV in both adults and children [15, 64, 65]. The genotype Ba HBV was reported to associate with the development of HCC in young non-cirrhotic patients in Taiwan, while the genotype Bj HBV does not correlate with increased HCC risk as compared with genotype C HBV infection in Japan [66].

7.3.2 HBV Mutants and Viremia Profile

Due to the lack of proofreading of the HBV polymerase, HBV is prone to development of various mutant strains under host immune selection pressure. Wild-type HBV is the dominant strain during the natural infection. Approximately 10–24% of children develop HBV precore mutants before HBeAg seroconversion, and around 50% of children develop these mutants after HBeAg seroconversion [67, 68].

Mutations of the core promoter at nucleotide positions A1752G, A1775G, and G1799C correlate significantly with the occurrence of HBeAg seroconversion; the precore stop codon G1896A mutant exists in 50% of chronic HBV-infected children after HBeAg seroconversion [68]. Genotype C HBV is associated with BCP A1762T/G1764A mutations during HBeAg seroconversion [68]. The prevalence of HBV precore/core mutant strains increases significantly in the immune clearance/inflammatory phase compared to the immune-tolerant phase in patients with chronic HBV infection [69]. The presence of BCP A1762T/G1764A mutant strain was also demonstrated to be associated with the occurrence of HBeAg-negative hepatitis flare-up after HBeAg seroconversion in a pediatric chronic HBV cohort infected by genotypes B and C [15]. The increased proportion of BCP A1762T/G1764A mutant strains in adults chronically infected with genotype B or C was correlated with an increased risk of liver cirrhosis and HCC [70, 71]. A recent quantitative analysis of precore stop codon G1896A and BCP A1762T/G1764A mutants in interferon-treated patients showed that the distinct HBV evolution/mutation patterns during HBeAg seroconversion may present with different HBV viremia patterns after HBeAg seroconversion [72]. The presence of BCP A1762T/ G1764A mutants after HBeAg seroconversion was recently reported to associate with HBeAg-negative hepatitis and liver cirrhosis in later life [15, 73].

HBeAg seroconversion in young children with chronic HBV infection showed decreased viral loads, persistently normal ALT levels, lower risk of HBeAg-negative hepatitis, and uneventful courses after HBeAg seroconversion [15, 74]. HBeAg seroconversion beyond the fourth decade of life in adults is associated with an increased risk of liver cirrhosis and HCC occurrence [8, 9, 75]. These data implied that different immune mechanisms and perhaps different HBV mutants selected during the course of the immune clearance/inflammatory phase between young and old HBeAg seroconverters may lead to different consequences of chronic HBV infection.

HBV precore/core gene mutants which occurred during the immune clearance/inflammatory phase are known to be the result of viral escape mutations occurring under host immune selection pressure [10, 75]. Mutations in the HBV precore/core gene may change the amino acid sequence, protein structure, antigenicity, and the biological function of both HBeAg and HBcAg. The alteration of HBcAg sequence and structure may change the stability of HBV nucleocapsid, the HBV pre-genomic RNA (pgRNA) packaging, and the efficacy and accuracy of HBV replication [76–78]. A previous study showed that subjects carrying the IL-10-1082 polymorphism site *G/G* genotype exhibited high HBV P135Q mutations during the immune clearance/inflammatory phase and decreased HBV viral load after HBeAg seroconversion [69]. The HBV core protein P135Q mutant and the precore stop codon G1896A mutant were the most prevalent mutants before HBeAg seroconversion in genotype B and C subjects with chronic HBV infection [69, 78]. The HBV P135Q mutant strain was further demonstrated to alter the HBV capsid assembly and the HBeAg biosynthesis and to reduce human immune responses after HBeAg seroconversion [78–80].

7.3.3 Pediatric HCC

The age at HBeAg seroconversion and the severity of liver damage during the immune clearance/inflammation phase are both important outcome predictors during the chronic course of HBV infection [81–84]. Extremely early HBeAg seroconversion before 3 years of age, in an immature liver, with severe liver damage was regarded to increase the risk of childhood HCC [85–91]. The pre-S2 deletion of HBV genome was reported in nearly half of children with HBV-related HCC [92–99].

7.3.4 De Novo HBV Infection After Liver Transplantation

The shortage of liver donors leads to the use of HBsAg-negative and anti-HBc-positive liver allografts for patients in need of orthotopic liver transplantation (OLT) in HBV-endemic areas, while occult HBV infection (OBI) in these grafts may lead to de novo HBV infection after liver transplantation [100–103]. Without adequate prophylaxis in liver recipients receiving a graft from an HBsAg-negative/anti-HBc-positive donor, the incidence of de novo HBV infection in pediatric OLT recipients is up to 15.3% in HBV-endemic areas [102]. An anti-HB titer of >200 mIU/mL prior to liver transplant and the usage of hepatitis B immunoglobulin (HBIG) and antiviral agents may effectively reduce the risk of de novo HBV infection in liver recipients receiving HBsAg-negative/anti-HBc-positive liver allografts [101–104]. In a recent systematic review, de novo infection rates were 19%, 2.6%, and 2.8% in HBsAg-negative recipients under HBIG, lamivudine, and combination of the two, respectively [104]. Mutations in the major S gene (681 base pairs) were discovered in 88.9% of de novo HBV-infected children after liver transplant [105]. The majority of them harbored mutations within the *a* determinant region (codons 124–147) [105].

7.3.5 Future Prospects in Pediatric HBV

HBV infection remains one of the most common pathogens of viral hepatitis globally to date. Universal HBV vaccination eliminated a vast majority of chronic HBV infection in the world, but vaccination failure in newborn born to a mother with high viremia still existed [106, 107]. After universal vaccination in HBV-endemic areas, the transmission of HBV from mothers with high HBV viremia and incomplete immunization was associated with breakthrough infection and the development of HCC [95, 106].

Vaccine escape mutants may develop after immunoprophylaxis, and their long-term impact on the clinical course of chronic HBV seemed to be milder but needs further investigation [85–88].

7.4 Summary

The viral factors (genotype, viral load, mutant strains, etc.), host factors (hormone, adaptive immunity, innate immunity, etc.), and host-virus interactions all act together to modulate the natural course of chronic HBV infection [15, 17, 23, 108]. The early childhood events of chronic HBV infection, reflecting the complex interactions between the host and HBV, are early key predictors of the late outcomes of chronic HBV infection.

Careful monitoring of host and viral biomarkers and providing adequate and effective therapeutic interventions may improve the long- term outcome of patients with chronic HBV infection. Elucidation of the mechanisms triggering liver inflammation and their long-term impact may enhance the development of better and earlier therapeutic strategies for children with chronic HBV infection.

References

1. Stevens CE, Beasley RP, Tsui J, Lee WC (1975) Vertical transmission of hepatitis B antigen in Taiwan. N Engl J Med 292:771–774
2. Lok AS, McMahon AJ (2007) Chronic hepatitis B. Hepatology 45:507–539
3. Beasley RP (2009) Rocks along the road to the control of HBV and HCC. Ann Epidemiol 19:231–234
4. Ni YH, Huang LM, Chang MH, Yen CJ, Lu CY, You SL, Kao JH, Lin YC, Chen HL, Hsu HY, Chen DS (2007) Two decades of universal hepatitis B vaccination in Taiwan: impact and implication for future strategies. Gastroenterology 132:1287–1293
5. Chu CM, Hung SJ, Lin J, Tai DI, Liaw YF (2004) Natural history of hepatitis B e antigen to antibody seroconversion in patients with normal serum aminotransferase levels. Am J Med 116:829–834
6. Chu CM, Liaw YF (2007) Chronic hepatitis B virus infection acquired in childhood: special emphasis on prognostic and therapeutic implication of delayed HBeAg seroconversion. J Viral Hepat 14:147–152
7. Yang HI, Lu SN, Liaw YF, You SL, Sun CA, Wang LY et al (2002) Hepatitis B e antigen and the risk of hepatocellular carcinoma. N Engl J Med 347:168–174
8. Chang ML, Liaw YF (2014) Hepatitis B flares in chronic hepatitis B: pathogenesis, natural course, and management. J Hepatol 61:1407–1417
9. Chen YC, Chu CM, Liaw YF (2010) Age-specific prognosis following spontaneous hepatitis B e antigen seroconversion in chronic hepatitis B. Hepatology 51:435–444
10. Lim SG, Cheng Y, Guindon S, Seet BL, Lee LY, Hu P et al (2007) Viral quasi-species evolution during hepatitis be antigen seroconversion. Gastroenterology 133:951–958
11. Lin CL, Liao LY, Liu CJ, Yu MW, Chen PJ, Lai MY (2007) Hepatitis B viral factors in HBeAg-negative carriers with persistently normal serum alanine aminotransferase levels. Hepatology 45:1193–1198
12. Chen DS (1993) From hepatitis to hepatoma: lessons from type B viral hepatitis. Science 262:369–370
13. Kao JH, Chen DS (2002) Global control of hepatitis B virus infection. Lancet Infect Dis 2:395–403
14. Wu JF, Su YR, Chen CH, Chen HL, Ni YH, Hsu HY, Wang JL, Chang MH (2012) Predictive effect of serial serum alanine aminotransferase levels on spontaneous HBeAg seroconversion in chronic genotypes B and C HBV-infected children. J Pediatr Gastroenterol Nutr 54:97–100
15. Wu JF, Chiu YC, Chang KC, Chen HL, Ni YH, Hsu HY, Chang MH (2016) Predictors of hepatitis B e antigen-negative hepatitis in chronic hepatitis B virus infected patients from childhood to adulthood. Hepatology 63:74–82
16. Chiu YC, Liao SF, Wu JF, Lin CY, Lee WC, Chen HL, Ni YH, Hsu HY, Chang MH (2014) Factors affecting the natural decay of hepatitis B surface antigen in children with chronic hepatitis B virus infection during long-term follow-up. J Pediatr 165:767–772
17. Wu JF, Hsu HY, Chiu YC, Chen HL, Ni YH, Chang MH (2015) The effects of cytokines on spontaneous hepatitis B surface antigen seroconversion in chronic hepatitis B virus infection. J Immunol 194:690–696
18. Wu JF, Chang MH (2015) Natural history of chronic hepatitis B virus infection from infancy to adult life – the mechanism of inflammation triggering and long-term impacts. J Biomed Sci 22:92
19. Watashi K, Urban S, Li W, Wakita T (2014) NTCP and beyond: opening the door to unveil hepatitis B virus entry. Int J Mol Sci 15:2892–2905
20. Yan H, Peng B, Liu Y, Xu G, He W, Ren B, Jing Z, Sui J, Li W (2014) Viral entry of hepatitis B and D viruses and bile salts transportation share common molecular determinants on sodium taurocholate cotransporting polypeptide. J Virol 88:3273–3284
21. Hu HH, Liu J, Lin YL, Luo WS, Chu YJ, Chang CL, Jen CL, Lee MH, Lu SN, Wang LY, You SL, Yang HI, Chen CJ, REVEAL-HBV Study Group (2016) The rs2296651 (S267F) variant on NTCP (SLC10A1)

is inversely associated with chronic hepatitis B and progression to cirrhosis and hepatocellular carcinoma in patients with chronic hepatitis B. Gut 65:1514–1521

22. Chang MH, Sung JL, Lee CY, Chen CJ, Chen JS, Hsu HY et al (1989) Factors affecting clearance of hepatitis B e antigen in hepatitis B surface antigen carrier children. J Pediatr 115:385–390
23. Wu JF, Tsai WY, Hsu HY, Ni YH, Chen HL, Tsuei DJ, Chang MH (2010) The effect of puberty onset on spontaneous hepatitis B virus e antigen seroconversion in men. Gastroenterology 138:942–948
24. Wu JF, Tsai WY, Tung YC, Chen HL, Ni YH, Hsu HY, Chang MH (2014) Effect of menarche onset on the clinical course in females with chronic hepatitis B virus infection. J Pediatr 165:534–538
25. Schuurs AH, Verheul HA (1990) Effects of gender and sex steroids on the immune response. J Steroid Biochem Mol Biol 35:157–175
26. Guerra-Silveira F, Abad-Franch F (2013) Sex bias in infectious disease epidemiology: patterns and processes. PLoS One 8:e62390
27. Wang SH, Yeh SH, Lin WH, Wang HY, Chen DS, Chen PJ (2009) Identification of androgen response elements in the enhancer I of hepatitis B virus: a mechanism for sex disparity in chronic hepatitis B. Hepatology 50:1392–1402
28. Chen PJ, Yeh SH, Liu WH, Lin CC, Huang HC, Chen CL et al (2012) Androgen pathway stimulates microRNA-216a transcription to suppress the tumor suppressor in lung cancer-1 gene in early hepatocarcinogenesis. Hepatology 56:632–643
29. Wang SH, Yeh SH, Lin WH, Yeh KH, Yuan Q, Xia NS et al (2012) Estrogen receptor a represses transcription of HBV genes via interaction with hepatocyte nuclear factor 4a. Gastroenterology 142:989–998
30. Wu JF, Tsai WY, Tung YC, Chen HL, Ni YH, Hsu HY, Chang MH (2014) Role of serum dehydroepiandrosterone sulfate level on the clearance of chronic hepatitis B virus infection. J Gastroenterol 49:900–906
31. Nawata H, Yanase T, Goto K, Okabe T, Nomura M, Ashida K et al (2004) Andropause. Horm Res 62:110–114
32. Hazeldine J, Arlt W, Lord JM (2010) Dehydroepiandrosterone as a regulator of immune cell function. J Steroid Biochem Mol Biol 120:127–136
33. Chittiprol S, Kumar AM, Shetty KT, Kumar HR, Satishchandra P, Rao RS et al (2009) HIV-1 clade C infection and progressive disruption in the relationship between cortisol, DHEAS and CD4 cell numbers: a two-year follow-up study. Clin Chim Acta 409:4–10
34. de la Torre B, von Krogh G, Svensson M, Holmberg V (1997) Blood cortisol and ehydroepiandrosterone sulfate (DHEAS) levels and CD4 T cell counts in HIV infection. Clin Exp Rheumatol 15:87–90
35. Kutlu NO, Akinci A, Sönmezgöz E, Temel I, Evliyaoğlu E (2003) The effects of androstenediol and dehydroepiandrosterone on the immune response to BCG at puberty. J Trop Pediatr 49:181–185
36. Kao PC, Wu JF, Ni YH, Lin YT, Chen HL, Hsu SH, Hsu HY, Chang MH (2010) Tumour necrosis factor-α promoter region polymorphisms affect the course of spontaneous HBsAg clearance. Liver Int 30:1448–1453
37. Wu JF, Wu TC, Chen CH, Ni YH, Chen HL, Hsu HY, Chang MH (2010) Serum levels of interleukin 10 and 12 predict early, spontaneous hepatitis B virus e antigen seroconversion. Gastroenterology 138:165–172
38. Rigopoulou EI, Suri D, Chokshi S et al (2005) Lamivudine plus interleukin-12 combination therapy in chronic hepatitis B, antiviral and immunological activity. Hepatology 42:1028–1036
39. Santin AD, Hermonat PL, Ravaggi A et al (2000) Interleukin-10 increases Th1 cytokine production and cytotoxic potential in human papilloma-virus-specific CD8+ cytotoxic T lymphocytes. J Virol 74:4729–4737
40. Bertoni R, Sidney J, Fowler P, Chesnut RW, Chisari FV, Sette A (1997) Human histocompatibility leukocyte antigen-binding supermotifs predict broadly cross-reactive cytotoxic T lymphocyte responses in patients with acute hepatitis. J Clin Invest 100:503–513
41. Wu JF, Hsu HY, Ni YH, Chen HL, Wu TC, Chang MH (2012) Suppression of furin by interferon-γ and the impact on hepatitis B virus antigen biosynthesis in human hepatocytes. Am J Pathol 181:19–25
42. Chou HH, Chien WH, Wu LL, Cheng CH, Chung CH, Horng JH, Ni YH, Tseng HT, Wu D, Lu X, Wang HY, Chen PJ, Chen DS (2015) Age-related immune clearance of hepatitis B virus infection requires the establishment of gut microbiota. Proc Natl Acad Sci U S A 112:2175–2180
43. Mühlbauer M, Fleck M, Schütz C, Weiss T, Froh M, Blank C, Schölmerich J, Hellerbrand C (2006) PD-L1 is induced in hepatocytes by viral infection and by interferon-alpha and -gamma and mediates T cell apoptosis. J Hepatol 45:520–528
44. Pesu M, Watford WT, Wei L, Xu L, Fuss I, Strober W, Andersson J, Shevach EM, Quezado M, Bouladoux N, Roebroek A, Belkaid Y, Creemers J, O'Shea JJ (2008) T-cell-expressed proprotein convertase furin is essential for maintenance of peripheral immune tolerance. Nature 455:246–250
45. Lei RX, Shi H, Peng XM, Zhu YH, Cheng J, Chen GH (2009) Influence of a single nucleotide polymorphism in the P1 promoter of the furin gene on transcription activity and hepatitis B virus infection. Hepatology 50:763–771
46. Yang HY, Zheng NQ, Li DM, Gu L, Peng XM (2014) Entecavir combined with furin inhibitor simultaneously reduces hepatitis B virus replication and e antigen secretion. Virol J 11:165. https://doi.org/10.1186/1743-422X-11-165

47. Evans A, Riva A, Cooksley H, Phillips S, Puranik S, Nathwani A, Brett S, Chokshi S, Naoumov NV (2008) Programmed death 1 expression during antiviral treatment of chronic hepatitis B: impact of hepatitis B e-antigen seroconversion. Hepatology 48:759–769
48. Peng G, Li S, Wu W, Tan X, Chen Y, Chen Z (2008) PD-1 upregulation is associated with HBV-specific T cell dysfunction in chronic hepatitis B patients. Mol Immunol 45:963–970
49. Fisicaro P, Valdatta C, Massari M, Loggi E, Biasini E, Sacchelli L, Cavallo MC, Silini EM, Andreone P, Missale G, Ferrari C (2010) Antiviral intrahepatic T-cell responses can be restored by blocking programmed death-1 pathway in chronic hepatitis B. Gastroenterology 138:682–693
50. Zhang Z, Zhang JY, Wherry EJ, Jin B, Xu B, Zou ZS, Zhang SY, Li BS, Wang HF, Wu H, Lau GK, Fu YX, Wang FS (2008) Dynamic programmed death 1 expression by virus-specific CD8 T cells correlates with the outcome of acute hepatitis B. Gastroenterology 134:1938–1949
51. Isogawa M, Furuichi Y, Chisari FV (2005) Oscillating CD8(+) T cell effector functions after antigen recognition in the liver. Immunity 23:53–56
52. Mühlbauer M, Fleck M, Schütz C, Weiss T, Froh M, Blank C, Schölmerich J, Hellerbrand C (2006) PD-L1 is induced in hepatocytes by viral infection and by interferon-alpha and -gamma and mediates T cell apoptosis. J Hepatol 45:520–528
53. Thursz MR, Kwiatkowski D, Allsopp CE, Greenwood BM, Thomas HC, Hill AV (1995) Association between an MHC class II allele and clearance of hepatitis B virus in the Gambia. N Engl J Med 332:1065–1069
54. Hohler T, Gerken G, Notghi A, Lubjuhn R, Taheri H, Protzer U et al (1997) HLA-DRB1*1301 and *1302 protect against chronic hepatitis B. J Hepatol 26:503–507
55. Ahn SH, Han KH, Park JY, Lee CK, Kang SW, Chon CY et al (2000) Association between Hepatitis B virus infection and HLA-DR type in Korea. Hepatology 31:1371–1373
56. Almarri A, Batchlor JR (1994) HLA and hepatitis B infection. Lancet 344:1994–1995
57. Wu YF, Wang LY, Lee TD, Lin HH, Hu CT, Cheng ML et al (2004) HLA phenotypes and outcomes of hepatitis B virus infection in Taiwan. J Med Virol 72:17–25
58. Nishida N, Sawai H, Matsuura K, Sugiyama M, Ahn SH, Park JY, Hige S, Kang JH, Suzuki K, Kurosaki M, Asahina Y, Mochida S, Watanabe M, Tanaka E, Honda M, Kaneko S, Orito E, Itoh Y, Mita E, Tamori A, Murawaki Y, Hiasa Y, Sakaida I, Korenaga M, Hino K, Ide T, Kawashima M, Mawatari Y, Sageshima M, Ogasawara Y, Koike A, Izumi N, Han KH, Tanaka Y, Tokunaga K, Mizokami M (2012) Genome-wide association study confirming association of HLA-DP with protection against chronic hepatitis B and viral clearance in Japanese and Korean. PLoS One 7:e39175
59. Wu JF, Chen CH, Hsieh RP, Shih HH, Chen YH, Li CR, Chiang CY, Shau WY, Ni YH, Chen HL, Hsu HY, Chang MH (2006) HLA typing associated with hepatitis B e antigen seroconversion in children with chronic hepatitis B virus infection: a prospective sibling cohort study in Taiwan. J Pediatr 148:647–651
60. Hsu HY, Chang MH, Ni YH, Lee PI (1999) Cytokine release of peripheral blood mononuclear cells in children with chronic hepatitis B virus infection. J Pediatr Gastroenterol Nutr 29:540–545
61. Wu JF, Chen CH, Ni YH, Lin YT, Chen HL, Hsu HY, Chang MH (2012) Toll-like receptor and hepatitis B virus clearance in chronic infected patients: a long-term prospective cohort study in Taiwan. J Infect Dis 206:662–668
62. Lange NE, Zhou X, Lasky-Su J et al (2011) Comprehensive genetic assessment of a functional TLR9 promoter polymorphism: no replicable association with asthma or asthma-related phenotypes. BMC Med Genet 12:26
63. Thakur V, Guptan RC, Kazim SN, Malhotra V, Sarin SK (2002) Profile, spectrum and significance of HBV genotypes in chronic liver disease patients in the Indian subcontinent. J Gastroenterol Hepatol 17:165–170
64. Kao JH, Chen PJ, Lai MY, Chen DS (2000) Hepatitis B genotypes correlate with clinical outcomes in patients with chronic hepatitis B. Gastroenterology 118:554–559
65. Ni YH, Chang MH, Wang KJ, Hsu HY, Chen HL, Kao JH, Yeh SH, Jeng YM, Tsai KS, Chen DS (2004) Clinical relevance of hepatitis B virus genotype in children with chronic infection and hepatocellular carcinoma. Gastroenterology 127:1733–1738
66. Orito E, Ichida T, Sakugawa H et al (2001) Geographic distribution of hepatitis B virus (HBV) genotype in patients with chronic HBV infection in Japan. Hepatology 34:590–594
67. Chang MH (2006) Hepatitis B virus mutation in children. Indian J Pediatr 73:803–807
68. Ni YH, Chang MH, Hsu HY, Tsuei DJ (2004) Longitudinal study on mutation profiles of core promoter and precore regions of the hepatitis B virus genome in children. Pediatr Res 56:396–399
69. Wu JF, Ni YH, Lin YT, Lee TJ, Hsu HJ, Chen HL, Tsuei DJ, Hsu HY, Chang MH (2011) Human interleukin-10 genotypes are associated with different precore/core gene mutation patterns in children with chronic hepatitis B virus infection. J Pediatr 158:808–813
70. Tseng TC, Liu CJ, Yang HC, Chen CL, Yang WT, Tsai CS, Kuo SF, Verbree FC, Su TH, Wang CC, Liu CH, Chen PJ, Chen DS, Kao JH (2015) Higher proportion of viral basal core promoter mutant increases the risk of liver cirrhosis in hepatitis B carriers. Gut 64:292–302

71. Liu CJ, Chen BF, Chen PJ, Lai MY, Huang WL, Kao JH, Chen DS (2006) Role of hepatitis B virus precore/core promoter mutations and serum viral load on noncirrhotic hepatocellular carcinoma: a case-control study. J Infect Dis 194:594–599
72. Yang HC, Chen CL, ShenYC PCY, Liu CJ, Tseng TC, Su TH, Chuang WL, Yu ML, Dai CY, Liu CH, Chen PJ, Chen DS, Kao JH (2013) Distinct evolution and predictive value of hepatitis B virus precore and basal core promoter mutations in interferon-induced hepatitis B e antigen seroconversion. Hepatology 57:934–943
73. Tseng TC, Liu CJ, Yang HC, Chen CL, Yang WT, Tsai CS, Kuo SF, Verbree FC, Su TH, Wang CC, Liu CH, Chen PJ, Chen DS, Kao JH (2015) Higher proportion of viral basal core promoter mutant increases the risk of liver cirrhosis in hepatitis B carriers. Gut 64:292–302
74. Ni YH, Chang MH, Chen PJ, Tsai KS, Hsu HY, Chen HL, Tsuei DJ, Chen DS (2007) Viremia profiles in children with chronic hepatitis B virus infection and spontaneous e antigen seroconversion. Gastroenterology 132:2340–2345
75. Chang MH, Hsu HY, Ni YH, Tsai KS, Lee PI, Chen PJ et al (1998) Precore stop codon mutant in chronic hepatitis B virus infection in children: its relation to hepatitis B e antigen seroconversion and maternal hepatitis B surface antigen. J Hepatol 28:915–922
76. Schlicht HJ, Wasenauer G (1991) The quaternary structure, antigenicity, and aggregational behavior of the secretory core protein of human hepatitis B virus are determined by its signal sequence. J Virol 65:6817–6825
77. Wynne SA, Crowther RA, Leslie AGW (1999) The crystal structure of the human hepatitis B virus capsid. Mol Cell 3:771–780
78. Wu JF, Ni YH, Chen HL, Hsu HY, Chang MH (2014) The impact of hepatitis B virus precore/core gene carboxyl terminal mutations on viral biosynthesis and the host immune response. J Infect Dis 209:1374–1381
79. Hsu HY, Chang MH, Chen DS, Lee CY, Sung JL (1986) Baseline seroepidemiology of hepatitis B virus infection in children in Taipei, 1984: a study just before mass hepatitis B vaccination program in Taiwan. J Med Virol 18:301–307
80. Ni YH, Chang MH, Wu JF, Hsu HY, Chen HL, Chen DS (2012) Minimization of hepatitis B infection by a 25-year universal vaccination program. J Hepatol 57:730–735
81. Ni YH, Chang MH, Jan CF, Hsu HY, Chen HL, Wu JF, Chen DS (2016) Continuing decrease in hepatitis B virus infection 30 years after initiation of infant vaccination program in Taiwan. Clin Gastroenterol Hepatol 14:1324–1330
82. Wen WH, Chen HL, Ni YH, Hsu HY, Kao JH, Hu FC, Chang MH (2011) Secular trend of the viral genotype distribution in children with chronic hepatitis B virus infection after universal infant immunization. Hepatology 53:429–436
83. Poovorawan Y, Chongsrisawat V, Theamboonlers A, Leroux-Roels G, Crasta PD, Hardt K (2012) Persistence and immune memory to hepatitis B vaccine 20 years after primary vaccination of Thai infants, born to HBsAg and HBeAg positive mothers. Hum Vaccin Immunother 8:896–904
84. Lin YC, Chang MH, Ni YH, Hsu HY, Chen DS (2003) Long-term immunogenicity and efficacy of universal hepatitis B virus vaccination in Taiwan. J Infect Dis 187:134–138
85. Hsu HY, Chang MH, Ni YH, Lin HH, Wang SM, Chen DS (1997) Surface gene mutants of hepatitis B virus in infants who develop acute or chronic infections despite immunoprophylaxis. Hepatology 26:786–791
86. Hsu HY, Chang MH, Liaw SH, Ni YH, Chen HL (1999) Changes of hepatitis B surface antigen variants in carrier children before and after universal vaccination in Taiwan. Hepatology 30:1312–1317
87. Hsu HY, Chang MH, Ni YH, Chiang CL, Chen HL, Wu JF, Chen PJ (2010) No increase in prevalence of hepatitis B surface mutant in a population of children and adolescents who were fully covered by universal infant immunization. J Infect Dis 201:1192–1200
88. Hsu HY, Chang MH, Ni YH, Jeng YM, Chiang CL, Chen HL, Wu JF, Chen PJ (2013) Long-term follow-up of children with postnatal immunoprophylaxis failure who were infected with hepatitis B virus surface antigen gene mutant. J Infect Dis 207:1047–1057
89. Komatsu H, Inui A, Umetsu S, Tsunoda T, Sogo T, Konishi Y, Fujisawa T (2016) Evaluation of the G145R mutant of the hepatitis B virus as a minor strain in mother-to-child transmission. PLoS One 11:e0165674
90. Chang MH, Hsu HY, Hsu HC, Ni YH, Chen JS, Chen DS (1995) The significance of spontaneous hepatitis B e antigen sero-conversion in childhood: with special emphasis of the clearance of hepatitis B e antigen before 3 years of age. Hepatology 22:1387–1392
91. Tseng YR, Wu JF, Kong MS, Hu FC, Yang YJ, Yeung CY, Huang FC, Huang IF, Ni YH, Hsu HY, Chang MH, Chen HL (2014) Infantile hepatitis B in immunized children: risk for fulminant hepatitis and long-term outcomes. PLoS One 9:e111825
92. Huang HP, Hsu HY, Chen CL, Ni YH, Wang HY, Tsuei DJ, Chiang CL, Tsai YC, Chen HL, Chang MH (2010) Pre-S2 deletions of hepatitis B virus and hepatocellular carcinoma in children. Pediatr Res 67:90–94
93. Teng YC, Neo JC, Wu JC, Chen YF, Kao CH, Tsai TF (2016) Expression of a hepatitis B virus pre-S2 deletion mutant in the liver results in hepatomegaly and hepatocellular carcinoma in mice. J Pathol 241:463. https://doi.org/10.1002/path.4850
94. Chang MH, Chen CJ, Lai MS, Hsu HM, Wu TC, Kong MS, Liang DC, Shau WY, Chen DS (1997) Universal hepatitis B vaccination in Taiwan and the

incidence of hepatocellular carcinoma in children. Taiwan Childhood Hepatoma Study Group. N Engl J Med 336:1855–1859
95. Chang MH, You SL, Chen CJ, Liu CJ, Lai MW, Wu TC, Wu SF, Lee CM, Yang SS, Chu HC, Wang TE, Chen BW, Chuang WL, Soon MS, Lin CY, Chiou ST, Kuo HS, Chen DS, Taiwan Hepatoma Study Group (2016) Long-term effects of hepatitis B immunization of infants in preventing liver cancer. Gastroenterology 151:472–480
96. McMahon BJ, Bulkow LR, Singleton RJ, Williams J, Snowball M, Homan C, Parkinson AJ (2011) Elimination of hepatocellular carcinoma and acute hepatitis B in children 25 years after a hepatitis B newborn and catch-up immunization program. Hepatology 54:801–807
97. Chang MH, You SL, Chen CJ, Liu CJ, Lee CM, Lin SM, Chu HC, Wu TC, Yang SS, Kuo HS, Chen DS, Taiwan Hepatoma Study Group (2009) Decreased incidence of hepatocellular carcinoma in hepatitis B vaccinees: a 20-year follow-up study. J Natl Cancer Inst 101:1348–1355
98. Chang MH, Chen TH, Hsu HM, Wu TC, Kong MS, Liang DC, Ni YH, Chen CJ, Chen DS, Taiwan Childhood HCC Study Group (2005) Prevention of hepatocellular carcinoma by universal vaccination against hepatitis B virus: the effect and problems. Clin Cancer Res 11:7953–7957
99. Ni YH, Chen DS (2010) Hepatitis B vaccination in children: the Taiwan experience. Pathol Biol (Paris) 58:296–300
100. Hsu HY, Chang MH, Ni YH, Chiang CL, Wu JF, Chen HL (2015) Universal infant immunization and occult hepatitis B virus infection in children and adolescents: a population-based study. Hepatology 61:1183–1191
101. Su WJ, Ho MC, Ni YH, Chen HL, Hu RH, Wu YM, Chang MH, Lee PH (2009) High-titer antibody to hepatitis B surface antigen before liver transplantation can prevent de novo hepatitis B infection. J Pediatr Gastroenterol Nutr 48:203–208
102. Yu AS, Vierling JM, Colquhoun SD, Arnaout WS, Chan CK, Khanafshar E, Geller SA, Nichols WS, Fong TL (2001) Transmission of hepatitis B infection from hepatitis B core antibody – positive liver allografts is prevented by lamivudine therapy. Liver Transpl 7:513–517
103. Loss GE, Mason AL, Blazek J, Dick D, Lipscomb J, Guo L, Perrillo RP, Eason JD (2001) Transplantation of livers from hbc Ab positive donors into HBc Ab negative recipients: a strategy and preliminary results. Clin Transpl 15(Suppl 6):55–58
104. Cholongitas E, Papatheodoridis GV, Burroughs AK (2010) Liver grafts from anti-hepatitis B core positive donors: a systematic review. J Hepatol 52:272–279
105. Su WJ, Ho MC, Ni YH, Wu JF, Jeng YM, Chen HL, Wu YM, Hu RH, Chang MH, Lee PH (2010) Clinical course of de novo hepatitis B infection after pediatric liver transplantation. Liver Transpl 16:215–221
106. Chen HL, Lin LH, Hu FC, Lee JT, Lin WT, Yang YJ, Huang FC, Wu SF, Chen SC, Wen WH, Chu CH, Ni YH, Hsu HY, Tsai PL, Chiang CL, Shyu MK, Lee PI, Chang FY, Chang MH (2012) Effects of maternal screening and universal immunization to prevent mother-to-infant transmission of HBV. Gastroenterology 142:773–781
107. Liaw YF, Kao JH, Piratvisuth T et al (2012) Asia-Pacific consensus statement on the management of chronic hepatitis B: a 2012 update. Hepatol Int 6:531–561
108. Hsu HC, Su IJ, Lai MY, Chen DS, Chang MH, Chuang SM et al (1987) Biologic and prognostic significance of hepatocyte hepatitis B core antigen expressions in the natural course of chronic hepatitis B virus infection. J Hepatol 5:45–50

Immune Tolerance and Hepatitis B

8

Michelle Hong and Antonio Bertoletti

Abstract

Chronic hepatitis B (CHB) infection is the major cause of liver cirrhosis and hepatocellular carcinoma. Current treatment for CHB aims to suppress viral replication with little emphasis on viral eradication, and lifelong therapy is required in the majority of infected patients. CHB infection is, particularly in Asia, the result of virus transmission from HBV^+ mothers to their infants/children. HBV is thought to exploit the immaturity of the host immune system by inducing a state of immune tolerance that facilitates HBV persistence. Consequently, treatment is generally not recommended in "immunotolerant" children or young patients due to the presumably lack of disease/immune activity and poor treatment responses. However, recent advances in our understanding of the immunopathological manifestations of the disease challenge the concept of a generic immunotolerant state in CHB-infected children/young patients, with immunological, histological, and virological evidence supporting an underlying active disease. Thus, we propose a need to redefine the major phases of CHB infection, with the "high replicative, low inflammatory" phase replacing the classical "immune tolerant" phase. With many new and exciting HBV therapeutic strategies in the development pipeline, together with our changing perceptions of the disease, we address the potential to consider earlier therapeutic intervention in young patients to better harness their immune system to achieve a "functional cure."

Keywords

Hepatitis B · Vertical transmission · Immune tolerance · HBV-specific T cells · Trained immunity · Antiviral therapy · Immunomodulator

M. Hong (✉)
Emerging Infectious Diseases (EID) Program, Duke-NUS Medical School, Singapore, Singapore
e-mail: gmshong@nus.edu.sg

A. Bertoletti
Emerging Infectious Diseases (EID) Program, Duke-NUS Medical School, Singapore, Singapore

Singapore Immunology Network, Agency for Science, Technology & Research (A*STAR), Singapore, Singapore
e-mail: antonio@duke-nus.edu.sg

8.1 Global Importance of Hepatitis B

The World Health Organization (WHO) estimates that approximately 240 million people, or about 4% of the global population, are chronically infected with hepatitis B virus (HBV) representing a major public health problem [1, 2]. About half of the world's population with chronic

M.-H. Chang, K. B. Schwarz (eds.), *Viral Hepatitis in Children*,
https://doi.org/10.1007/978-981-13-0050-9_8

HBV lives in areas of high endemicity, including Asia and sub-Saharan Africa, and the development of chronicity, particularly in Asia, is usually the result of virus transmission from HBV^+ mothers to their infants. Despite the development of an effective HBV prophylactic vaccine since the 1980s [3, 4], the prevalence of the virus continues to increase, and liver-related morbidity and mortality due to chronic hepatitis B (CHB) including cirrhosis and hepatocellular carcinoma account for more than 600,000 deaths per year [5].

Hepatitis B virus is a hepatotropic, non-cytopathic, DNA virus that causes acute or chronic liver diseases characterized by different levels of liver inflammation and viral replication. An acute HBV infection is often self-limited and resolves without any clinical symptoms or with acute liver inflammation (acute hepatitis). Other patients fail to clear the virus and develop chronic infection. Persistent HBV infection can cause minimal pathological manifestations or trigger chronic liver inflammation that develops into liver cirrhosis or cancer [2]. These different clinical and virological profiles are determined by a complex interplay of host and viral factors including host genetic background, dose or route of infection, viral genotype, and age of the patient at the time of infection [6, 7]. The natural history of chronic HBV is considered to evolve through a number of distinct disease phases reflecting different points in the host-virus relationship. Thus, understanding the concept of these different phases not only sheds light on the pathogenesis of chronic HBV infection but also helps determine the optical timing and strategy of antiviral therapy toward the ultimate goal of HBV cure.

8.2 Revisiting the Natural History of Chronic Hepatitis B

Classically, the natural history of CHB is divided into four distinct chronological phases: immune tolerance, immune clearance, inactive carrier, and reactivation phases. In recent years, our understanding of HBV immunopathogenesis and virology has improved considerably. This has prompted researchers into redefining the phases of infection during the natural course of CHB, given that the classical definition of disease phases may not accurately reflect the true immunological status of patients in each phase. The course of HBV infection depends largely on the age of the patient at the time of infection, with more than 90% chronicity following vertical or perinatal transmission, 20–30% between the ages of 1–5 years, and less than 5% in immunocompetent adults [8, 9]. Based on our newfound knowledge on the immunopathogenesis and virology of the disease, we propose an alternative interpretation of the natural history of CHB: high replicative low inflammatory or HRLI (previously known as "immune tolerance"), low replicative high inflammatory or LRHI (previously known as "immune clearance"), non-replicative or NR (previously known as "inactive carrier"), and reactivation phase (Fig. 8.1). It is important to note that CHB is a dynamic disease and the stages of infection are not always sequential, with the possibility of transition from one phase to another in any direction [10]. It should also be noted that not all patients will go through all four phases, and arguments against such new definitions have raised an interesting debate [11].

Nevertheless, what we proposed to define as the initial "high replicative, low inflammatory" or HRLI phase (previously termed "immune tolerance") is characteristically associated with perinatal infection or infection acquired during early childhood, the predominant mode of HBV transmission in Asia or Africa [4]. In patients infected perinatally or during early childhood, there is commonly a prolonged period of high serum HBV DNA levels, positive hepatitis B e antigen (HBeAg) in the sera, normal or low serum alanine aminotransferase (ALT) levels, and minimal or no liver inflammation that usually lasts from a few years to several decades without disease progression [6, 8, 12]. It is thought that the establishment of persistent infection is due to immaturity of the neonatal immune system, i.e., the inability to mount a virus-specific immune response [7], or deletion/exhaustion of HBV-specific T cells *in utero* due to high levels of viral antigenemia from the mother [13]. CHB is believed to run a benign

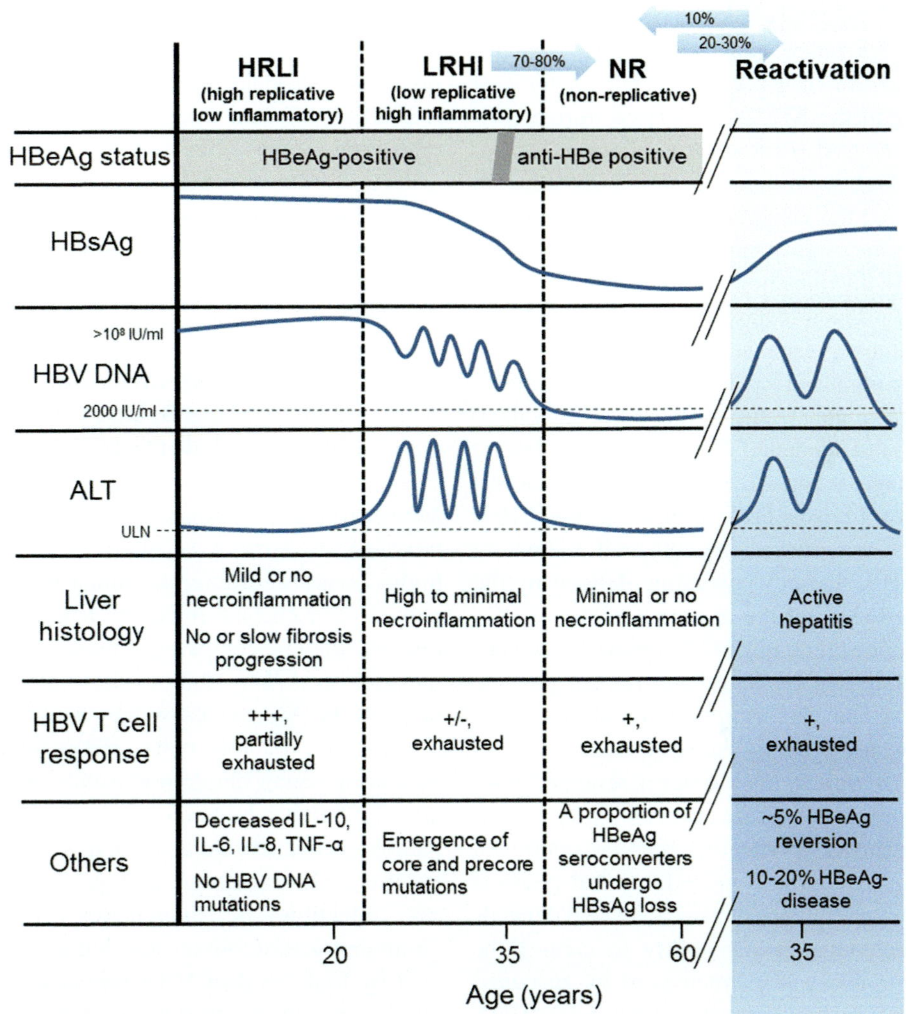

Fig. 8.1 Proposed new representations of the major phases of chronic hepatitis B infection. We propose to redefine the natural history of CHB into four major phases: high replicative, low inflammatory (HRLI); low replicative, high inflammatory (LRHI); non-replicative (NR); and reactivation. The corresponding virological, serological, biochemical, histological, and immunological characteristics are shown in the figure. These phases do not occur in all patients, and transitions between them are dynamic and can be non-sequential. ULT – upper limit of normal

course in children and young adults [14, 15], and therefore antiviral therapy is generally not recommended during this phase. However, the concept that this disease phase remains quiescent in children and young adults is now increasingly being challenged (refer next Sects. 8.3 on **Vertical Transmission of Hepatitis B: Does It Induce Immune Tolerance?** and 8.4 **Immunological and Virological Parameters During the HRLI Phase of HBV Infection**).

The transition from HRLI phase to the low replicative, high inflammatory phase or LRHI (previously known as "immune clearance") is characterized by HBeAg positivity at the outset and fluctuating levels of serum HBV DNA and ALT. ALT levels are persistently or intermittently elevated, reflecting immune activity against the virus. Consequently, HBV DNA levels fluctuate, decreasing from high (>20,000 IU/ml) to low or undetectable levels (>2000 IU/ml). Similarly,

Alt levels eventually decline to normal levels (<25 U/l for males and < 22 U/l for females or < 33 U/l for males and < 24 U/l for females according to the NHANES-derived normal values [16] and CALIPER study [17], respectively). There is high to minimal necroinflammation in the liver and the emergence of core and precore mutations in some patients. The mechanism(s) involved in the transition from the HRLI phase to the LRHI phase remains largely unknown, but it is thought to represent an "awakening" or activation of the immune response to actively "combat" HBV infection [7] and is therefore associated with immune-mediated liver injury leading to liver damage, progressive disease, and the development of fibrosis [18]. Following the LRHI phase, the majority of patients will eventually undergo HBeAg seroconversion, defined by the loss of HBeAg and the appearance of anti-HBe antibody. The remaining 10% of patients encounter recurrent hepatic flares and remain positive for HBeAg and often require antiviral therapy.

Following HBeAg seroconversion, about 70–80% of patients then enter a residual "non-replicative" or NR phase (previously known as "inactive carrier"), reflecting immune control of the virus. Transition from LRHI to NR phase is not a definite sequence of events, since it depends on the individual host's ability to control the virus. This phase is characterized by sustained low (<2000 IU/ml) or undetectable HBV DNA levels, normalization of ALT, and minimal or no hepatic necroinflammation. A small proportion of HBeAg seroconverters will eventually undergo spontaneous HBsAg loss, which may indicate either (1) the resolution of CHB, and such patients usually have good clinical outcome provided there is no underlying cirrhosis, or (2) occult HBV infection, in which there is loss of HBsAg but intrahepatic persistence of the entire viral genome as free episomal forms and, in particular, the persistence of viral cccDNA as stable chromatinized episomes. There is detectable HBV DNA in the liver and very low or undetectable HBV DNA in the serum, and in certain cases all serum HBV markers are negative [19].

A proportion of patients with HBeAg seroconversion may develop disease reactivation, with 5% experiencing HBeAg reversion [2, 20] and 10–20% of them encounter reactivation of hepatitis with elevated serum HBV DNA level (>2000 IU/ml) and fluctuations in ALT despite remaining negative for HBeAg. This phase of disease is referred as HBeAg-negative CHB, and these patients usually have low rates of spontaneous remission, with high risk of HBV complications if left untreated [21–23].

8.3 Vertical Transmission of Hepatitis B: Does It Induce Immune Tolerance?

Mother-to-child transmission (or vertical transmission) of viruses is often associated with higher levels of viral replication, a greater risk of persistent or chronic infection, and more severe disease outcome compared to those acquired during adulthood [24]. Chronic HBV infection, particularly in Asia, is caused by mother-to-child transmission of the virus. HBV infection in infants or young children is usually asymptomatic until late adulthood, when it causes liver pathologies (cirrhosis and hepatocellular carcinoma) [2]. To explain this dichotomy, HBV vertical infection is thought to induce an "immunotolerant phase" of disease, characterized by high level of HBV replication and low incidence of liver inflammatory events.

This immunotolerance hypothesis is mainly supported by data from experimental animal models (i.e., HBV transgenic animals) that showed the presence of immunological defects which impair HBV-specific T- and B cell priming in neonatal animals [13, 25, 26], thus predisposing to HBV chronicity. A recent study in 2016 by Tian et al. [27] investigated the immunological mechanisms contributing to the ability of HBV to establish chronicity after vertical infection using a mouse model of HBV persistence. The authors found qualitative and quantitative defects in HBV-specific $CD8^+$ T cells in mice born to HBeAg-transgenic mothers, and these defects were associated with the expression of the co-inhibitory ligand PD-L1 on HBeAg-conditioned macrophages. As a result, mice born to $HBeAg^+$

mothers failed to clear HBV from the liver following hydrodynamic transfection. While these data are methodologically robust, their significance in relation to HBV pathogenesis should be taken with caution, since the data supporting such immunological features are derived exclusively from HBV transgenic animals that do not support natural HBV infection. Instead, HBV virions are produced from HBV transgenes introduced into the mouse genome under the control of hepatocyte-specific promoter and as such cannot fully recapitulate the natural course of HBV infection. Therefore, a lack of appropriate animal models represents a major hurdle to study immunotolerance in HBV [28].

The concept of immunological tolerance, the basis of which the disease is managed and treatment decisions are made, is increasingly being challenged. Although the immunological data both during and after natural vertical HBV infection is limited, several epidemiological and experimental evidences can be used to challenge this concept of immunotolerance during vertical HBV infection. For example, the functionality of dendritic cells, immune cells important for the presentation and maturation of HBV-specific T cells, are intact or minimally altered in neonates of HBV^+ mothers [29–31]. Furthermore, a better analysis of T cells during natural vertical HBV infection has demonstrated that both core- and polymerase-specific T cells can be detected in HBsAg-negative children born to HBV^+ mothers in two independent studies [32, 33]. This shows that neonates born to HBV^+ mothers do not necessarily harbor defects in T cell priming and that they have the ability to mount HBV-specific T cell responses. Analysis of HBV quasispecies in children with a clinical profile labeled as immunotolerant showed a high HBV diversity [34], a virological profile that is compatible with the presence of an active immune pressure and not with complete immune tolerance during this initial phase of infection.

Furthermore, the efficacy of HBV vaccination at birth in HBV^+ children [35, 36] raises doubts that the state of complete HBV immune tolerance and the broad defects in T- and B cell interaction detected in murine models exist during natural infection. The dogma of immunotolerance in vertical HBV-infected children is also in contrast to epidemiological observations showing that HBV-related fulminant hepatitis is more frequent in infants <1 year of age compared to older subjects [37] or with the observations obtained from malaria-HBV coinfected young patients in whom reduced parasitemia [38] and increased incidences of cerebral malaria [39], a Th1-mediated malaria complication, have been reported. Such observations are more in line with the possibility of an alternative relationship between HBV and humans during early life.

The concept that the neonatal immune response is somehow "defective" or "immature" is also changing, and there is mounting evidence showing that the neonatal immune responses defy such simple categorization. Recent findings have provided new insights that the immune effectors as well as regulatory responses are already in place during early fetal life [40, 41]. Newborns have also been shown to have the ability to mount virus-specific T cell response toward viral infections in early life [42–44]. Besides, exposure of the newborn immune system toward microbes at birth can also alter the maturation status of the newborn infant. For instance, epidemiological and experimental evidences have shown that exposure to bacterial or viral infections after birth and vaccination with live vaccines can protect infants against unrelated pathogens by inducing an increased functional efficiency of their innate immune system. Such nonspecific enhancement of innate immune functionality against reinfection has been termed "trained immunity" [45]. All these earlier reports show that the immune system of newborns and infants is not "immature" or "defective" per se. Rather, it appears to be less prone to trigger a full-blown pro-inflammatory reaction, likely as an evolutionary adaptation to prevent undesirable immune reactions *in utero*.

We have recently performed a detailed characterization of the immunological parameters in the cord blood of newborns of HBV^+ mothers. Contrary to the dogma of generic immunotolerance, we found that HBV exposure *in utero* triggers a state of "trained immunity," characterized

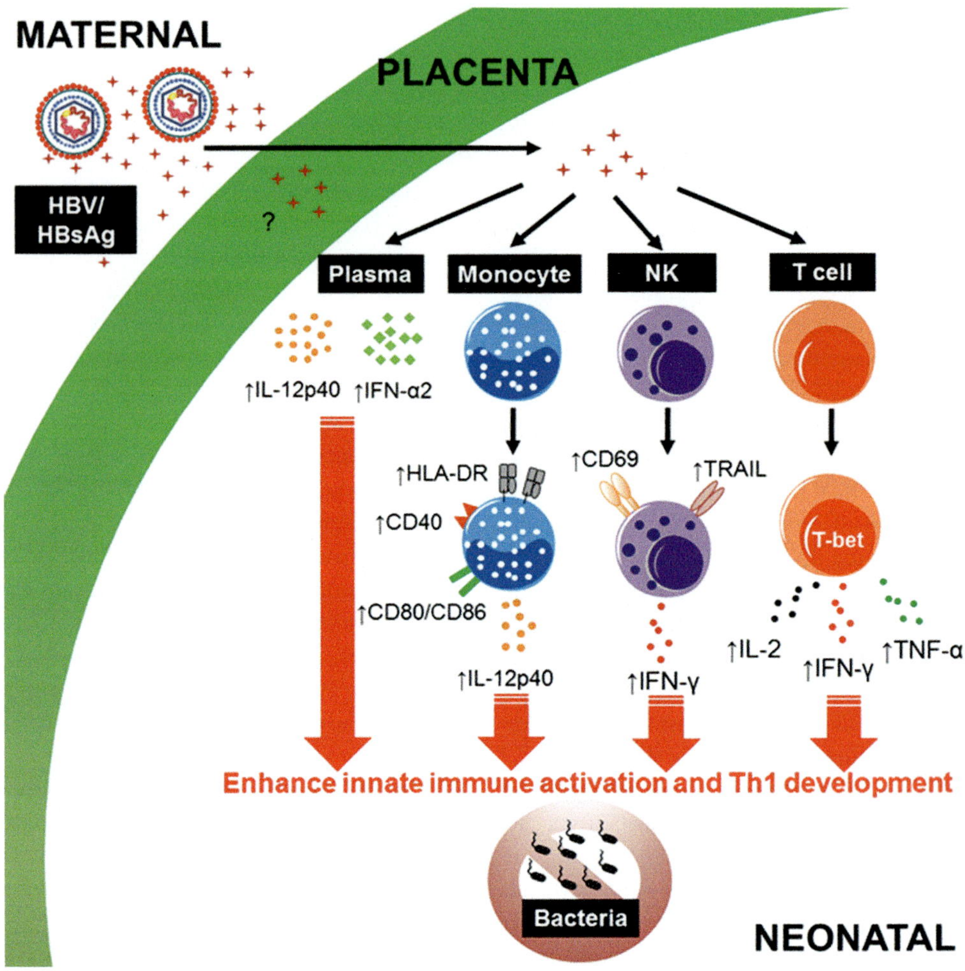

Fig. 8.2 Trained immunity in neonates of HBV⁺ mothers. HBsAg⁺ cells could be detected in the neonatal cord blood of HBV-infected mothers, demonstrating *in utero* exposure to viral products. These HBsAg⁺ cells could be due to transplacental passage of maternal HBsAg⁺ cells or active uptake of serum HBsAg by neonatal cells. HBV exposure *in utero* was associated with significantly elevated plasma levels of the antiviral cytokine IL-12p40 and, in some cases, IFN-α2. Exposure to HBV *in utero* also induced innate immune cell (including monocytes and NK cells) maturation/activation, and enhanced Th1 T cell development. Importantly, this heightened state of innate immune functionality results in a stronger ability of neonatal immune cells to respond to unrelated pathogen challenge, in a process known as "trained immunity"

by increased innate immune cell activation and Th1 development, which in turn enhances the ability of HBV-exposed cord blood immune cells to respond to bacterial infection *in vitro* [46] (Fig. 8.2). These training effects are associated with alterations in the cytokine environment. Specifically, cytokine analysis in the sera of neonates born to HBV⁺ mothers revealed a cytokine signature compatible with a Th1-like response with higher production of IL-12p40, and in some cases IFN-α2, and lower production of IL-10 and pro-inflammatory cytokines (such as IL-6, IL-8, TNF-α). This Th1 cytokine signature is more suggestive of a symbiotic relationship between HBV and humans during early life, similar to that already demonstrated in murine models of herpesvirus persistent infection [47] than to the induction of a tolerogenic response. Various attempts to detect HBV-specific T cells in cord blood of HBV^+ mothers were unsuccessful, supporting the hypothesis that HBV vertical infection can preferentially tolerize HBV-specific immunity. Nonetheless, whether the absence of HBV-specific T cells in cord blood is really linked to genuine features of immunotolerance is questionable since it is difficult to study, due to ethical constraints, whether these neonates are infected by HBV (i.e., HBV replication in the hepatocytes) or are only exposed to it (i.e., HBV is present in the circulation but is not able to establish a productive infection in hepatocytes). Nevertheless, the induction of a trained immunity profile with a general Th1 response and suppression of pro-inflammatory events in HBV-exposed neonates show that the neonatal immune system can be "trained" by HBV exposure and further activated to possibly counteract unrelated pathogens during early life.

8.4 Immunological and Virological Parameters During the HRLI Phase of HBV Infection

Most of the evidence supporting an immunotolerance disease phase of HBV infection during early childhood is based on clinical and virological parameters. HBV is not directly cytopathic, and HBV-specific $CD8^+$ T cells control virus replication by recognizing and killing HBV-infected hepatocytes [48]. As a consequence, ALT is released from dying hepatocytes leading to a rise in serum ALT levels. Therefore, serum ALT is interpreted as a marker of immune activity, i.e., the presence or absence of ALT fluctuations correlates with the presence or absence of HBV-specific T cells. In this context, normal or minimal alterations in ALT levels, detectable in the majority of HBV-infected children, have been perceived as an indication of lack of HBV-specific T cell response. On the other hand, fluctuations in the levels of ALT and HBV DNA replication, more commonly observed during adulthood, are interpreted as an "awakening" of HBV-specific immunity.

In reality, both experimental data in animal models and in humans during natural HBV infection have shown that ALT measurement cannot be used as a reliable surrogate of a virus-specific T cell response. Studies performed in adenovirus-infected mice revealed that T cell immunity against hepatocytes could occur without elevation in serum ALT level [49]. Furthermore, adoptive transfer of HBV-specific T cells can lead to substantial inhibition of HBV replication without increase in serum ALT through cytokine-mediated non-cytopathic effects [50]. Direct quantification of HBV-specific T cells in the blood and liver of CHB patients has shown that, in contrast to patients with acute hepatitis B [51], the quantity of HBV-specific T cells does not correlate with ALT levels [52, 53]. Instead, robust inflammatory events in the liver causing fluctuations in ALT levels, demonstrated both in adult mice and in patients, are associated with intrahepatic recruitment of granulocytes, monocytes, and non-antigen-specific T cells [52, 54, 55].

The concept of immune tolerance phase being a quiescent disease phase with an absence of virus-specific T cells and minimal changes in liver histology is now increasingly being challenged. Our recent study of chronic hepatitis B-infected children and young adults with a clinical and virological profile labeled as "immunotolerant" showed the existence of HBV-specific T cell responses that is less compromised than that observed in CHB-infected adult patients in the "immune clearance" phase [56]. A further demonstration that these patients do not display any generic state of immunotolerance was exemplified by the superior ability of circulating T cells from young IT patients with CHB to produce type 1 T-helper cytokines including TNF-α and IFN-γ, compared to age-matched healthy controls. Besides, the production of immunosuppressive cytokines including IL-10 and IL-4 was not increased in these patients. Detailed analysis of the phenotype of T cells in these patients showed that young IT patients with CHB have increased frequency of T cells with an exhausted/inhibitory phenotype, characterized by the expression of the co-inhibitory receptor programmed death 1 (PD-1). This expression of

PD-1 is interpreted as a marker of immune activity since T cell exhaustion is a consequence of repetitive activation of reactive T cells. The frequency of exhausted T cells ($CD8^+$ T cells that are $PD\text{-}1^+$ and $CD127^{lo}$) increases with age in CHB patients, reflecting a progressive state of T cell exhaustion over time during the course of CHB infection. In this context, children and young adults were found to exhibit a partially exhausted T cell profile, compared to adult patients with a more exhausted T cell profile. This could explain why older patients have a less favorable response to therapy and suggest that earlier therapeutic intervention may be more advantageous in young people who lack a fully exhausted T cell profile.

In addition, there is mounting evidence that surrogate markers such as ALT that suggest quiescent disease might not reflect the true disease status and what constitutes a normal or healthy ALT level has been the subject of much discussion. The new cutoff value for adults recommended as healthy by Prati et al. [57], i.e., ≤30 U/l for men and ≤ 19 U/l for women, is lower than the traditional cutoff value of 40 U/l. For children, the cutoff values for ALT are <25 U/l for males and < 22 U/l for females according to the NHANES-derived normal values [16] or < 33 U/l for males and < 24 U/l for females according to the CALIPER study [17]. Indeed, a study by Seto et al. reported that substantial fibrosis and necroinflammatory activity already exist in the liver biopsy of some patients in the HRLI phase with the traditional normal ALT value of ~40 U/l [58]. Similarly, a recent study by Mason et al. further strengthens the concept that ongoing disease activity exists in the liver of CHB patients during the HRLI phase [59]. In this study, the immunopathological profiles of patients with HRLI disease were compared to patients with $HBeAg^+$ disease or those in the immune clearance phase. The authors showed by inverse polymerase chain reaction (PCR) that an unexpectedly high number of HBV DNA integration sites were randomly distributed across the human chromosome in all three groups of patients. These results imply that HBV DNA integration occurs not only in the later active disease phase but also during the initial, presumably quiescent, disease phase. Viral DNA integration and the resulting genomic instability are associated with the risk of developing hepatocarcinogenesis, with 80% of HBV-related HCC demonstrating clonal integrated HBV sequences [60]. Therefore, these results signify that genetic alterations promoting HCC development already exist in the initial HRLI phase, which is in agreement with previous findings suggesting the presence of viral integration even earlier at an acute phase of infection [61] or in $HBsAg^+$ children with hepatocellular carcinoma [62].

In addition to HBV DNA integration, clonal hepatocyte expansion was also detected in patients with HRLI disease at an unexpectedly high rate [59]. Clonal expansion of hepatocytes, a risk factor for the development of HCC, probably occurs in response to hepatocyte turnover mediated by HBV-specific T cell killing of infected hepatocytes, since HBV-specific T cells were detected in the peripheral blood of these patients. Furthermore, the maximum hepatocyte clone size did not differ between patients with HRLI disease and those with $HBeAg^+$ disease or in the immune clearance phase. All these findings demonstrate that promoters of oncogenesis exist in all phases of CHB infection, even in patients at the early stage of CHB infection traditionally considered "immunotolerant." Collectively, these recent findings do not support the notion that the initial HRLI phase is completely devoid of markers of disease progression or that there is a lack of immune response during this initial disease phase.

8.5 Current Treatment Recommendations for Chronic HBV Patients (Please also Read Chap. 10)

Treatment objectives in CHB are constantly evolving. Historically, the goals of therapy for CHB patients are the reduction of viremia and amelioration of hepatic dysfunction, with the hope that this would delay progression to cirrhosis and the subsequent development of HCC [12]. While a "sterilizing cure" of HBV with the removal of cccDNA and integrated virus is difficult or impossible to achieve, most experts now agree that a "functional cure," whereby patients achieve sustained suppression of HBV viremia and loss of HBsAg after a defined course of therapy and returned to a state of health equivalent to a person who has recovered spontaneously from HBV infection, should at least be the goal of next wave of therapies [12].

Current first-line therapies for CHB remain limited to nucleos(t)ide analogues (NUCs) and pegylated IFN-α (pegIFN-α). NUCs target the reverse transcriptase function of the HBV polymerase and prevent the synthesis of viral DNA from pregenomic RNA. These antiviral agents are highly effective in suppressing viral replication, leading to ALT normalization, and more recently shown to reverse fibrosis [63]. However, they have limited effect on HBeAg seroconversion and rarely lead to HBsAg loss in the majority of patients. Furthermore, since NUCs do not directly target cccDNA, the chance of relapse after drug withdrawal is high. Consequently, lifelong therapy is usually required [64]. Another concern with long-term NUC therapy is the development of drug resistance mutations, which could lead to exacerbation of liver disease.

Conversely, pegIFN-α exhibits pleiotropic effects with antiviral, antiproliferative, and immunomodulatory properties, with the ability to halt the progression of fibrosis [65, 66]. Moreover, pegIFN-α offers the advantage of finite treatment duration (48 weeks) with the absence of antiviral resistance. Although pegIFN-α leads to slower clearance of HBV viremia, higher rates of HBeAg and HBsAg loss with anti-HBe and anti-HBs seroconversion, even though at modest levels, could be achieved [67]. However, the main disadvantages of pegIFN-α are the need for parenteral administration and the frequent side effects. Besides, pegIFN-α is contraindicated in patients with decompensated cirrhosis [68] or those undergoing immunosuppressive or cancer chemotherapy. Combination or sequential therapies with NUCs and pegIFN-α are rapidly evolving and may offer the promise of achieving higher rates of HBeAg seroconversion and HBsAg decline.

8.6 Novel Treatment Strategies in Chronic HBV Patients (Please also Read Chap. 16)

The key challenges in achieving sustained virologic control or functional cure of CHB are the persistence of nuclear HBV cccDNA and the ability of HBV to evade the host immune response recognition [69]. Exciting progress has been made in the preclinical development of new class of antivirals with novel mechanisms of action with the focus on strategies targeting cccDNA and the development of novel immune-based strategies to better harness the immune system for effective off-treatment responses.

8.6.1 Novel Antivirals Against Chronic Hepatitis B

Putative new antivirals targeting various steps of the HBV life cycle are under investigations, including viral entry inhibitors, core/capsid inhibitors, targets against cccDNA (including rcDNA-cccDNA conversion inhbitors, DNA cleavage enzymes, and small interfering RNA or siRNA-based strategies), apoptosis inducers, and HBV secretion inhibitors (Table 8.1). Viral entry inhibitor such as the well-known pre-S1-derived lipopeptide Myrcludex B targets the HBV entry receptor NTCP, thus preventing viral entry and viral replication [70–72]. Furthermore, Myrcludex B was shown, in a humanized mouse model, to reduce cccDNA formation in hepatocytes without overt cytotoxicity and pathology [73]. This makes Myrcludex B a promising candidate in targeting both active viral replication and persistence. Myrcludex B is currently being evaluated in a phase II clinical trial in Russia.

Multiple capsid inhibitors are in the pipeline, and they work by interfering with HBV RNA packaging and capsid assembly, resulting in lower intracellular capsids and ultimately undetectable HBV DNA [74, 75]. Some capsid inhibitors have been shown to interfere directly with cccDNA transcription and stability or indirectly with cccDNA formation by preventing the recycling of capsids into the nucleus to replenish cccDNA [12].

Table 8.1 Novel antivirals against chronic HBV

Type	Target	Compounds	Stage of development	References
Entry inhibitor	NTCP	HBV preS1-derived lipopeptide	Myrcludex B in phase II	[70–73]
		Cyclosporine A, ezetimibe	FDA approved but not tested for HBV	
Capsid inhibitor	HBV capsid	Phenylpropenamide derivatives	Preclinical and early clinical phase	[74, 75]
		Heteroaryl-dihydropyrimidines	Morphothiadine mesilate (GLS4) in phase II	
	rcDNA-cccDNA conversion	Disubstituted sulfonamide	Preclinical	[76]
	cccDNA	DNA cleavage enzymes	Preclinical	[77–85]
	HBV RNA	siRNA	ARC-520 in phase II	[86]
		Antisense	ISIS-HBVRx in phase I	
Apoptotic inducer	Cellular inhibitor of apoptosis proteins	Birinapant	Preclinical	[87]
Secretion inhibitor	HBV secretion and budding	Benzimidazole BM601	Preclinical	[88]

Novel therapies directly targeting cccDNA are the focus of current therapeutics, which may show promise in the treatment of CHB. Some examples include disubstituted sulfonamide (DSS) compounds that inhibit the conversion of rcDNA to cccDNA [76] and DNA cleavage enzymes such as zinc finger nucleases, homing endonucleases, and transcription activator-like effector nucleases that directly degrades cccDNA [77–80]. A therapeutic strategy that has generated great interest is the development of the CRISPR-Cas9 genome editing tool, which has shown promise in removing cccDNA *in vitro* [81, 82] and recently in HBV-infected mice [83–85]. However, both theoretical and practical considerations have to be taken into consideration for future therapeutic application in CHB patients. Another direct antiviral strategy against cccDNA is based on RNA interference (RNAi). A phase II study performed in HBeAg- CHB patients showed that the combination of entecavir and the HBV siRNA ARC-520 resulted in 50% reduction in HBsAg levels in treated patients compared to placebo [86] and similar success has been demonstrated with other siRNA platforms in preclinical models.

In addition to interfering with cccDNA formation and stability, novel drugs targeting other host cell pathways are being developed. This includes a new class of antivirals that target the apoptotic mechanism of infected hepatocytes, leading to cytolysis and clearance of HBV. An example is birinapant (TL32711), a second mitochondrial-derived activator of caspases (SMAC) mimetic that antagonizes the cellular inhibitor of apoptosis proteins. Birinapant has been shown to improve TNF-mediated killing of HBV-infected hepatocytes and reduce HBV DNA load and HBsAg production in a mouse model [87], suggesting the potential to translate this drug from treating cancers to CHB. Lastly, several inhibitors of HBV secretion have been described that could decrease HBV DNA levels and interfere with HBsAg release, thereby restoring antiviral immunity. The benzimidazole BM601 has been reported to selectively inhibit HBsAg relocalization to the Golgi, thus decreasing HBsAg release, HBV maturation, and secretion [88]. However, the drawback of such inhibitors is the accumulation of HBsAg leading to storage diseases, and the blockage of mature virion release could increase intracellular cccDNA pools.

8.6.2 Immunomodulators

A different therapeutic area for CHB is the development of immunotherapies that (1) activate

Table 8.2 Immunomodulators against chronic HBV

Type	Target	Compounds	Stage of development	References
Innate immune system modulator	TLR7 activation	GS-9620	Phase II	[90–92]
	RIG-I and NOD2 activation	SB-9200	Phase II	[94, 95]
	T cell, NK activator, cytokine production	Thymosin-α1	Phase IV	[96, 97]
	Protein kinase activation	Nitazoxanide	Phase I	[98]
Therapeutic vaccine	T cell	Recombinant HBsAg/HBcAg	ABX 203 in phase II/III	[99]
		Recombinant HBsAg	Engerix-B in phase I/IV	
		Fusion X-S-Core proteins	GS-4774 in phase II	[104]
		HBV CTL epitope	CY-1899 in pilot study	[100]
		HBV DNA	DV-601 in phase I	[101–103]
			DNA vaccine pCMVS2.S in phase I/II	
		Autologous monocytes	*In vitro*	[105]
Adaptive immune system modulator	PD-1 blockade	Nivolumab	Phase II	[107]
	Genetically modified T cells	Engineered HBV-specific T cells using CAR or HLA-restricted TCR	CAR T cells in preclinical	[109–111]
			HLA-restricted TCR-redirected T cells in phase I	
Inflammation modulator	Antiplatelet	Aspirin/clopidogrel	Preclinical	[113]

intrahepatic antiviral immunity and (2) restore HBV-specific T- and B cell immunity. Immunomodulatory compounds exhibiting activity against HBV in preclinical or clinical development include TLR agonists, therapeutic vaccines, immune checkpoint inhibitors, and engineered T cells (Table 8.2).

Agonists of TLRs 3, 8, 7, and 9 have been shown to have anti-HBV effects in animal models [89]. Of these, GS-9620, an oral TLR7 agonist, has been shown to reduce HBV DNA levels in serum and livers of chronic HBV-infected woodchucks and chimpanzees [90, 91]. Upon stimulation of TLR7, plasmacytoid dendritic cells produce high levels of IFN-α and other cytokines, resulting in activation of natural killer cells and cytotoxic T lymphocytes. Despite its success in preclinical setting, a recent clinical trial testing the efficacy of low-dose TLR7 agonist in CHB patients showed lack of clinical efficacy, even though treatment was safe and well tolerated [92]. The use of another TLR agonist, such as TLR8, may be a potential new therapeutic target since it has been reported that activation of TLR8 efficiently triggered IFN-ɣ production in human intrahepatic environment [93]. In addition to TLR agonists, other small molecule modulators of innate immunity are being tested for their anti-HBV effects: SB-9200, which activates the RIG-I/NOD2 pathway [94, 95], and thymosin α1 [96, 97] and nitazoxanide [98], which induce the production of IFN and/or activation of T- and B cells.

Numerous therapeutic vaccine approaches for CHB have been explored, including antigen-based vaccines [99], CTL epitope vaccine [100], and DNA-based vaccines [101–103]. Although these strategies demonstrated good safety and tolerability profiles with robust immunogenicity, they do not show significant clinical benefit in chronic hepatitis B patients [104]. One likely explanation is the exhaustion of HBV-specific T cells caused by prolonged exposure to high levels of soluble HBV antigens. Therefore, factors that are known to impair the effectiveness of therapeutic vaccines need to be reversed, at least partially, to increase the efficacy of therapeutic vaccines. As an alternative to vaccine therapy, an interesting approach to consider is the use of autologous monocytes to present personalized HBV antigens in CHB patients [105].

T cell exhaustion is a hallmark of human chronic viral infections and is characterized by the increased expression of various inhibitory receptors such as programmed death-1 (PD-1) and cytotoxic T-lymphocyte antigen-4 (CTLA-4), among others [106]. PD-1 is strongly upregulated in circulating HBV-specific T cells in CHB patients, and blockade of this inhibitory signal restores HBV-specific T cell functionality. A recent phase I/II trial of nivolumab, an anti-PD-1 monoclonal antibody, in HCC patients infected with HBV showed some clinical benefit, suggesting the potential to use such therapy in patients with HBV-related HCC [107]. Another underlying molecular defect of exhausted HBV-specific T cells was recently reported in the mitochondria, which showed defects in depolarization [108]. The cytokine IL-12 was shown to recover mitochondrial potential and oxidative phosphorylation of HBV-specific T cells *in vitro*, highlighting the prospect of targeting mitochondrial or other metabolic defects as novel therapeutic approaches to restore antiviral T cell responses.

Another exciting approach to immunotherapy is to engineer patients' immune cells, such as T cells to eliminate HBV-infected hepatocytes. This could be achieved via the expression of chimeric antigen receptors (CARs) or HLA-restricted T cell receptors (TCRs) on T cells that enable HLA-independent or HLA-dependent recognition and killing of HBV-infected hepatocytes. CAR-engineered T cells were recently shown to have potential promise in mouse models of HBV [109], but no human data are available, whereas T cells engineered to overexpress HBV-specific TCR have been shown to recognize HBV-infected hepatoma cells *in vitro* and *in vivo* [110] and can significantly reduce HBsAg levels in a patient with HBV-associated hepatocellular carcinoma [111]. Newer approaches utilizing mRNA electroporation, instead of retroviral vectors, to overexpress HBV-specific TCRs are underway. These electroporated T cells have been successful in reducing tumor growth in HCC mouse models [112] and have unique antiviral effects *in vitro* without overt cytotoxicity. Thus, this highly individualized therapy could become a feasible option in advancing therapies for CHB patients.

Finally, CHB can be viewed not only as a viral disease but also a necroinflammatory disease. To this end, anti-inflammatory agents designed to inhibit liver inflammatory events such as antiplatelet therapy to inhibit the development of hepatocellular carcinoma in transgenic mice [113] may prove to be important in controlling CHB infection. Thus, the goals of immunotherapy are to increase antiviral immunity and to reduce the chronic inflammatory process with the ultimate aim of achieving a reliable cure for HBV.

8.7 Future Treatment Strategies for Chronic Hepatitis B: Can We Treat Earlier or at a Younger Age?

With major advances in HBV therapeutics in recent years, together with our increased scientific insights into the pathogenesis of CHB, it is now an exciting moment for the treatment of CHB patients. However, it remains debated whether young CHB patients in the initial HRLI disease phase are indicated for treatment. Current guidelines from the international liver associations recommend treatment for CHB patients only when they show signs of clinically active disease or development of fibrosis, typically after the age of 30 years old. Yet, symptoms of advanced disease often appear later in life, at a stage when little can be done to alter the disease course. This could explain the poor response rate to therapies observed in adult patients, thus highlighting the limitations of current practice and the need to better define the optimal timing for treatment. The recent new findings discussed above challenge the concept of immunotolerance from HBV-exposed newborn infants to children and young adults and provide further support for considering earlier therapeutic treatment in young patients with CHB, a patient cohort currently excluded from treatment consideration.

A point to note is that there is a paucity of data on the treatment of children and young adults, the patient population which is highly viremic and infectious with the highest risk of disease progression and HCC development [114]. A small pilot study by D'Antiga et al. [115] investigated the effect of combination therapy with lamivudine and pegIFN-α in children with HRLI disease. The results were encouraging, evidenced by a beneficial response to early treatment in a proportion of young patients. These beneficial responses were associated with an increase in HBV-specific T cell proliferation, reduction in HBV DNA levels, and notable increase in HBsAg seroconversion, thus providing further support for the potential benefit of early treatment in CHB patients [115, 116]. Similar studies performed in CHB-infected children have demonstrated that IFN-α was well tolerated and children less than 5 years of age may have an enhanced response to IFN-α [117]. Likewise, the efficacy of tenofovir disoproxil fumarate was comparable between CHB-infected adolescents (<18 years old) with that observed in adult subjects [118]. Nonetheless, extended longitudinal follow-up observations of these young patients will undoubtedly provide more insights on the rates of HBeAg and HBsAg loss as well as the rates of seroconversion, in order to determine whether earlier treatment is genuinely associated with better treatment outcomes.

The emerging concept of "trained immunity" discussed above [46] also has significant therapeutic implications. Rather than being immature or tolerized, we should keep in mind that the immune system of neonates or even young children is already "trained" or "matured" following birth and is actually capable of responding immunologically with broad cross-protective responses toward viral antigens. In this context, therapies that reduce viral protein expression may "release the brakes" on the immune system of these young patients, allowing it to be fully competent to achieve long-term suppression of HBV. On the other hand, our findings that young CHB patients in the initial HRLI phase have a less compromised HBV-specific T cell response compared to adult patients in the LRHI phase [56] suggest that therapeutic interventions aimed at enhancing HBV-specific immunity are likely to be more effective in young CHB patients compared to adult patients.

8.8 Summary

CHB infection is a complex dynamic disease where the timing and most appropriate treatments continue to be debated. We have shown that CHB-infected children and young adults, a patient population historically considered to be "immunotolerant," are less likely to run a benign course of disease since liver histology, T cell responses, DNA integration, and hepatocyte clonal expansion all point toward underlying disease and immune activity. A better understanding of trained immunity and how HBV establishes a permissive state in the host may pave the way for better development of therapies that is targeted toward these group of patients currently not indicated for treatment. This could potentially result in expanding therapeutic options to more patients, including treating at a younger age and at a much earlier stage of disease. If earlier treatment is advocated, careful consideration should be taken into account for pediatric patients, in whom the safety, efficacy, and adverse effect profiles of NUCs have not been well established compared to the adult population.

References

1. El-Serag HB (2012) Epidemiology of viral hepatitis and hepatocellular carcinoma. Gastroenterology 142(1264–1273):e1261
2. Liaw YF, Chu CM (2009) Hepatitis B virus infection. Lancet 373:582–592

3. Hilleman MR, Buynak EB, Roehm RR, Tytell AA, Bertland AU, Lampson GP (1975) Purified and inactivated human hepatitis B vaccine: progress report. Am J Med Sci 270:401–404
4. Lavanchy D (2004) Hepatitis B virus epidemiology, disease burden, treatment, and current and emerging prevention and control measures. J Viral Hepat 11:97–107
5. Szpakowski JL, Tucker LY (2013) Causes of death in patients with hepatitis B: a natural history cohort study in the United States. Hepatology 58:21–30
6. Bertoletti A, Hong M (2014) Age-dependent immune events during HBV infection from birth to adulthood: an alternative interpretation. Front Immunol 5:441
7. Yim HJ, Lok AS (2006) Natural history of chronic hepatitis B virus infection: what we knew in 1981 and what we know in 2005. Hepatology 43:S173–S181
8. Bertoletti A, Kennedy PT (2015) The immune tolerant phase of chronic HBV infection: new perspectives on an old concept. Cell Mol Immunol 12:258–263
9. Protzer U, Knolle P (2016) "To be or not to be": Immune tolerance in chronic hepatitis B. Gastroenterology 151:805–806
10. McMahon BJ (2009) The natural history of chronic hepatitis B virus infection. Hepatology 49:S45–S55
11. Milich DR (2016) The concept of immune tolerance in chronic hepatitis B virus infection is alive and well. Gastroenterology 151:801–804
12. Gish RG, Given BD, Lai CL, Locarnini SA, Lau JY, Lewis DL, Schluep T (2015) Chronic hepatitis B: virology, natural history, current management and a glimpse at future opportunities. Antivir Res 121:47–58
13. Milich DR, Jones JE, Hughes JL, Price J, Raney AK, McLachlan A (1990) Is a function of the secreted hepatitis B e antigen to induce immunologic tolerance in utero? Proc Natl Acad Sci USA 87:6599–6603
14. Della Corte C, Comparcola D, Nobili V (2012) Hepatitis B virus infection in children. Clin Res Hepatol Gastroenterol 36:291–293
15. Gill US, Kennedy PT (2014) Chronic hepatitis B virus in young adults: the need for new approaches to management. Expert Rev Anti-Infect Ther 12:1045–1053
16. Schwimmer JB, Dunn W, Norman GJ, Pardee PE, Middleton MS, Kerkar N, Sirlin CB (2010) SAFETY study: alanine aminotransferase cutoff values are set too high for reliable detection of pediatric chronic liver disease. Gastroenterology 138:1357–1364, 364 e1351–1352
17. Shaw JL, Cohen A, Konforte D, Binesh-Marvasti T, Colantonio DA, Adeli K (2014) Validity of establishing pediatric reference intervals based on hospital patient data: a comparison of the modified Hoffmann approach to CALIPER reference intervals obtained in healthy children. Clin Biochem 47:166–172
18. Liaw YF, Chu CM, Su IJ, Huang MJ, Lin DY, Chang-Chien CS (1983) Clinical and histological events preceding hepatitis B e antigen seroconversion in chronic type B hepatitis. Gastroenterology 84:216–219
19. Pollicino T, Raimondo G (2014) Occult hepatitis B infection. J Hepatol 61:688–689
20. Hsu YS, Chien RN, Yeh CT, Sheen IS, Chiou HY, Chu CM, Liaw YF (2002) Long-term outcome after spontaneous HBeAg seroconversion in patients with chronic hepatitis B. Hepatology 35:1522–1527
21. Chen YC, Chu CM, Liaw YF (2010) Age-specific prognosis following spontaneous hepatitis B e antigen seroconversion in chronic hepatitis B. Hepatology 51:435–444
22. Chu CM, Hung SJ, Lin J, Tai DI, Liaw YF (2004) Natural history of hepatitis B e antigen to antibody seroconversion in patients with normal serum aminotransferase levels. Am J Med 116:829–834
23. Chu CM, Liaw YF (2007) Predictive factors for reactivation of hepatitis B following hepatitis B e antigen seroconversion in chronic hepatitis B. Gastroenterology 133:1458–1465
24. Prendergast AJ, Klenerman P, Goulder PJ (2012) The impact of differential antiviral immunity in children and adults. Nat Rev Immunol 12:636–648
25. Publicover J, Gaggar A, Nishimura S, Van Horn CM, Goodsell A, Muench MO, Reinhardt RL, van Rooijen N, Wakil AE, Peters M, Cyster JG, Erle DJ, Rosenthal P, Cooper S, Baron JL (2013) Age-dependent hepatic lymphoid organization directs successful immunity to hepatitis B. J Clin Invest 123:3728–3739
26. Publicover J, Goodsell A, Nishimura S, Vilarinho S, Wang ZE, Avanesyan L, Spolski R, Leonard WJ, Cooper S, Baron JL (2011) IL-21 is pivotal in determining age-dependent effectiveness of immune responses in a mouse model of human hepatitis B. J Clin Invest 121:1154–1162
27. Tian Y, Kuo CF, Akbari O, Ou JH (2016) Maternal-derived hepatitis B virus e antigen alters macrophage function in offspring to drive viral persistence after vertical transmission. Immunity 44:1204–1214
28. Bertoletti A, Gehring A (2007) Immune response and tolerance during chronic hepatitis B virus infection. Hepatol Res 37(Suppl 3):S331–S338
29. Guo J, Gao Y, Guo Z, Zhang LR, Wang B, Wang SP (2015) Frequencies of dendritic cells and Toll-like receptor 3 in neonates born to HBsAg-positive mothers with different HBV serological profiles. Epidemiol Infect 143:62–70
30. Koumbi LJ, Papadopoulos NG, Anastassiadou V, Machaira M, Kafetzis DA, Papaevangelou V (2010) Dendritic cells in uninfected infants born to hepatitis B virus-positive mothers. Clin Vaccine Immunol 17:1079–1085
31. Zhang Z, Chen D, Yao J, Zhang H, Jin L, Shi M, Zhang H, Wang FS (2007) Increased infiltration of intrahepatic DC subsets closely correlate with viral control and liver injury in immune active pediatric patients with chronic hepatitis B. Clin Immunol 122:173–180

32. Komatsu H, Inui A, Sogo T, Hiejima E, Tateno A, Klenerman P, Fujisawa T (2010) Cellular immunity in children with successful immunoprophylactic treatment for mother-to-child transmission of hepatitis B virus. BMC Infect Dis 10:103
33. Koumbi L, Bertoletti A, Anastasiadou V, Machaira M, Goh W, Papadopoulos NG, Kafetzis DA, Papaevangelou V (2010) Hepatitis B-specific T helper cell responses in uninfected infants born to HBsAg+/HBeAg- mothers. Cell Mol Immunol 7:454–458
34. Wang HY, Chien MH, Huang HP, Chang HC, Wu CC, Chen PJ, Chang MH, Chen DS (2010) Distinct hepatitis B virus dynamics in the immunotolerant and early immunoclearance phases. J Virol 84:3454–3463
35. Beasley RP, Hwang LY, Lee GC, Lan CC, Roan CH, Huang FY, Chen CL (1983) Prevention of perinatally transmitted hepatitis B virus infections with hepatitis B immune globulin and hepatitis B vaccine. Lancet 2:1099–1102
36. Mackie CO, Buxton JA, Tadwalkar S, Patrick DM (2009) Hepatitis B immunization strategies: timing is everything. CMAJ 180:196–202
37. Chen HL, Chang CJ, Kong MS, Huang FC, Lee HC, Lin CC, Liu CC, Lee IH, Wu TC, Wu SF, Ni YH, Hsu HY, Chen DS, Chang MH (2004) Pediatric fulminant hepatic failure in endemic areas of hepatitis B infection: 15 years after universal hepatitis B vaccination. Hepatology 39:58–63
38. Andrade BB, Santos CJ, Camargo LM, Souza-Neto SM, Reis-Filho A, Clarencio J, Mendonca VR, Luz NF, Camargo EP, Barral A, Silva AA, Barral-Netto M (2011) Hepatitis B infection is associated with asymptomatic malaria in the Brazilian Amazon. PLoS One 6:e19841
39. Thursz MR, Kwiatkowski D, Torok ME, Allsopp CE, Greenwood BM, Whittle HC, Thomas HC, Hill AV (1995) Association of hepatitis B surface antigen carriage with severe malaria in Gambian children. Nat Med 1:374–375
40. Mold JE, Venkatasubrahmanyam S, Burt TD, Michaelsson J, Rivera JM, Galkina SA, Weinberg K, Stoddart CA, McCune JM (2010) Fetal and adult hematopoietic stem cells give rise to distinct T cell lineages in humans. Science 330:1695–1699
41. Zhang X, Mozeleski B, Lemoine S, Deriaud E, Lim A, Zhivaki D, Azria E, Le Ray C, Roguet G, Launay O, Vanet A, Leclerc C, Lo-Man R (2014) CD4 T cells with effector memory phenotype and function develop in the sterile environment of the fetus. Sci Transl Med 6:238ra272
42. Luzuriaga K, Holmes D, Hereema A, Wong J, Panicali DL, Sullivan JL (1995) HIV-1-specific cytotoxic T lymphocyte responses in the first year of life. J Immunol 154:433–443
43. Marchant A, Appay V, Van Der Sande M, Dulphy N, Liesnard C, Kidd M, Kaye S, Ojuola O, Gillespie GM, Vargas Cuero AL, Cerundolo V, Callan M, McAdam KP, Rowland-Jones SL, Donner C, McMichael AJ, Whittle H (2003) Mature CD8(+) T lymphocyte response to viral infection during fetal life. J Clin Invest 111:1747–1755
44. Vermijlen D, Brouwer M, Donner C, Liesnard C, Tackoen M, Van Rysselberge M, Twite N, Goldman M, Marchant A, Willems F (2010) Human cytomegalovirus elicits fetal gammadelta T cell responses in utero. J Exp Med 207:807–821
45. Netea MG, Quintin J, van der Meer JW (2011) Trained immunity: a memory for innate host defense. Cell Host Microbe 9:355–361
46. Hong M, Sandalova E, Low D, Gehring AJ, Fieni S, Amadei B, Urbani S, Chong YS, Guccione E, Bertoletti A (2015) Trained immunity in newborn infants of HBV-infected mothers. Nat Commun 6:6588
47. Barton ES, White DW, Cathelyn JS, Brett-McClellan KA, Engle M, Diamond MS, Miller VL, Virgin HW t (2007) Herpesvirus latency confers symbiotic protection from bacterial infection. Nature 447:326–329
48. Thimme R, Wieland S, Steiger C, Ghrayeb J, Reimann KA, Purcell RH, Chisari FV (2003) CD8(+) T cells mediate viral clearance and disease pathogenesis during acute hepatitis B virus infection. J Virol 77:68–76
49. Stabenow D, Frings M, Truck C, Gartner K, Forster I, Kurts C, Tuting T, Odenthal M, Dienes HP, Cederbrant K, Protzer U, Knolle PA (2010) Bioluminescence imaging allows measuring CD8 T cell function in the liver. Hepatology 51:1430–1437
50. Guidotti LG, Ishikawa T, Hobbs MV, Matzke B, Schreiber R, Chisari FV (1996) Intracellular inactivation of the hepatitis B virus by cytotoxic T lymphocytes. Immunity 4:25–36
51. Dunn C, Peppa D, Khanna P, Nebbia G, Jones M, Brendish N, Lascar RM, Brown D, Gilson RJ, Tedder RJ, Dusheiko GM, Jacobs M, Klenerman P, Maini MK (2009) Temporal analysis of early immune responses in patients with acute hepatitis B virus infection. Gastroenterology 137:1289–1300
52. Maini MK, Boni C, Lee CK, Larrubia JR, Reignat S, Ogg GS, King AS, Herberg J, Gilson R, Alisa A, Williams R, Vergani D, Naoumov NV, Ferrari C, Bertoletti A (2000) The role of virus-specific CD8(+) cells in liver damage and viral control during persistent hepatitis B virus infection. J Exp Med 191:1269–1280
53. Webster GJ, Reignat S, Brown D, Ogg GS, Jones L, Seneviratne SL, Williams R, Dusheiko G, Bertoletti A (2004) Longitudinal analysis of CD8+ T cells specific for structural and nonstructural hepatitis B virus proteins in patients with chronic hepatitis B: implications for immunotherapy. J Virol 78:5707–5719
54. Ando K, Moriyama T, Guidotti LG, Wirth S, Schreiber RD, Schlicht HJ, Huang SN, Chisari FV (1993) Mechanisms of class I restricted immunopathology. A transgenic mouse model of fulminant hepatitis. J Exp Med 178:1541–1554

55. Sitia G, Isogawa M, Kakimi K, Wieland SF, Chisari FV, Guidotti LG (2002) Depletion of neutrophils blocks the recruitment of antigen-nonspecific cells into the liver without affecting the antiviral activity of hepatitis B virus-specific cytotoxic T lymphocytes. Proc Natl Acad Sci USA 99:13717–13722
56. Kennedy PT, Sandalova E, Jo J, Gill U, Ushiro-Lumb I, Tan AT, Naik S, Foster GR, Bertoletti A (2012) Preserved T-cell function in children and young adults with immune-tolerant chronic hepatitis B. Gastroenterology 143:637–645
57. Prati D, Taioli E, Zanella A, Della Torre E, Butelli S, Del Vecchio E, Vianello L, Zanuso F, Mozzi F, Milani S, Conte D, Colombo M, Sirchia G (2002) Updated definitions of healthy ranges for serum alanine aminotransferase levels. Ann Intern Med 137:1–10
58. Seto WK, Lai CL, Ip PP, Fung J, Wong DK, Yuen JC, Hung IF, Yuen MF (2012) A large population histology study showing the lack of association between ALT elevation and significant fibrosis in chronic hepatitis B. PLoS One 7:e32622
59. Mason WS, Gill US, Litwin S, Zhou Y, Peri S, Pop O, Hong ML, Naik S, Quaglia A, Bertoletti A, Kennedy PT (2016) HBV DNA integration and clonal hepatocyte expansion in chronic hepatitis B patients considered immune tolerant. Gastroenterology 151(986–998):e984
60. Hai H, Tamori A, Kawada N (2014) Role of hepatitis B virus DNA integration in human hepatocarcinogenesis. World J Gastroenterol 20:6236–6243
61. Kimbi GC, Kramvis A, Kew MC (2005) Integration of hepatitis B virus DNA into chromosomal DNA during acute hepatitis B. World J Gastroenterol 11:6416–6421
62. Chang MH, Chen PJ, Chen JY, Lai MY, Hsu HC, Lian DC, Liu YG, Chen DS (1991) Hepatitis B virus integration in hepatitis B virus-related hepatocellular carcinoma in childhood. Hepatology 13:316–320
63. Marcellin P, Gane E, Buti M, Afdhal N, Sievert W, Jacobson IM, Washington MK, Germanidis G, Flaherty JF, Aguilar Schall R, Bornstein JD, Kitrinos KM, Subramanian GM, McHutchison JG, Heathcote EJ (2013) Regression of cirrhosis during treatment with tenofovir disoproxil fumarate for chronic hepatitis B: a 5-year open-label follow-up study. Lancet 381:468–475
64. Perez-Cameo C, Pons M, Esteban R (2014) New therapeutic perspectives in HBV: when to stop NAs. Liver Int 34(Suppl 1):146–153
65. Kao JH (2014) HBeAg-positive chronic hepatitis B: why do I treat my patients with pegylated interferon? Liver Int 34(Suppl 1):112–119
66. Vlachogiannakos J, Papatheodoridis GV (2014) HBeAg-negative chronic hepatitis B: why do I treat my patients with pegylated interferon-alfa? Liver Int 34(Suppl 1):127–132
67. Fung J, Lai CL, Seto WK, Yuen MF (2011) Nucleoside/nucleotide analogues in the treatment of chronic hepatitis B. J Antimicrob Chemother 66:2715–2725
68. Jafri SM, Lok AS (2010) Antiviral therapy for chronic hepatitis B. Clin Liver Dis 14:425–438
69. Pham EA, Perumpail RB, Fram BJ, Glenn JS, Ahmed A, Gish RG (2016) Future therapy for hepatitis B virus: role of immunomodulators. Curr Hepatol Rep 15:237–244
70. Kim DH, Ni Y, Lee SH, Urban S, Han KH (2008) An anti-viral peptide derived from the preS1 surface protein of hepatitis B virus. BMB Rep 41:640–644
71. Ni Y, Lempp FA, Mehrle S, Nkongolo S, Kaufman C, Falth M, Stindt J, Koniger C, Nassal M, Kubitz R, Sultmann H, Urban S (2014) Hepatitis B and D viruses exploit sodium taurocholate co-transporting polypeptide for species-specific entry into hepatocytes. Gastroenterology 146:1070–1083
72. Petersen J, Dandri M, Mier W, Lutgehetmann M, Volz T, von Weizsacker F, Haberkorn U, Fischer L, Pollok JM, Erbes B, Seitz S, Urban S (2008) Prevention of hepatitis B virus infection in vivo by entry inhibitors derived from the large envelope protein. Nat Biotechnol 26:335–341
73. Volz T, Allweiss L, Ben MM, Warlich M, Lohse AW, Pollok JM, Alexandrov A, Urban S, Petersen J, Lutgehetmann M, Dandri M (2013) The entry inhibitor Myrcludex-B efficiently blocks intrahepatic virus spreading in humanized mice previously infected with hepatitis B virus. J Hepatol 58:861–867
74. Feld JJ, Colledge D, Sozzi V, Edwards R, Littlejohn M, Locarnini SA (2007) The phenylpropenamide derivative AT-130 blocks HBV replication at the level of viral RNA packaging. Antivir Res 76:168–177
75. King RW, Ladner SK, Miller TJ, Zaifert K, Perni RB, Conway SC, Otto MJ (1998) Inhibition of human hepatitis B virus replication by AT-61, a phenylpropenamide derivative, alone and in combination with (-)beta-L-2′,3′-dideoxy-3′-thiacytidine. Antimicrob Agents Chemother 42:3179–3186
76. Cai D, Mills C, Yu W, Yan R, Aldrich CE, Saputelli JR, Mason WS, Xu X, Guo JT, Block TM, Cuconati A, Guo H (2012) Identification of disubstituted sulfonamide compounds as specific inhibitors of hepatitis B virus covalently closed circular DNA formation. Antimicrob Agents Chemother 56:4277–4288
77. Bloom K, Ely A, Mussolino C, Cathomen T, Arbuthnot P (2013) Inactivation of hepatitis B virus replication in cultured cells and in vivo with engineered transcription activator-like effector nucleases. Mol Ther 21:1889–1897
78. Chen J, Zhang W, Lin J, Wang F, Wu M, Chen C, Zheng Y, Peng X, Li J, Yuan Z (2014) An efficient antiviral strategy for targeting hepatitis B virus genome using transcription activator-like effector nucleases. Mol Ther 22:303–311
79. Cradick TJ, Keck K, Bradshaw S, Jamieson AC, McCaffrey AP (2010) Zinc-finger nucleases as a novel therapeutic strategy for targeting hepatitis B virus DNAs. Mol Ther 18:947–954
80. Schiffer JT, Swan DA, Stone D, Jerome KR (2013) Predictors of hepatitis B cure using gene therapy to deliver DNA cleavage enzymes: a mathematical modeling approach. PLoS Comput Biol 9:e1003131

81. Karimova M, Beschorner N, Dammermann W, Chemnitz J, Indenbirken D, Bockmann JH, Grundhoff A, Luth S, Buchholz F, Schulze zur Wiesch J, Hauber J (2015) CRISPR/Cas9 nickase-mediated disruption of hepatitis B virus open reading frame S and X. Sci Rep 5:13734
82. Seeger C, Sohn JA (2014) Targeting hepatitis B virus with CRISPR/Cas9. Mol Ther Nucleic Acids 3:e216
83. Dong C, Qu L, Wang H, Wei L, Dong Y, Xiong S (2015) Targeting hepatitis B virus cccDNA by CRISPR/Cas9 nuclease efficiently inhibits viral replication. Antivir Res 118:110–117
84. Lin SR, Yang HC, Kuo YT, Liu CJ, Yang TY, Sung KC, Lin YY, Wang HY, Wang CC, Shen YC, Wu FY, Kao JH, Chen DS, Chen PJ (2014) The CRISPR/Cas9 system facilitates clearance of the intrahepatic HBV templates in vivo. Mol Ther Nucleic Acids 3:e186
85. White MK, Hu W, Khalili K (2015) The CRISPR/Cas9 genome editing methodology as a weapon against human viruses. Discov Med 19:255–262
86. Wooddell CI, Rozema DB, Hossbach M, John M, Hamilton HL, Chu Q, Hegge JO, Klein JJ, Wakefield DH, Oropeza CE, Deckert J, Roehl I, Jahn-Hofmann K, Hadwiger P, Vornlocher HP, McLachlan A, Lewis DL (2013) Hepatocyte-targeted RNAi therapeutics for the treatment of chronic hepatitis B virus infection. Mol Ther 21:973–985
87. Ebert G, Allison C, Preston S, Cooney J, Toe JG, Stutz MD, Ojaimi S, Baschuk N, Nachbur U, Torresi J, Silke J, Begley CG, Pellegrini M (2015) Eliminating hepatitis B by antagonizing cellular inhibitors of apoptosis. Proc Natl Acad Sci USA 112:5803–5808
88. Xu YB, Yang L, Wang GF, Tong XK, Wang YJ, Yu Y, Jing JF, Feng CL, He PL, Lu W, Tang W, Zuo JP (2014) Benzimidazole derivative, BM601, a novel inhibitor of hepatitis B virus and HBsAg secretion. Antivir Res 107:6–15
89. Chang J, Guo JT (2015) Treatment of chronic hepatitis B with pattern recognition receptor agonists: current status and potential for a cure. Antivir Res 121:152–159
90. Lanford RE, Guerra B, Chavez D, Giavedoni L, Hodara VL, Brasky KM, Fosdick A, Frey CR, Zheng J, Wolfgang G, Halcomb RL, Tumas DB (2013) GS-9620, an oral agonist of Toll-like receptor-7, induces prolonged suppression of hepatitis B virus in chronically infected chimpanzees. Gastroenterology 144:1508–1517, 1517 e1501–1510
91. Menne S, Tumas DB, Liu KH, Thampi L, AlDeghaither D, Baldwin BH, Bellezza CA, Cote PJ, Zheng J, Halcomb R, Fosdick A, Fletcher SP, Daffis S, Li L, Yue P, Wolfgang GH, Tennant BC (2015) Sustained efficacy and seroconversion with the Toll-like receptor 7 agonist GS-9620 in the Woodchuck model of chronic hepatitis B. J Hepatol 62:1237–1245
92. Gane EJ, Lim YS, Gordon SC, Visvanathan K, Sicard E, Fedorak RN, Roberts S, Massetto B, Ye Z, Pflanz S, Garrison KL, Gaggar A, Mani Subramanian G, McHutchison JG, Kottilil S, Freilich B, Coffin CS, Cheng W, Kim YJ (2015) The oral toll-like receptor-7 agonist GS-9620 in patients with chronic hepatitis B virus infection. J Hepatol 63:320–328
93. Jo J, Tan AT, Ussher JE, Sandalova E, Tang XZ, Tan-Garcia A, N. To, Hong M, Chia A, Gill US, Kennedy PT, Tan KC, Lee KH, De Libero G, Gehring AJ, Willberg CB, Klenerman P, Bertoletti A (2014) Toll-like receptor 8 agonist and bacteria trigger potent activation of innate immune cells in human liver. PLoS Pathog 10:e1004210
94. Korolowicz KE, Iyer RP, Czerwinski S, Suresh M, Yang J, Padmanabhan S, Sheri A, Pandey RK, Skell J, Marquis JK, Kallakury BV, Tucker RD, Menne S (2016) Antiviral efficacy and host innate immunity associated with SB 9200 treatment in the woodchuck model of chronic hepatitis B. PLoS One 11:e0161313
95. Suresh M, Korolowicz KE, Balarezo M, Iyer RP, Padmanabhan S, Cleary D, Gimi R, Sheri A, Yon C, Kallakury BV, Tucker RD, Afdhal N, Menne S (2017) Antiviral efficacy and host immune response induction during sequential treatment with SB 9200 followed by Entecavir in Woodchucks. PLoS One 12:e0169631
96. Goldstein AL, Goldstein AL (2009) From lab to bedside: emerging clinical applications of thymosin alpha 1. Expert Opin Biol Ther 9:593–608
97. Rasi G, Mutchnick MG, Di Virgilio D, Sinibaldi-Vallebona P, Pierimarchi P, Colella F, Favalli C, Garaci E (1996) Combination low-dose lymphoblastoid interferon and thymosin alpha 1 therapy in the treatment of chronic hepatitis B. J Viral Hepat 3:191–196
98. Korba BE, Montero AB, Farrar K, Gaye K, Mukerjee S, Ayers MS, Rossignol JF (2008) Nitazoxanide, tizoxanide and other thiazolides are potent inhibitors of hepatitis B virus and hepatitis C virus replication. Antivir Res 77:56–63
99. Chang KM, Liu M (2016) Chronic hepatitis B: immune pathogenesis and emerging immunotherapeutics. Curr Opin Pharmacol 30:93–105
100. Heathcote J, McHutchison J, Lee S, Tong M, Benner K, Minuk G, Wright T, Fikes J, Livingston B, Sette A, Chestnut R (1999) A pilot study of the CY-1899 T-cell vaccine in subjects chronically infected with hepatitis B virus. The CY1899 T Cell Vaccine Study Group. Hepatology 30:531–536
101. Fontaine H, Kahi S, Chazallon C, Bourgine M, Varaut A, Buffet C, Godon O, Meritet JF, Saidi Y, Michel ML, Scott-Algara D, Aboulker JP, Pol S, A. H. s. group (2015) Anti-HBV DNA vaccination does not prevent relapse after discontinuation of analogues in the treatment of chronic hepatitis B: a randomised trial–ANRS HB02 VAC-ADN. Gut 64:139–147
102. Godon O, Fontaine H, Kahi S, Meritet J, Scott-Algara D, Pol S, Michel M, Bourgine M (2014) Immunological and antiviral responses after therapeutic DNA immunization in chronic hepatitis B patients efficiently treated by analogues. Mol Ther 22:675–684

103. Yoon SK, Seo YB, Im SJ, Bae SH, Song MJ, You CR, Jang JW, Yang SH, Suh YS, Song JS, Kim BM, Kim CY, Jeong SH, Sung YC (2015) Safety and immunogenicity of therapeutic DNA vaccine with antiviral drug in chronic HBV patients and its immunogenicity in mice. Liver Int 35:805–815
104. Lok AS, Pan CQ, Han SH, Trinh HN, Fessel WJ, Rodell T, Massetto B, Lin L, Gaggar A, Subramanian GM, McHutchison JG, Ferrari C, Lee H, Gordon SC, Gane EJ (2016) Randomized phase II study of GS-4774 as a therapeutic vaccine in virally suppressed patients with chronic hepatitis B. J Hepatol 65:509–516
105. Gehring AJ, Haniffa M, Kennedy PT, Ho ZZ, Boni C, Shin A, Banu N, Chia A, Lim SG, Ferrari C, Ginhoux F, Bertoletti A (2013) Mobilizing monocytes to cross-present circulating viral antigen in chronic infection. J Clin Invest 123:3766–3776
106. Pauken KE, Wherry EJ (2015) Overcoming T cell exhaustion in infection and cancer. Trends Immunol 36:265–276
107. Moreno-Cubero E, Larrubia JR (2016) Specific CD8(+) T cell response immunotherapy for hepatocellular carcinoma and viral hepatitis. World J Gastroenterol 22:6469–6483
108. Schurich A, Pallett LJ, Jajbhay D, Wijngaarden J, Otano I, Gill US, Hansi N, Kennedy PT, Nastouli E, Gilson R, Frezza C, Henson SM, Maini MK (2016) Distinct metabolic requirements of exhausted and functional virus-specific CD8 T cells in the same host. Cell Rep 16:1243–1252
109. Krebs K, Bottinger N, Huang LR, Chmielewski M, Arzberger S, Gasteiger G, Jager C, Schmitt E, Bohne F, Aichler M, Uckert W, Abken H, Heikenwalder M, Knolle P, Protzer U (2013) T cells expressing a chimeric antigen receptor that binds hepatitis B virus envelope proteins control virus replication in mice. Gastroenterology 145:456–465
110. Gehring AJ, Xue SA, Ho ZZ, Teoh D, Ruedl C, Chia A, Koh S, Lim SG, Maini MK, Stauss H, Bertoletti A (2011) Engineering virus-specific T cells that target HBV infected hepatocytes and hepatocellular carcinoma cell lines. J Hepatol 55:103–110
111. Qasim W, Brunetto M, Gehring AJ, Xue SA, Schurich A, Khakpoor A, Zhan H, Ciccorossi P, Gilmour K, Cavallone D, Moriconi F, Farzhenah F, Mazzoni A, Chan L, Morris E, Thrasher A, Maini MK, Bonino F, Stauss H, Bertoletti A (2015) Immunotherapy of HCC metastases with autologous T cell receptor redirected T cells, targeting HBsAg in a liver transplant patient. J Hepatol 62:486–491
112. Koh S, Shimasaki N, Suwanarusk R, Ho ZZ, Chia A, Banu N, Howland SW, Ong AS, Gehring AJ, Stauss H, Renia L, Sallberg M, Campana D, Bertoletti A (2013) A practical approach to immunotherapy of hepatocellular carcinoma using T cells redirected against hepatitis B virus. Mol Ther Nucleic Acids 2:e114
113. Sitia G, Iannacone M, Guidotti LG (2013) Anti-platelet therapy in the prevention of hepatitis B virus-associated hepatocellular carcinoma. J Hepatol 59:1135–1138
114. Jonas MM, Block JM, Haber BA, Karpen SJ, London WT, Murray KF, Narkewicz MR, Rosenthal P, Schwarz KB, McMahon BJ, Hepatitis BF (2010) Treatment of children with chronic hepatitis B virus infection in the United States: patient selection and therapeutic options. Hepatology 52:2192–2205
115. D'Antiga L, Aw M, Atkins M, Moorat A, Vergani D, Mieli-Vergani G. Combined lamivudine/interferon-alpha treatment in "immunotolerant" children perinatally infected with hepatitis B: a pilot study. J Pediatr. 2006;148:228–33.
116. Carey I, D'Antiga L, Bansal S, Longhi MS, Ma Y, Mesa IR, Mieli-Vergani G, Vergani D. Immune and viral profile from tolerance to hepatitis B surface antigen clearance: a longitudinal study of vertically hepatitis B virus-infected children on combined therapy. J Virol. 2011;85:2416–28
117. Kobak GE, MacKenzie T, Sokol RJ, Narkewicz MR (2004) Interferon treatment for chronic hepatitis B: enhanced response in children 5 years old or younger. J Pediatr 145:340–345
118. Murray KF, Szenborn L, Wysocki J, Rossi S, Corsa AC, Dinh P, McHutchison J, Pang PS, Luminos LM, Pawlowska M, Mizerski J (2012) Randomized, placebo-controlled trial of tenofovir disoproxil fumarate in adolescents with chronic hepatitis B. Hepatology 56:2018–2026

Prevention of Viral Hepatitis B and Related Complications

9

Mei-Hwei Chang

Abstract

Hepatitis B virus (HBV) infection is a major global health problem, which may cause acute or fulminant hepatitis, chronic hepatitis, liver cirrhosis, and/or hepatocellular carcinoma (HCC). Transmission of HBV is through either horizontal or mother-to-infant route. In endemic areas maternal transmission is the major route of transmission.

Early diagnosis and management of HBV, particularly in children, are not easily achieved worldwide. The rate of HBV elimination by currently available antiviral agents is very low. Prevention by HBV immunization, either with vaccination alone or in combination with HBIG, is the best way to eliminate HBV infection and its related diseases. The impact of universal HBV immunization is remarkable. It has effectively reduced the rate of acute and fulminant hepatitis B, chronic hepatitis B, and HCC. The long-term data revealed that approximately 90% of chronic hepatitis B and 70% of HCC are reduced in the vaccinated birth cohorts, in comparison with the unvaccinated birth cohorts.

In spite of the great success, around 10% of chronic HBV infections could not be prevented by current HBV immunization. This vaccine failure occurred mainly (~90%) in infants of highly infectious mothers with positive serum hepatitis B e antigen (HBeAg) and hepatitis B surface antigen (HBsAg) and high-serum HBV-DNA levels $>10^6$ IU/mL. Furthermore, the vaccination coverage rate is not high enough in areas with limited resources. To achieve elimination of hepatitis B and related complications, further efforts are needed to prevent vaccine failure and to increase global vaccine coverage.

Keywords

Hepatitis B virus · Hepatitis B immunization · Vaccine failure · Hepatocellular carcinoma · Cancer prevention

9.1 Hepatitis B Virus Infection Is a Global Health Problem

Hepatitis B virus (HBV) infection can cause acute, fulminant, or chronic hepatitis, liver cirrhosis, and hepatocellular carcinoma (HCC). It is a potentially life-threatening infection and is a major global health problem. Liver cirrhosis is a

M.-H. Chang (✉)
Department of Pediatrics, National Taiwan University, Taipei, Taiwan
e-mail: changmh@ntu.edu.tw

M.-H. Chang, K. B. Schwarz (eds.), *Viral Hepatitis in Children*,
https://doi.org/10.1007/978-981-13-0050-9_9

common precancerous lesion, accounting for approximately 80% of patients with HCC, including children [29]. This sequel usually results from severe liver injury caused by chronic HBV infection. HCC is one of the most common causes of cancer death worldwide because of a poor prognosis and a high recurrence rate after curative therapy. Around one third of chronically infected patients will eventually develop cirrhosis and HCC. Liver injury caused by chronic HBV infection is the most important initiation event of hepatocarcinogenesis. The role of HBV in tumor formation appears to be complex and may involve both direct and indirect mechanisms of carcinogenesis. The outcome of persistent HBV infection is affected by the interaction of host, virus, and environmental factors. As evidenced by the large population infected with HBV in the developing world, HBV remains the most prevalent oncogenic virus for HCC in humans. HBV is estimated to cause around 55–70% of HCC worldwide [8].

In spite of the progress of antiviral therapy to suppress HBV replication and reduce liver injury in people with chronic hepatitis B, a cure for HBV infection is still almost impossible. To eliminate hepatitis B, prevention is more effective than therapy. The HBV vaccine was developed using hepatitis B surface antigen (HBsAg) as the immunogen to induce protective antibody (hepatitis B surface antibody, anti-HBs) against HBV infection. During the past three decades, HBV has proved to be safe and successful in preventing HBV infection and the related diseases worldwide.

9.2 Transmission Routes of HBV Infection

HBV infection is most prevalent in Asia-Pacific and sub-Saharan African regions, where the HBsAg-positive rate in the general population is more than 8% [43]. The age and source of primary HBV infection are important factors affecting the outcome of infection. HBV infection is transmitted through either the horizontal or mother-to-infant route. To prevent HBV infection effectively, it is crucial to understand its route of transmission.

9.2.1 Mother-to-Infant Transmission

In endemic areas of HBV infection, HBV infection occurs mainly during infancy and early childhood. Perinatal mother-to-infant transmission is the main route of transmission. Maternal serum HBsAg and hepatitis B e antigen (HBeAg) status affect the outcome of HBV infection in their offspring. In Asia and many other endemic areas in the world, perinatal transmission through HBsAg carrier mothers accounts for 40–50% of HBsAg carriers in the era before universal HBV immunization. Irrespective of the extent of HBsAg carrier rate in the population, around 85–90% of the infants of HBeAg-seropositive carrier mothers became HBsAg carriers [57]. A study in Taiwan revealed that most chronic HBV infection resulted from infections before 2 years of age [28].

HBV infection during infancy and early childhood as compared to infection in adults results in a much higher rate of persistent infection and long-term serious complications, such as liver cirrhosis and HCC [12]. Those with positive maternal serum HBsAg have a 30 times higher risk of developing HCC than those with negative maternal HBsAg [14]. HBeAg is a soluble antigen produced by HBV. It can cross the placenta from the mother to the infant and induce a specific unresponsiveness of helper T cells to HBeAg and HBcAg in neonates born to HBeAg-positive HBsAg carrier mothers [30]. This may help to explain why most infants of HBeAg-positive carrier mothers became persistently infected [3] while only approximately $<=5\%$ of the infants of HBeAg-negative HBsAg carrier mothers became persistently infected. Such immune tolerance state persists for years to decades after neonatal HBV infection.

9.2.2 Horizontal Transmission of HBV

Horizontal transmission, which accounts for another half of the transmission route in the era before the universal HBV vaccination program, was mainly through the use of unsterile needles or medical equipment, unsafe blood product or transfusions, unprotected sex, unsterile skin piercing, or other intrafamilial close contact. In Africa, where HBV infection is also endemic, horizontal infection during early childhood is the main route of transmission. In rural Senegal, by the age of 2 years, 25% of children are infected, while at age 15, the HBV infection rate rises to 80% [23].

9.2.3 Transmission Route and Age at Infection Affect the Outcome of Infection

Age at infection and source of infection affect the outcome of HBV infection [2]. The younger the age at infection, the higher the chronicity rate. In the era with no immune prophylaxis, perinatal transmission from highly infectious (HBeAg-positive) hepatitis B carrier mothers resulted in chronic infection in 85–90% of their infants [57]. In contrast, only <=5% of infants of HBeAg-negative HBsAg carrier mothers become chronic carriers, and a small number may develop acute or fulminant hepatitis B [11, 56]. Approximately 25% of HBV-infected 2–4-year-old toddlers will become chronic carriers [4]. In contrast, only 2.7% of the newly HBV-infected 18–19-year-old university students became chronic carriers [5].

9.3 Prevention Is the Best Way to Control Hepatitis B Virus Infection and Its Complication

Prevention, screening/early diagnosis, and treatment are the main strategies to control HBV infection and its related diseases and complication. In spite of the development of new antiviral therapies for hepatitis B patients, elimination of HBV by antiviral agent(s) is still not possible in most cases. In addition, HBV cannot be eradicated by a passive immune response [52]. Therefore, prevention is the best way to control HBV infection and complications. In order to successfully prevent HBV infection, blocking the transmission routes of HBV is mandatory. Strategies for preventing HBV infection include immunization and other methods. Universal HBV vaccination is the most effective way for long-term prevention against HBV infection. Other methods such as safe blood products, safe injections, and avoidance of risky behaviors to prevent horizontal transmission are also very helpful and complementary to immunization to prevent HBV infection (Table 9.1).

9.3.1 HBV Immunization in Infancy

HBV immunization can be classified into passive immunization and active immunization. Passive immunization using hepatitis B immunoglobulin (HBIG) provides temporary immunity, whereas active immunization by the vaccine yields long-term immunity. In endemic areas, the main infection route is mother-to-infant transmission from highly infectious mothers. So the best timing of initiating HBV vaccination should be within 24 h after birth (the birth dose), followed by subsequent doses of HBV vaccine during infancy. Universal HBV vaccination in infancy is more effective than selective immunization for high-risk groups. Previous HBV immunization programs for adolescents were not as successful as the program in infancy.

9.3.1.1 Hepatitis B Vaccine

Two kinds of HBV vaccine, the plasma-derived vaccine (the first generation vaccine) and the recombinant vaccine (the second generation vaccine), have been used widely for infant vaccination. Plasma-derived HBV vaccine is an HBsAg-based highly purified and inactivated vaccine made from serum of chronic HBV-infected subjects [27]. In order to produce a safe

Table 9.1 Prevention strategies against HBV infection include hepatitis B immunization by vaccine and/or HBIG, providing safe blood products, safe injection procedures, and avoidance of risky behaviors

Prevention strategies	Main targeting subjects	Effect and main transmission route to be prevented
Immunization		
1. HBV vaccine >= three doses (active)	1. For all infants starting from birth dose	The most effective strategy which provides long-term protection
2. HBIG[a] (passive)	2. To neutralize HBV in exposed subjects	Can prevent both mother-to-infant transmission and horizontal transmission
3. Combining HBV vaccine + HBIG	3. For infants of highly infectious mothers	
Blood safety, injection safety, and avoidance of risky behaviors		
1. Screening blood product	1. For people who require blood product	Prevent horizontal transmission in the risky condition of infection
2. Implementation of injection safety by proper sterilization of injection needles and syringes	2. For people who receive injection therapy, health-care worker, or parenteral drug abuser	
3. Avoidance of risky behaviors	3. Parenteral drug abuser, people who intend to have tattoo, skin piercing, etc.	

[a] *HBIG* hepatitis B immunoglobulin

vaccine, stringent treatments with pepsin, urea, and formaldehyde and rigorous filtration destroy all viruses, and chimpanzee tests were conducted during the production process of plasma vaccine [9]. With good protective efficacy, the plasma vaccine was approved by FDA of the USA in 1981 [45].

In order to avoid using serum from chronic HBV-infected subjects as the material to produce HBV vaccine, the recombinant HBV vaccine was developed and was licensed in 1986 [26]. The recombinant vaccine was produced by inserting and expressing the gene encoding HBsAg in yeast [63]. Gradually, recombinant vaccine replaced plasma vaccine, and became the main vaccine used worldwide.

Active immunization with three or four doses of HBV vaccine without HBIG was proved to be immunogenic in more than 90% of infants of non-carrier mothers or HBeAg-negative HBsAg carrier mothers. A pilot clinical trial revealed that for infants of HBsAg-negative mothers, the first dose of vaccine at 1 week stimulated anti-HBs within 1 month in 48% of the neonates. By the age of 6 months and 7 months, 96% and 100% of vaccines developed anti-HBs after a third dose, respectively [38].

For infants of highly infectious mothers seropositive for both HBeAg and HBsAg, the HBsAg-positive rate was very high (88%) in their unvaccinated infants. After three doses of HBV plasma vaccine, HBsAg-positive rate reduced to 23%, with a prevention rate of approximately 75% (Beasley et al. Unpublished data). The results implicated that, for infants of highly infectious mothers, a better strategy is needed to further improve the prevention efficacy of using vaccine only.

9.3.1.2 Hepatitis B Immunoglobulin (HBIG)

HBIG is used for postexposure prophylaxis (passive immunoprophylaxis) of HBV infection. It is prepared from the pooled plasma of donors who have high levels of anti-HBs. Viruses are inactivated during the process of extraction for anti-HBs. HBIG was given immediately after birth to infants of HBeAg-positive HBsAg carrier mothers to prevent transmission of HBV to infants from highly infectious mothers. Comparing to the 91% of HBsAg carrier rate among infants without immunoprophylaxis, the HBsAg carrier rate was 26% among infants who received three doses of HBIG at birth, 3 and 6 months old, and was 54% in those who received a single 1.0 ml dose of HBIG at birth. Without HBV vaccine, the prevention efficacy was 45% by one dose of 1.0 ml HBIG at birth and 75% by three doses of HBIG starting from birth, respectively [6].

9.3.1.3 Combining Active and Passive Immunization to Prevent HBV Transmission from Highly Infectious Mothers with Positive Serum HBeAg and HBsAg

Pilot studies combined HBIG immediately after birth followed by HBV vaccination using plasma-derived vaccine for infants of HBeAg-positive HBsAg carrier mothers. The prevention efficacy was 94%, which is superior than HBIG alone (71%) or vaccination alone (74%) [7]. This excellent prevention result established the basis of the current universal HBV immunization strategies to prevent perinatal transmission of HBV infection by highly infectious mothers. A similar efficacy was obtained in a subsequent study using HBIG at birth and three doses of recombinant HBV vaccine [58].

9.3.2 Universal Hepatitis B Immunization Program in Infancy

The world's first universal hepatitis B vaccination program was launched in Taiwan [16]. Pregnant women were screened for both serum HBsAg and HBeAg. All infants were covered by the HBV vaccination. Infants of mothers negative for HBeAg or HBsAg received three or four

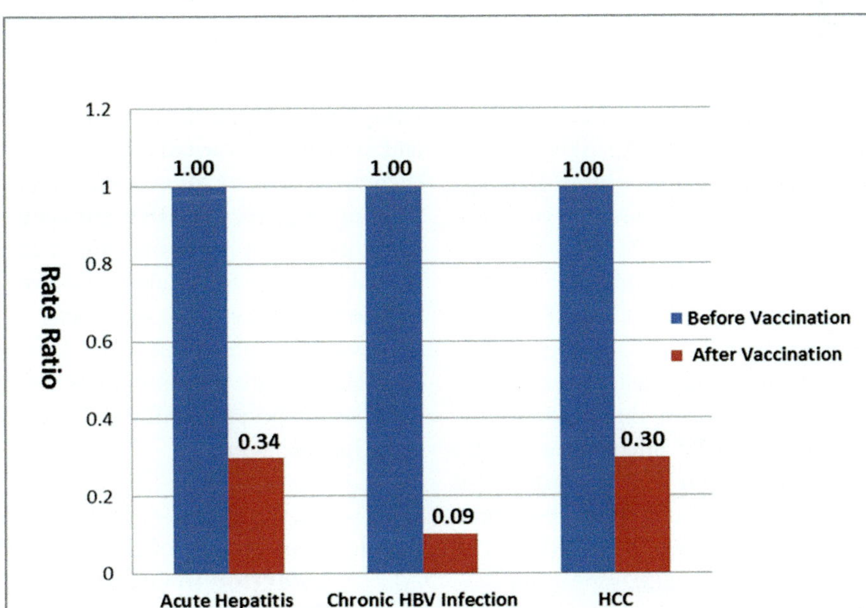

Fig. 9.1 Comparing with the cohorts born before the hepatitis B immunization program (rate ratio as 1.00), the rate ratios of the incidence rate of acute hepatitis B, the prevalence rate of chronic hepatitis B virus (HBV) infection, and the incidence rate of hepatocellular carcinoma (HCC) were reduced to 0.34, 0.09, and 0.30 in children and adolescents born after the vaccination program in Taiwan

doses of hepatitis B vaccine (Fig. 9.1). Infants of highly infectious mothers with positive HBeAg and HBsAg received HBIG within 24 h after birth, in addition to the hepatitis B vaccine. The coverage rate of hepatitis B vaccine for neonates was around 94% in the initial years and increased to 99% recently.

9.3.2.1 Different Strategies of Universal HBV Immunization in the World: Maternal Screening and Infant Immunization Programs

There are several strategies of universal infant immunization programs in the world depending largely on resources and prevalence of HBV infection. In countries with better resources, screening of maternal HBsAg is conducted during pregnancy. In some of those countries with a high prevalence of HBV infection like Taiwan, both HBsAg and HBeAg were screened, and HBIG was given only to newborns of HBeAg-positive HBsAg carrier mothers immediately after birth, and all infants received three doses of the HBV vaccine [19]. In some other countries of low HBV infection prevalence and good resources, pregnant women are screened for HBsAg only but not HBeAg. HBIG is given to newborns of HBsAg-positive mothers, and all infants receive three doses of the HBV vaccine [55]. This strategy saves the cost and labor of maternal HBeAg screening but increases the cost of HBIG, which is very expensive.

To save the costs of maternal screening and HBIG, most countries with intermediate/low prevalence of chronic HBV infection or limited resources do not screen HBV markers in pregnant women, and all infants receive three doses of HBV vaccine without HBIG. The efficacy of protecting the infants from chronic infection seems satisfactory. For infants of highly infectious mothers with seropositive HBeAg, this latter strategy offers a prevention efficacy of around 75% to 80%. Using this strategy, the cost of maternal screening and HBIG can be saved [54].

9.3.2.2 WHO's Recommendation and Global Infant HBV Immunization Status

In 2009, the World Health Organization (WHO) recommended that all infants receive hepatitis B vaccine as early as possible after birth, preferably within 24 hours. The birth dose should be followed by two or three doses of HBV vaccine in infancy. In 1992, the World Health Assembly passed a resolution to recommend global vaccination against hepatitis B. Hepatitis B vaccine for infants had been introduced nationwide in 185 countries by the end of 2015. Global coverage with three doses of hepatitis B vaccine is estimated at 83%. In addition, 96 countries introduced one dose of hepatitis B vaccine to newborns within the first 24 hours of life, and the global coverage is 39%. (http://www.who.int/mediacentre/factsheets/fs378/en/) (accessed January 31, 2017).

9.3.3 HBV Prevention Strategies Other Than Immunization

Other prevention strategies, such as screening of blood products, implementation of injection safety by proper sterilization of injection needles and syringes, and avoidance of risky behaviors, such as parenteral drug abuse, tattoo, or skin piercing, may prevent HBV horizontal transmission. Education to avoid high-risk behaviors should be advocated in addition to vaccination. In addition to the program for infants, many countries with low prevalence of HBV infection also have HBV vaccination programs for adolescents to prevent exposure to HBV by sexual contacts or other risk behaviors.

9.3.4 Prevention of De Novo HBV Infection in Organ Transplant Recipients

De novo HBV infection is defined as infection occurring in HBsAg-negative patients who become HBsAg positive after organ transplantation. With three or more doses of HBV vaccine during infancy in most children recipients (81%), de novo HBV infection after orthotopic liver transplantation (OLT) occurred mostly (89%) in those who received allografts from HBsAg-negative and anti-HBc-positive donors. Pre-OLT anti-HBs titers were < 200 mIU/mL in most patients with de novo HBV infection [59]. Pretransplantation HBV vaccination was helpful for achieving a posttransplantation vaccine response. Giving pretransplantation booster doses of HBV vaccine to increase the titer of anti-HBs to >200 mIU/mL is helpful to prevent de novo HBV infection in HBsAg-negative recipients. In addition, giving HBIG routinely in the pretransplantation and posttransplantation periods and subcutaneous vaccination with recombinant HBV vaccine concomitant with HBIG until acquisition of active immunization was reported to provide an effective strategy for preventing de novo hepatitis B infection after liver transplantation in recipients with anti-HBc-positive liver grafts [51].

9.4 The Effect of HBV Immunization on Reduction of HBV Infection and Related Complications

Universal hepatitis B immunization has successfully reduced acute, fulminant, and chronic hepatitis B and hepatocellular carcinoma [21]. HBV-associated membranous nephropathy in the vaccinated children also decreased remarkably, most likely due to the reduction in horizontal transmission of HBV infection after universal HBV vaccination [40].

9.4.1 Prevention of Acute HBV Infection

After universal HBV immunization, the incidence of acute hepatitis B declined worldwide substantially [46, 67]. Routine infant vaccination for HBV has been recommended in the USA since 1991. A trend toward reduction in acute hepatitis B among children aged <15 years has been noted in the USA with a remarkable fall in the incidence of acute HBV by 80% over 10 years [67, 72].

Acute hepatitis B among vaccinated children, adolescents, and young adults was also markedly reduced after universal HBV immunization in Taiwan. However, owing to breakthrough HBV infection from mother-to-infant transmission, vaccinated infants had higher rates of acute HBV infection than those aged 1–14 years old [60] (Fig. 9.1).

9.4.2 Prevention of Fulminant Hepatitis B

After initiation of the HBV immunization program. HBV rarely caused fulminant hepatitis in children older than 12 months old, but remained a significant cause of fulminant hepatitis in infants. HBV-positive fulminant hepatitis was prone to develop in infants born to HBeAg-

Table 9.2 Reduction of mortality rate associated with fulminant hepatitis (FH) in children after universal hepatitis B vaccination in Taiwan

Before vs. after the HBV vaccination program	Average annual mortality rate with FH per 100,000 infants	Mortality rate ratio in birth cohort before vs. after the HBV vaccination program	P value
<1 year old[a]			
Before (1975 to 1984)	5.36	1	
After (1985 to 1998)	1.71	0.32	<0.001
1–15 years old[b]			
Before (1980 to 1984)	0.27	1	<0.01
After (1985 to 1999)	0.10	0.37	

[a]Ref. [36]
[b]Ref. [18]

may help to reduce anxiety about the risks of the vaccine and enhance the HBV vaccine coverage rate. Furthermore, the HBV immunization program in some low-prevalence countries is not included in the routine infant immunization program, but is only focused on the prevention of perinatal infection and routine vaccination of adolescents [1]. In some other developed countries, under the competition from other new vaccines, HBV vaccination has not captured sufficient attention from the government [64].

9.6.3 Vaccine Failure

The causes of breakthrough HBV infection in the vaccinated subjects include high maternal viral load, intrauterine infection [41, 61], HBV surface gene mutants [31], genetic hyporesponsiveness to the vaccine [37], and immune compromised hosts (Table 9.3). In the era of post-HBV vaccination, even after complete immunization, vaccine failure still occurs. The leading cause of HBV vaccine failure is the mother-to-infant transmission of HBV from highly infectious mothers [19].

9.6.3.1 Mother-to-Infant Transmission of HBV (Also Refer to Chap. 4)

Infants of HBsAg carrier mothers with positive HBeAg and high viral load are the high-risk group of breakthrough HBV infection, despite immune prophylaxis with a combination of HBIG and vaccination. In children born to HBeAg-seropositive HBsAg carrier mothers, despite HBIG and three or four doses of the HBV vaccine, 9.26% still became HBsAg positive [19]. The predictive infection rates of vaccinated infants at maternal viral load levels of 7, 8, and 9 log10 copies/mL were 6.6%, 14.6%, and 27.7%, respectively [68].

9.6.3.2 Hepatitis B Surface Gene *a* Determinant Mutation

Vaccine failure has been attributed to hepatitis B surface gene mutants. Compared to the prevalence rate of hepatitis B surface gene mutants in unvaccinated subjects (7.8%), the rate of surface gene mutant among vaccinated HBsAg carrier children and adolescents increased to 22–28%. However, the prevalence rates of the surface gene mutants among the total vaccinated children and adolescents in the population have remained stationary for at least 20 years after the implementation of the universal hepatitis B immunization program. This most likely is due to the reduction of the total HBsAg seropositive rate in the vaccinated population. Recombinant vaccine uses less infectivity of mutant G145R, and mutant loss with older age seems to decrease the mutant prevalence in an immunized population over time [31, 32].

Table 9.3 Causes of HBV vaccine failure and strategies to overcome the problems

Problems	Descriptions	Strategies to overcome the problem
Maternal factor	Mother-to-infant transmission	1. Maternal screening for HBV markers
		2. Birth dose HBV vaccine
		3. Complete > = three doses of HBV vaccination on schedule in infancy
		4. HBIG at birth for infants of highly viremic mothers
		5. Antiviral therapy during last trimester for highly viremic mothers
Viral factor	Vaccine escape HBV surface gene mutant	Develop effective vaccine against HBV surface gene mutant(s)
Host factor	1. Genetic Hyporesponsiveness	1. High-dose vaccine or future better vaccine
	2. Immune compromised host	2. Complete vaccination before immunosuppression

9.6.4 Duration of Protection After HBV Vaccination in Infancy

After HBV immunization in infancy, anti-HBs titers gradually decline with age, even in those who received a booster dose during childhood [66]. In a study of post-one booster dose of HBV vaccine, the proportion of anti-HBs titer <10 mIU/mL among 15–20-year-olds were 24–28% [34]. In another study, a booster dose of HBV vaccination was administered to 1974 HBsAg- and anti-HBs-negative subjects. The proportions of post booster anti-HBs titer <10 mIU/ mL were 27.9% [74]. Even if studies show a loss of immune memory by this method, this does not necessarily mean that booster doses are required [24].

In a prospective long-term follow-up study of vaccinated 7–16-year-old subjects in the general population, the annual new anti-HBc seropositive rate was low (0.13%) and no new chronic HBV infection was detected. The decay rate of anti-HBs titer during age 7–16 years was approximately 20% of the titer of the previous year. Among the uninfected children who had anti-HBs <10 mIU/mL, the boosted and non-boosted children developed new anti-HBc positivity at a similar rate, implicating that a vaccine booster at this age is not mandatory [42].

How long can the protection by HBV vaccination last remains to be elucidated. Our recent evidence showed that up to 30 years after the infant universal HBV vaccination program, there had been no increase of HBsAg seropositive rates in cohorts born after the HBV vaccination program, as found in the seven consecutive surveys in Taiwan [50]. Loss of antibody among those who received HBV vaccination during infancy may not indicate loss of immunity or protection. For those who had received vaccinations in infancy, routine booster vaccination may not be required to protect against chronic HBV infection at least before 30 years of age. But a booster dose for high-risk subjects is indicated.

The complete vaccine series induces protective antibody levels in more than 95% of infants, children, and young adults. Protection lasts at least 30 years and is probably lifelong. Thus, WHO does not recommend booster vaccination for persons who have completed the three-dose vaccination schedule. The WHO also suggested that routine universal boosters are not recommended for children or adolescents. Nevertheless, it should be considered for those at high risk of HBV infection with anti-HBs < 10 mIU/mL after primary HBV vaccination. (www.who.int/mediacentre/factsheets/fs204/en/).

9.7 Strategies Toward the Success of Hepatitis B Prevention

9.7.1 Strategies to Enhance the Success of HBV Vaccination

In order to eliminate HBV infection, the preventive efficacy against HBV infection needs to be further enhanced. Strategies to increase the global HBV vaccine coverage rate and to eliminate vaccine failure are the key missions to be accomplished.

9.7.1.1 Increasing Vaccine Coverage Rate

Further increase of the global coverage rates of infant HBV vaccination is a critical issue toward a better control of hepatitis B and HCC. It is of vital importance to convince the government of countries without a universal HBV vaccination program to implement such a program and to help the countries with insufficient coverage rate to improve their vaccination programs. Coverage of the expenses of HBV vaccination in countries by the government or establishing a vaccine fund is very helpful to expand the HBV vaccine coverage. It is particularly urgent in areas where HBV infection and HCC are endemic [39].

9.7.1.2 Combating Vaccine Failure (Table 9.3)

In endemic areas, transmission of HBV infection is mainly from HBV-infected mothers to their infants during the perinatal period. Preventing mother-to-infant transmission of HBV is the most important strategy to overcome vaccine failure and to enhance the success of HBV prevention. Effective strategies, including screening HBV markers for pregnant women at their first prenatal visit; delivering the first dose of HBV vaccine to the infant within 24 hours of birth, and for infants of highly infectious mothers, adding HBIG at birth in addition to HBV vaccine, are of vital importance to prevent maternal transmission. In areas where a large proportion of births occur outside of health-care facilities, further efforts to overcome the difficulty of vaccine delivery for the birth dose of HBV vaccine are mandatory. In addition, a high coverage rate of three doses of HBV vaccine on schedule in infancy is also essential to induce long-term protection against HBV infection.

Development of new preventive methods to overcome vaccine failure in current HBV immunization program is anticipated. Pilot studies using antiviral therapy (lamivudine or telbivudine) during the last trimester of pregnancy to prevent mother-to-infant transmission have been reported [25, 65, 75]. Further successful prevention results were reported in a prospective, multicenter trial in HBsAg-positive and HBeAg-positive pregnant women with high-serum HBV-DNA levels. Treatment with tenofovir disoproxil fumarate for highly viremic mothers significantly reduced their infants' HBV-DNA positive rate at birth and HBsAg positivity at 6 months old and ameliorated maternal ALT elevations [20].

The development of better HBV vaccines to overcome the vaccine failure caused by HBV surface gene mutants and to protect immune compromised hosts is also anticipated. Before the start of immunosuppressive therapy or organ transplantation, HBV vaccination should be completed, and booster dose(s) may be needed to achieve adequate protective levels of anti-HBs in those who have low-anti-HBs levels.

9.7.2 Improving Blood Safety and Injection Safety and Reducing Risky Behaviors

Continuous efforts of infection control, which include improving blood safety by introducing effective screening methods for blood products, implementation of safe injection measures in health-care and community settings, and reducing risky behaviors, will reduce transmission of HBV. WHO recommends that all activities related to blood collection, testing, processing, storage, and distribution be coordinated at the national level through effective organization and integrated blood supply networks. The national blood system should be governed by national blood policy and legislative framework to promote uniform implementation of standards and consistency in the quality and safety of blood and blood products. (www.who.int/mediacentre/factsheets/fs279/en/) (accessed January 31, 2017).

9.7.3 World Health Organization (WHO) Global Heath Sector Strategy on Viral Hepatitis 2016–2021 – Toward Ending Viral Hepatitis

In 2014, the World Health Assembly in resolution WHA67.6 requested that WHO examine the feasibility of viral hepatitis elimination. WHO has defined the elimination of viral hepatitis as a public health threat as achieving a 90% reduction in new chronic infections and a 65% reduction in mortality. WHO Global Heath Sector Strategy on Viral Hepatitis 2016-2021 was proposed in June 2016. It is the first global health sector strategy on viral hepatitis, a strategy that contributes to the achievement of the 2030 Agenda for Sustainable Development. The goal is to eliminate viral hepatitis as a major public health threat by 2030 [73]. (http://apps.who.int/iris/bitstream/10665/246177/1/WHO-HIV-2016.06-eng.pdf) (accessed on January 31, 2017).

The strategy calls for an increase in global routine childhood HBV vaccine third-dose coverage to 90% by 2020 and 2030 and emphasizes that birth dose vaccination is a key intervention for prevention of HBV infection in infants. The target is to prevent mother-to-child transmission of HBV for 90% by 2030. Regarding blood safety, blood donation screened in a quality-assured manner is targeted to be 100% in 2030, and safe injection device and manner are targeted to be in 90% by 2030.

9.8 Summary

Prevention is better than therapy for the successful elimination of HBV infection. It is particularly important in countries where HBV infection, chronic liver diseases, and HCC are prevalent. Hepatitis B vaccination is the most effective way to prevent HBV infection and its complications. To achieve better results of HBV prevention worldwide, higher global coverage rates of HBV vaccination, better strategies against vaccine failure and non-responsiveness, and good long-term protection effect are needed. Advocating broadly the accurate concept of HBV prevention including vaccination and enhancing blood product safety and injection safety and reducing risky behaviors to the general population and obtaining the support from the government are of vital importance to the success of hepatitis B prevention.

The WHO Global Health Sector Strategy on Viral Hepatitis 2016–2021 has provided clear strategies and future targets for the world people and government to work forward. When the high expected coverage rate of the universal hepatitis B vaccination program starting from birth in most countries is achieved, HBV infection and its sequelae will be further prevented or even eradicated in the future. Furthermore, the successful cancer preventive effect provided by HBV vaccination can serve as a model for the cancer preventive vaccine of other virus or bacteria-related cancers in human.

References

1. Alter MJ (2003) Epidemiology and prevention of hepatitis B. Semin Liver Dis 23:39–46
2. Beasley RP (2009) Rocks along the road to the control of HBV and HCC. Ann Epidemiol 19:231–234
3. Beasley RP, Trepo C, Stevens CE, Szmuness W (1977) The e antigen and vertical transmission of hepatitis B surface antigen. Am J Epidemiol 105:94–98
4. Beasley RP, Hwang LY, Lin CC, Leu ML, Stevens CE, Szmuness W, Chen KP (1982) Incidence of hepatitis B virus infections in preschool children in Taiwan. J Infect Dis 146:198–204
5. Beasley RP, Hwang LY, Lin CC, Ko YC, Twu SJ (1983a) Incidence of hepatitis among students at a university in Taiwan. Am J Epidemiol 117:213–222
6. Beasley RP, Hwang LY, Stevens CE et al (1983b) Efficacy of hepatitis B immune globulin for prevention of perinatal transmission of the hepatitis B virus carrier state: final report of a randomized double-blind, placebo- controlled trial. Hepatology 3:135–141
7. Beasley RP, Hwang LY, Lee GC et al (1983c) Prevention of perinatally transmitted hepatitis B virus infections with hepatitis B immune globulin and hepatitis B vaccine. Lancet 2:1099–1102
8. Bosch FX, Ribes J (2002) The epidemiology of primary liver cancer: global epidemiology. In: Tabor E (ed) Viruses and liver cancer. Elsevier, Amsterdam, pp 1–16
9. Buynak EB, Roehm RR, Tytell AA, Bertland AU 2nd, Lampson GP, Hilleman MR (1976) Vaccine against human hepatitis B. JAMA 235:2832–2834
10. Chang MH (2003) Decreasing incidence of hepatocellular carcinoma among children following universal hepatitis B immunization. Liver Int 23:309–314
11. Chang MH, Lee CY, Chen DS, Hsu HC, Lai MY (1987) Fulminant hepatitis in children in Taiwan: the important role of hepatitis B virus. J Pediatr 111:34–39
12. Chang MH, Chen DS, Hsu HC, Hsu HY, Lee CY (1989) Maternal transmission of hepatitis B virus in childhood hepatocellular carcinoma. Cancer 64:2377–2380
13. Chang MH, Chen CJ, Lai MS, Hsu HM, Wu TC, Kong MS, Liang DC, Shau WY, Chen DS, Taiwan Childhood Hepatoma Study Group (1997) Universal hepatitis B vaccination in Taiwan and the incidence of hepatocellular carcinoma in children. N Engl J Med 336:1855–1859
14. Chang MH, You SL, Chen CJ, Liu CJ, Lee CM, Lin SM, Chu HC, Wu TC, Yang SS, Kuo HS et al (2009) Decreased incidence of hepatocellular carcinoma in hepatitis B vaccinees: a 20-year follow-up study. J Natl Cancer Inst 101:1348–1355
15. Chang MH, You SL, Chen CJ, Liu CJ, Lai MW, Wu TC et al (2016) Long-term effects of hepatitis B immunization of infants in preventing liver cancer. Gastroenterology 151:472–480

16. Chen DS, Hsu NHM, Sung JL, Hsu TC, Hsu ST, Kuo YT, Lo KJ, Shih YT (1987) The hepatitis steering committee, the hepatitis control committee: a mass vaccination program in Taiwan against hepatitis B virus infection in infants of hepatitis B surface antigen carrier-mothers. JAMA 257:2597–2603
17. Chen HL, Chang MH, Ni YH, Hsu HY, Lee PI, Lee CY, Chen DS (1996) Seroepidemiology of hepatitis B virus infection in children: ten years of mass vaccination in Taiwan. JAMA 276:906–908
18. Chen HL, Chen HL, Chang CJ, Kong MS et al (2004) Pediatric fulminant hepatic failure in endemic areas of hepatitis B infection: 15 years after universal hepatitis B vaccination. Hepatology 39:58–63
19. Chen HL, Lin LH, Hu FC, Lee JT, Lin WT, Yang YJ, Huang FC, Wu SF, Chen SC, Wen WH, Chu CH, Ni YH, Hsu HY, Tsai PL, Chiang CL, Shyu MK, Lee PI, Chang FY, Chang MH (2012) Effects of maternal screening and universal immunization to prevent mother-to-infant transmission of HBV. Gastroenterology 142:773–781
20. Chen HL, Lee CN, Chang CH, Ni YH, Shyu MK, Chen SM et al (2015) Efficacy of maternal tenofovir disoproxil fumarate in interrupting other-to-infant transmission of HBV. Hepatology 62:375–386
21. Chiang CJ, YangYW YSL, Lai MS, Chen CJ (2013) Thirty year outcomes of the national hepatitis B immunization program in Taiwan. JAMA 310:974–976
22. Da Villa G, Picciottoc L, Elia S, Peluso F, Montanaro F, Maisto T (1995) Hepatitis B vaccination: universal vaccination of newborn babies and children at 12 years of age versus high risk groups – a comparison in the field. Vaccine 13:1240–1243
23. Feret E, Larouze B, Diop B, Sow M, London WT, Blumberg BS (1987) Epidemiology of hepatitis B virus infection in the rural community of tip, Senegal. Am J Epidemiol 125:140–149
24. Hall AJ (2010) Boosters for hepatitis B vaccination? Need for an evidence-based policy. Hepatology 51:1485–1486
25. Han GR, Cao MK, ZhaoW JHX, Wang CM, Bai SF, Yue X, Wang GJ, Tang X, Fang ZX (2011) A prospective and open-label study for the efficacy and safety of telbivudine in pregnancy for the prevention of perinatal transmission of hepatitis B virus infection. J Hepatol 55:1215–1221
26. Hilleman MR (1987) Yeast recombinant hepatitis B vaccine. Infection 15:3–7
27. Hilleman MR (2002) Overview of the needs and realities for developing new and improved vaccines in the 21st century. Intervirology 45:199–211
28. Hsu HY, Chang MH, Chen DS, Lee CY, Sung JL (1986) Baseline seroepidemiology of hepatitis B virus infection in children in Taipei, 1984: a study just before mass hepatitis B vaccination program in Taiwan. J Med Virol 18:301–307
29. Hsu HC, Lin YH, Chang MH, Su IJ, Chen DS (1988) Pathology of chronic hepatitis B virus infection in children: with special reference to the intrahepatic expression of hepatitis B virus antigens. Hepatology 8:378–382
30. Hsu HY, Chang MH, Hsieh KH, Lee CY, Lin HH, Hwang LH, Chen PJ, Chen DS (1992) Cellular immune response to HBcAg in mother-to-infant transmission of hepatitis B virus. Hepatology 15:770–776
31. Hsu HY, Chang MH, Ni YH, Chiang CL, Chen HL, Wu JF, Chen PJ (2010) No increase in prevalence of hepatitis B surface antigen mutant in a population of children and adolescents who were fully covered by universal infant immunization. J Infect Dis 201:1192–1200
32. Hsu HY, Chang MH, Ni YH, Jeng YM, Chiang CL, Chen HL, Wu JF, Chen PJ (2013) Long-term follow-up of children with postnatal immunoprophylaxis failure who were infected with hepatitis B virus surface antigen gene mutant. J Infect Dis 207:1047–1057
33. Hsu HY, Chang MH, Ni YH, Chiang CL, Wu JF, Chen HL (2015) Universal infant immunization and occult hepatitis B virus infection in children and adolescents: a population-based study. Hepatology 61:1183–1191
34. Jan CF, Huang KC, Chien YC, Greydanus DE, Davies HD, Chiu TY, Huang LM, Chen CJ, Chen DS (2010) Determination of immune memory to hepatitis B vaccination through early booster response in college students. Hepatology 51:1547–1554
35. Jang MK, Lee JY, Lee JH, Kim YB, Kim HY, Lee MS, Park CK, Yoo JY (2001) Seroepidemiology of HBV infection in South Korea, 1995 through 1999. Korean J Intern Med 16:153–159
36. Kao JH, Hsu HM, Shau WY, Chang MH, Chen DS (2001) Universal hepatitis B vaccination and the decreased mortality from fulminant hepatitis in infants in Taiwan. J Pediatr 139:349–352
37. Kruskall MS, Alper CA, Awdeh Z, Yunis EJ, Marcus-Bagley D (1992) The immune response to hepatitis B vaccine in humans: inheritance patterns in families. J Exp Med 175:495–502
38. Lee GC, Hwang LY, Beasley RP, Chen SH, Lee TY (1983) Immunogenicity of hepatitis B virus vaccine in healthy Chinese neonates. J Infect Dis 148:526–529
39. Lerkhachonsuk AA, Yip CH, Khuhaprema T, Chen DS, Piummer M, Jee SH, Toi M, Willailak S, Summit AO (2013) Cancer prevention in Asia: resource stratified guidelines from the Asian oncology summit 2013. Lancet Oncol 14:497–507
40. Liao MT, Chang MH, Lin FG, Tsai IJ, Chang YW, Tsau YK (2011) Universal hepatitis B vaccination reduces childhood hepatitis B virus-associated membranous nephropathy. Pediatrics 128:e600–e604
41. Lin HH, Lee TY, Chen DS, Sung JL, Ohto H, Etoh T, Kawana T, Mizuno M (1987) Transplacental leakage of HBeAg positive maternal blood as the most likely route in causing intrauterine infection with hepatitis B virus. J Pediatr 111:877–881
42. Lin YC, Chang MH, Ni YH, Hsu HY, Chen DS (2003) Long term immunogenicity and efficacy of universal

hepatitis B virus vaccination in Taiwan. J Infect Dis 187:134–138
43. MacLachlan JH, Cowie BC (2015) Hepatitis B virus epidemiology. Cold Spring Harb Perspect Med 5:a021410
44. Martínez-Sernández V, Figueiras A (2013) Central nervous system demyelinating diseases and recombinant hepatitis B vaccination: a critical systematic review of scientific production. J Neurol 260:1951–1959
45. Maupas P, Chiron JP, Barin F, Coursaget P, Goudeau A, Perrin J, Denis F, Mar ID (1981) Efficacy of hepatitis B vaccine in prevention of earl HBsAg carrier state in children. Controlled trial in an endemic area (Senegal). Lancet i:289–292
46. McMahon BJ, Bulkow LR, Singleton RJ, Williams J, Snowball M, Homan C, Parkinson AJ (2011) Elimination of hepatocellular carcinoma and acute hepatitis B in children 25 years after a hepatitis B newborn and catch-up immunization program. Hepatology 54:801–807
47. Montesano R (2011) Preventing primary liver cancer: the HBV vaccination project in the Gambia (West Africa). Environ Health 10(Suppl 1):S6
48. Ni YH, Chang MH, Huang LM, Chen HL, Hsu HY, Chiu TY, Tsai KS, Chen DS (2001) Hepatitis B virus infection in children and adolescents in a hyperendemic area: 15 years after mass hepatitis B vaccination. Ann Intern Med 135:796–800
49. Ni YH, Huang LM, Chang MH, Yen CJ, Lu CY, You SL, Kao JH, Lin YC, Chen HL, Hsu HY, Chen DS (2007) Two decades of universal hepatitis B vaccination in Taiwan: impact and implication for future strategies. Gastroenterology 132:1287–1293
50. Ni YH, Chang MH, Jan CF, Hsu HY, Chen HL, Wu JF, Chen DS (2016) Continuing decrease in hepatitis B virus infection 30 years after initiation of infant vaccination program in Taiwan. Clin Gastroenterol Hepatol 14:1324–1330
51. Ohno Y, Mita A, Ikegami T, Masuda Y, Urata K, Nakazawa Y, Urata K, Nakazawa Y, Kobayashi A, Miyagawa S (2014) Successful active immunization using a hepatitis B virus vaccination protocol for a recipient with hepatitis B core antibody- positive liver graft. Transplant Proc 46:721–725
52. Orlando R, Foggia M, Maraolo AE, Mascolo S, Palmiero G, Tambaro O, Tosone G (2015) Prevention of hepatitis B virus infection: from the past to the future. Eur J Clin Microbiol Infect Dis 34:1059–1070
53. Peto TJ, Mendy ME, Lowe Y, Webb EL, Whittle HC, Hall AJ (2014) Efficacy and effectiveness of infant vaccination against chronic hepatitis B in the Gambia hepatitis intervention study (1986–90) and in the nationwide immunization program. BMC Infect Dis 14:7
54. Poovorawan Y, Sanpavat S, Pongpunlert W, Chumdermpadetsuk S, Sentrakul P, Safary A (1989) Protective efficacy of a recombinant DNA hepatitis B vaccine in neonates of HBe antigen-positive mothers. JAMA 261:3278–3281
55. Shepard CW, Simard EP, Finelli L, Fiore AE, Bell BP (2006) Hepatitis B virus infection: epidemiology and vaccination. Epidemiol Rev 28:112–125
56. Shiraki K, Yoshihara N, Sakurai M, Eto T, Kawana T (1980) Acute hepatitis B in infants born to carrier mother with the antibody to hepatitis B e antigen. J Pediatr 97:768–770
57. Stevens CE, Beasley RP, Tsui J, LeeWC (1975) Vertical transmission of hepatitis B antigen in Taiwan. N Engl J Med 292:771–774
58. Stevens CE, Taylor PE, Tong MJ, Toy PT, Vyas GN, Nair PV, Weissman JY, Krugman S (1987) Yeast-recombinant hepatitis B vaccine. Efficacy with hepatitis B immune globulin in prevention of perinatal hepatitis B virus transmission. JAMA 257:2612–2616
59. Su WJ, Ho MC, Ni YH, Chen HL, Hu RH, Wu YM, Chang MH, Lee PH (2009) High- titer antibody to hepatitis B surface antigen before liver transplantation can prevent de novo hepatitis B infection. J Pediatr Gastroenterol Nutr 48:203–208
60. Su WJ, Liu CC, Liu DP, Chen SF, Huang JJ, Chan TC, Chang MH (2012) Effect of age on the incidence of acute hepatitis B after 25 years of a universal newborn hepatitis B immunization program in Taiwan. J Infect Dis 205:757–762
61. Tang JR, Hsu HY, Lin HH, Ni YH, Chang MH (1998) Hepatitis B surface antigenemia at birth: a long-term follow up study. J Pediatr 133:374–377
62. Tsen YJ, Chang MH, Hsu HY, Lee CY, Sung JL, Chen DS (1991) Seroprevalence of hepatitis B virus infection in children in Taipei, 1989: five years after a mass hepatitis B vaccination program. J Med Virol 34:96–99
63. Valenzuela P, Medina A, Rutter WJ, Ammerer G, Hall BD (1982) Synthesis and assembly of hepatitis B virus surface antigen particles in yeast. Nature 298:347–350
64. van Herck K, Vorsters A, Van Damme P (2008) Prevention of viral hepatitis (B and C) reassessed. Best Pract Res Clin Gastroenterol 22:1009–1029
65. van Zonneveld M, van Nunen AB, Niesters HG, de Man RA, Schalm SW, Janssen HL (2003) Lamivudine treatment during pregnancy to prevent perinatal transmission of hepatitis B virus infection. J Viral Hepat 10:294–297
66. Wang CW, Wang LC, Chang MH, Ni YH, Chen HL, Hsu HY, Chen DS (2005) Long- term follow-up of hepatitis B surface antibody levels in subjects receiving universal hepatitis B vaccination in infancy in an area of hyperendemicity: correlation between radioimmunoassay and enzyme immunoassay. Clin Diagn Lab Immunol 12:1442–1447
67. Wasley A, Miller JT, Finelli L, Centersfor Disease Control, Prevention (CDC) (2007) Surveillance for

acute viral hepatitis-United States, 2005. MMWR Surveill Summary 56:1–24
68. Wen WH, Chang MH, Zhao LL, Ni YH, Hsu HY, Wu JF, Chen PJ, Chen DS, Chen HL (2013) Mother-to-infant transmission of hepatitis B virus infection: significance of maternal viral load and strategies for intervention. J Hepatol 59:24–30
69. Whittle HC, Maine N, Pilkington J, Mendy M, Fortuin M, Bunn J, Allison L, Howard C, Hall A (1995) Long-term efficacy of continuing hepatitis B vaccination in infancy in two Gambian villages. Lancet 345:1089–1092
70. Whittle H, Jaffar S, Wansbrough M, Mendy M, Dumpis U, Collinson A, Hall A (2002) Observational study of vaccine efficacy 14 years after trial of hepatitis B vaccination in Gambian children. BMJ 325:569
71. Wichajarn K, Kosalaraksa P, Wiangnon S (2008) Incidence of hepatocellular carcinoma in children in Khon Kaen before and after national hepatitis B vaccine program. Asian Pac J Cancer Prev 9:507–509
72. Williams A (2002) Reduction in the hepatitis B related burden of disease- measuring the success of universal immunisation programs. Commun Dis Intell Q Rep 26:458–460
73. World Health Organization (WHO) 2016 Global health sector strategy on viral hepatitis 2016–2021-Towards ending viral hepatitis. June 2016. http://apps.who.int/iris/bitstream/10665/246177/1/WHO-HIV-2016.06-eng.pdf. Accessed on 31 Jan 2017.
74. Wu TW, Lin HH, Wang LY (2013) Chronic hepatitis B infection in adolescents who received primary infantile vaccination. Hepatology 57:37–45
75. Xu WM, Cui YT, Wang L, Yang H, Liang ZQ, Li XM, Zhang SL, Qiao FY, Campbell F, Chang CN, Gardner S, Atkins M (2009) Lamivudine in late pregnancy to prevent perinatal transmission of hepatitis B virus infection: a multicentre, randomized, double-blind, placebo-controlled study. J Viral Hepat 16:94–103

Viral Hepatitis B: Management in Children

10

Christine K. Lee and Maureen M. Jonas

Abstract

The natural history of chronic hepatitis B virus (HBV) infection in children varies with age at infection, acquisition, ethnicity, and endemic region. Around the world, most chronic hepatitis B virus (HBV) infection is transmitted perinatally or during early childhood. The risk of chronic infection when acquired in infancy is 90% versus 30% when acquired during the first 5 years of life and <5% in older childhood and adulthood (McMahon BJ, Alward WL, Hall DB, Heyward WL, Bender TR, Francis DP, Maynard JE. J Infect Dis 151:599–603, 1985). Loss of hepatitis B e antigen (HBeAg) or seroconversion to anti-HBe can occur spontaneously, and the annual rate differs by age (<2% in children <3 years, 4–5% after age 3), with higher rates during puberty (Chang MH, Sung JL, Lee CY, Chen CJ, Chen JS, Hsu HY et al. J Pediatr 115(3):385–390, 1989; Liaw YF, Chu CM, Lin DY, Sheen IS, Yang CY, Huang MJ. J Med Virol 13(4):385–391, 1984). Children from non-endemic areas are less likely to have been perinatally infected and will often undergo HBeAg seroconversion in the first two to three decades of life (Bortolotti F, Cadrobbi P, Crivellaro C, Guido M, Rugge M, Noventa F et al. Gastroenterology 99:805–810, 1990).

With cessation of active HBV replication, serum alanine aminotransferase (ALT) is normalized, HBeAg is lost with or without development of anti-HBe, and there is improvement in liver histology. Due to persistence of covalently closed circular DNA (cccDNA), the transcriptional template of HBV, in the nucleus of hepatocytes, patients who have undergone HBeAg seroconversion cannot be considered "cured" (Moraleda G, Saptuelli J, Aldrich CE, Averett D, Condreay L, Mason WS. J Virol 71:9392–9399, 1997; Wong DK, Seto WK, Fung J, Ip P, Huang FY, Lai CL et al. Clin Gastroenterol Hepatol 11:1004–1010. el, 2013). These patients are at lifelong risk for reactivation of infection. If patients lose the hepatitis B surface antigen (HBsAg), typically with persistent HBV DNA suppression, this is considered to be an "immunological cure." This is true whether seroconversion occurs spontaneously or as a result of treatment.

The most serious sequelae of chronic hepatitis B (CHB), cirrhosis and hepatocellular carcinoma (HCC), are not commonly seen during childhood and adolescence. In a study of 292 consecutive HBsAg positive children with elevated ALT levels, 10 patients (3%) had cirrhosis (Bortolotti F, Calzia R, Cadrobbi P, Giacchini R, Ciravegna B, Armigliato M. J

C. K. Lee · M. M. Jonas (✉)
Division of Gastroenterology, Hepatology and Nutrition, Boston Children's Hospital, Boston, MA, USA
e-mail: maureen.jonas@childrens.harvard.edu

M.-H. Chang, K. B. Schwarz (eds.), *Viral Hepatitis in Children*,
https://doi.org/10.1007/978-981-13-0050-9_10

Pediatr 108:224–227, 1986). In adults, HCC is thought to be related to the HBV DNA levels, degree of liver injury, and duration of infection. HCC can occur in children who have had HBeAg seroconversion, indicating that risk of HCC may continue even after viral replication is ceased (Livingston SE, Simonetti JP, McMahon BJ, Bulkow LR, Hurlburt KJ, Homan CE et al. J Infect Dis 195:5–11, 2007). Nonetheless, the goal of treatment of HBV in childhood is to decrease the morbidity and mortality of CHB later in life by using the surrogate endpoints of HBeAg seroconversion and ALT normalization.

10.1 Indication for Treatment

Selecting patients who can benefit from treatment and determining the optimal time for treatment are important decisions in order to maximize benefit while limiting duration of therapy and minimize the risk for antiviral drug resistance later in life. Most children with HBV have persistently normal ALT levels, high HBV DNA levels, and HBeAg in keeping with an immune-tolerant state, but immune activation can occur [1].

Children with ALT levels ≤1.5–2 times the upper limit of normal (ULN), positive HBeAg, and high HBV DNA levels (>10 million IU/ml) are likely in the immune-tolerant phase of HBV infection. These children are typically not ideal for treatment because current therapies have not been shown to induce HBeAg seroconversion when compared with no treatment. Thus, the American Association for the Study of Liver Diseases (AASLD) recommends against the use of therapy in these children, regardless of the HBV DNA level [1]. In addition, children with ALT values greater than ten times the ULN may be in the process of spontaneous HBeAg seroconversion and should be observed for several months before the decision to proceed with treatment is finalized. For patients with DNA level <10^4 IU/mL but elevated ALT, therapy can be deferred until other etiologies of liver disease and spontaneous HBeAg seroconversion are evaluated.

The AASLD recommends treatment for children ages 2 to <18 years who are HBeAg positive with persistently elevated ALT (>1.5 times the ULN at least 2 occasions over at least 6 months in HBeAg+ or 12 months in HBeAg− children) and HBV DNA levels of ≥2000 IU/ml [1]. The 2015 World Health Organization (WHO) and 2013 European Society of Pediatric Gastroenterology, Hepatology, and Nutrition (ESPGHAN) guidelines state that treatment priority should be given to children with clinical evidence of compensated or decompensated cirrhosis, regardless of ALT levels, HBeAg status, or HBV DNA levels [2, 3]. In addition to these considerations, treatment of patients with advanced inflammation or fibrosis or family history of HCC should also be considered [4].

10.2 Treatment Options, Mechanism of Action, and Therapeutic Studies

Therapies studied in children with chronic hepatitis B include one biologic preparation (interferon-alfa) and oral nucleoside (lamivudine, entecavir) and nucleotide (adefovir dipivoxil and tenofovir disoproxil fumarate) analogs (NA). There are currently five agents (interferon-α-2b, lamivudine, adefovir, tenofovir disoproxil fumarate, entecavir) approved for treatment for children or adolescents in the United States by the Food and Drug Administration.

Treatment studies in children have included HBeAg-positive patients with at least mildly elevated ALT (>1.3 times the ULN with the usual ULN of 30 U/L). Since endpoints such as cirrhosis, HCC, and death are rare in children, treatment studies in children typically invoked other intermediate endpoints including normalization of ALT, HBV DNA clearance/suppression, HBeAg loss and seroconversion, or a combination of these factors. Studies used different assays for the measurement of HBV DNA level, but all studies included only HBeAg-positive patients. There have been no studies of therapy for HBeAg-negative children, since this is rare during childhood and adolescence.

A recent meta-analysis examined randomized controlled trials (RCT) and observational studies of children <18 years with chronic HBV infection [4]. After searching 2321 citations, 14 qualifying studies with children were identified, in which some of the patients were followed for up to 15 years. Twelve of the RCTs studied intermediate treatment endpoints: ALT normalization, HBV DNA suppression, HBeAg/HBsAg seroconversion, and HBeAg/ HBsAg loss. Looking at all RCTs with posttreatment follow-up both <12 months and ≥12 months, antiviral treatment was more effective than placebo to achieve all intermediate endpoints: ALT normalization, HBeAg clearance loss, HBV DNA suppression, HBeAg seroconversion, and HBsAg clearance.

10.2.1 Interferon-Alfa(α)

Interferon (IFN) is a cytokine with immunomodulatory and antiviral properties [5]. IFN-α affects HBV by binding to its cellular receptor and activates secondary messengers which then help promote defense of the cell against viruses. IFN-α also enhances immunomodulation by increased antigen presentation to the immune system, activation of natural killer cells, and increased production of cytokines. Antiviral effects include degradation of viral mRNA, inhibition of viral protein synthesis, and prevention of cell infection.

The only drug studied in an RCT evaluating for the primary endpoints of HCC and cirrhosis was IFN-α. In these studies, IFN-α did not significantly reduce the risk of either HCC (RR 0.3) or cirrhosis (RR 0.2) [6, 7]. In RCTs looking at <12-month follow-up from therapy, patients treated with IFN-α were found to have statistically improved HBeAg clearance/loss (RR 3.2) [8, 9] and HBV DNA suppression (RR 2.2) [8–13] compared to no treatment. However, IFN-α treatment did not result in ALT normalization (RR 1.4) [8–10, 13], HBeAg seroconversion (RR 2.8) [11], or HBsAg clearance (RR 7.4) [10]. When followed for ≥12 months post IFN-α treatment, there was improved HBeAg clearance/loss (RR 2.0) [8, 11, 13–15] and HBeAg seroconversion (RR 3.1) [11, 15], but not ALT normalization (RR 1.4) [14], HBV DNA suppression(RR 1.5) [8, 9, 11, 12, 15], HBsAg clearance (RR 3.3) [14, 15], or HBsAg seroconversion (RR 2.5) [14, 15].

10.2.2 Lamivudine

Lamivudine is a nucleoside analog reverse transcriptase inhibitor with anti-HIV and anti-HBV properties. Inside the cell, it is converted into a form which can incorporate into a growing HBV DNA chain and then act as a chain terminator [16]. It can also inhibit viral DNA synthesis, halt the recycling of virions to the nucleus, and slow the formation of cccDNA [17, 18]. With lower levels of circulating HBV DNA, there is a concomitant increase in the clearance of HBeAg from the circulation [18–20].

There was one RCT which studied lamivudine treatment for 48 weeks. Patients treated with lamivudine were found to have significant advantage in three of the intermediate endpoints including ALT normalization (RR 4.5), HBeAg clearance/loss (RR 1.8), and HBV DNA suppression (RR 3.9) but not HBeAg seroconversion (RR 1.7) or HBsAg clearance (RR 3.5) [21]

In adults, monotherapy with lamivudine confers a high risk for resistance, with 20% of patients developing resistance at 1 year and 70% after 5 years [22, 23]. In children, resistance to lamivudine developed in 19% at 1 year [21] of therapy and 67% after 2 years [24]. For this reason, lamivudine is not considered a first-line agent, since long-duration therapy is typically required for most patients. The lamivudine-resistant HBV variant is sensitive to adefovir and tenofovir.

10.2.3 Adefovir

Adefovir dipivoxil is a nucleotide analog. Once inside the cell, it is phosphorylated to the active form which acts as a chain terminator of the HBV DNA chain and/or a competitive inhibitor of the substrate dATP [7]. When used for 48 weeks, it has been shown to decrease both cccDNA and HBsAg levels in HBeAg-positive patients [25].

In one RCT of pediatric patients treated for 48 weeks, adefovir was found to produce a higher rate of ALT normalization (RR 2.7) and HBV DNA suppression (RR 11.1) but not HBeAg seroconversion (RR 3, 95% CI 0.9–9.9) when compared to placebo treatment [24]. When the same cohort of patients was followed in an open-label study for 192 weeks, adefovir-treated patients showed continued viral suppression and ALT normalization [26]. Adefovir is approved for the treatment of adolescents (≥12 years of age) in the United States. Nonetheless, since adefovir has less potent antiviral activity than other currently available agents, its use is now very limited.

The rate of development of adefovir resistance mutations is lower than those reported for lamivudine. It has been predicted to be 5% at 12 months and 17% at 24 months in adults [27]. Adefovir-resistant variants are sensitive to tenofovir and other L-nucleoside analogs, lamivudine and entecavir.

10.2.4 Entecavir

Entecavir is a guanosine nucleoside analog active against HBV polymerase. Similar to the other nucleoside analogs, entecavir is phosphorylated to its active form intracellularly. It inhibits the HBV DNA polymerase by interfering with the priming of the polymerase, is a competitive inhibitor of dGTP, and acts as a chain terminator at three major steps of HBV replication [28, 29].

When entecavir was studied in children for 48 weeks, compared to placebo, treated patients had higher rates of ALT normalization (RR 2.9), HBV DNA suppression (RR 14.8), and HBeAg seroconversion (RR 2.4) [30]. The only statistically significant difference with treatment at 96 weeks was for HBeAg seroconversion.

The likelihood for entecavir resistance is low due to a high genetic barrier. Entecavir-resistant variants are seen almost exclusively in lamivudine-experienced patients; when entecavir is used in that setting, a higher dose (double) is recommended.

10.2.5 Tenofovir

Tenofovir disoproxil fumarate (TDF) has been shown to have effects against wild-type and lamivudine-resistant HBV strains. Tenofovir DF is phosphorylated into the active form with a long half-life [31]. Like the other NAs, it also functions as a chain terminator but also is a poor substrate for cellular DNA polymerase [32]. Tenofovir DF is well tolerated with a similar safety profile to adefovir but is more potent.

When TDF treatment was studied in an adolescent RCT for 72 weeks, in comparison with placebo, there were higher rates of ALT normalization (RR 2) and HBV DNA suppression (RR 92.4) but no difference in the rate of HBeAg clearance/loss (RR 1.4) [33]. TDF is approved for use in adolescents ≥12 years of age in the United States. Long-term studies of TDF in adults have not reported detectable resistance [34].

10.3 Clinical Management

AASLD [1], WHO [2], European Association for the Study of the Liver (EASL) [35], and the ESPGHAN [3] guidelines all agree that the goal of treatment is to improve long-term survival and decrease the morbidity associated with chronic HBV infection. Although these guidelines also agree that the optimal endpoint of treatment is persistent HBsAg clearance, which indicates a halting of disease progression and thereby a reduction in the risk for HCC, this endpoint occurs rarely in treated patients. If this is not attained, the next goal of therapy is to reach sustained undetectable HBV DNA levels and anti-HBe seroconversion in patient who was previously HBeAg positive. Alternatively, undetectable HBV DNA while under prolonged antiviral therapy is also a reasonable goal.

Current treatment options for children are limited but hopefully will continue to expand (Table 10.1). The currently approved treatments have acceptable safety profiles in children. Prior to treatment, patients and their caregivers should be counseled on the indications of treatment and possible benefits and side effects. Practitioners should also assess their understanding for the

Table 10.1 Approved antiviral therapies in children in the United States

Drug	Age	Dose	Possible side effects	Monitoring while on treatment
Interferon-α-2b	≥1–18 years	6 million IU/m^2 TIW	Flu-like symptoms Fatigue Mood changes Cytopenias Autoimmune disorders	CBC (q 1–3 months) TSH (q 3 months) Monitor for autoimmune, ischemic, neuropsychiatric, and infectious issues
Lamivudine	≥2 years	3 mg/kg daily (max 100 mg)	Lactic acidosis Pancreatitis	Amylase/lipase if symptoms are concerning for pancreatitis Lactic acid level if concerned
Entecavir	≥2 years	**For treatment naïve** For 10–30 kg, there is weight-based dosing 0.15 mg (10–11 kg) 0.2 mg (>11–14 kg) 0.25 mg (>14–17 kg) 0.3 mg (>17–20 kg) 0.35 mg (>20–23 kg) 0.4 mg (>23–26 kg) 0.45 mg (>26–30 kg) 0.5 mg (>30 kg) For *lamivudine experienced* 0.3 mg (10–11 kg) 0.4 mg (>11–14 kg) 0.5 mg (>14–17 kg) 0.6 mg (>17–20 kg) 0.7 mg (>20–23 kg) 0.8 mg (>23–26 kg) 0.9 mg (>26–30 kg) 1 mg (>30 kg)	Lactic acidosis	Lactic acid levels if concerned
Adefovir	≥12 years	10 mg daily	Acute renal failure Fanconi syndrome Nephrogenic diabetes insipidus Lactic acidosis	CrCl at baseline If at risk for renal impairment, CrCl, serum phosphorus, urine glucose, and protein yearly In patients with fractures or risk for osteopenia, bone density at baseline and during treatment Lactic acid levels if concerned
Tenofovir DF	≥12 years	300 mg daily	Nephropathy Fanconi syndrome Osteomalacia, decrease in bone density Lactic acidosis	CrCl at baseline If at risk for renal impairment, CrCl, serum phosphorus, urine glucose, and protein yearly In patients with fractures or risk for osteopenia, bone density at baseline and during treatment Lactic acid levels if concerned

Abbreviations: *CBC* complete blood counts, *TSH* thyroid-stimulating hormone, *CrCl* creatinine clearance need and willingness for long-term treatment and regular monitoring. Additional counseling on lifestyle choices and hepatitis A vaccination should also be considered in all patients.

In the United States, for children older than 1 year of age, interferon-α-2b is approved for a course of 24 weeks. The major advantage of interferon treatment is the lack of resistance and the possibility of off-treatment sustained virological response, chance of HBsAg loss, and undetectable HBV DNA. Like in adults, children can experience flu-like symptoms with interferon treatment. Body weight and growth have also been reported to be influenced transiently in children [36]. In addition, the three-times-per-week injection schedule can be more challenging in children. There are several relative contraindications for its use in patients with decompensated cirrhosis, hypersplenism, thyroid disease, autoimmune disease, severe coronary artery disease, renal transplant status, pregnancy, seizures, psychiatric illness, thrombocytopenia, leucopenia, and retinopathy and certain concomitant medication use [2]. Although not approved for chronic hepatitis B infection, PEGylated interferon-α-2a once weekly therapy is approved for adults with hepatitis B and for chronic hepatitis C in children 5 years and older. Clinicians can potentially consider this drug for chronic HBV.

The oral antiviral therapies approved for children in the United States are lamivudine, adefovir, tenofovir DF, and entecavir. The main advantage for the NA over IFN is the once-daily oral dosing and tolerability. Disadvantages of NAs are that they may require long-term, potentially lifelong therapy, with high long-term costs and the risk of developing drug resistance [2]. In addition, all NAs carry a black box warning from the US FDA for lactic acidosis, although this is exceedingly rare in CHB. NAs are primarily renally excreted, and dose adjustments are necessary with renal functional impairment. The cost of therapy is also quite variable especially in resource-poor areas with higher cost of TDF and entecavir in these areas. Regardless of oral NA chosen, treatment with oral antivirals has been studied for 1–4 years with the main therapeutic endpoint in children of HBeAg seroconversion. An additional 12 months of consolidation therapy (after HBeAg seroconversion) is recommended, as in adults. Once therapy is completed, monitoring every 3 months for the 1st year is recommended for signs of recurrent viremia, ALT elevations, and decompensation of clinical status.

Like in adults, lamivudine and adefovir are also associated with high viral resistance rates in children [37] and thus are not used as first-line therapy. Lamivudine and entecavir are approved for children 2 years and older. Adefovir and TDF are approved only for use in children 12 years and older. However, in adults, TDF has been reported to cause renal dysfunction, hypophosphatemia and Fanconi syndrome (glycosuria, hypophosphatemia, metabolic acidosis), and the associated reduced bone density and osteomalacia/osteoporosis [38]. The AASLD practice guidelines recommend that patients on TDF should be assessed for renal safety with serum creatinine, phosphorus, urine glucose, and urine protein before treatment initiation and at least annually or more frequently during treatment [1]. There is insufficient evidence to recommend monitoring of bone mineral density for patients on TDF. There are no specific monitoring recommendations for children, but it seems prudent to consider evaluation for these events in adolescents receiving this agent.

In November 2016, the FDA approved tenofovir alafenamide (TAF), the prodrug of TDF, for use in adults with chronic HBV. It is reported to have similar efficacy but with greater plasma stability. Thus, the effective dose of TAF is much lower than TDF, resulting in lower rates of renal and bone adverse effects. Like other NAs, TAF also carries a black box warning for lactic acidosis but also carries an additional warning for hepatomegaly with steatosis. Though not studied in children yet, this offers hope that this may be an option for children in the future.

10.4 Summary

Though most children with chronic hepatitis B infection typically do not develop advanced liver disease, complications such as HCC and cirrhosis are reported in childhood. The literature on antiviral therapy for chronic HBV infection in children shows the improvement of intermediate outcomes including ALT normalization, HBeAg loss, HBV DNA suppression, HBeAg seroconversion, and HBsAg loss when compared to no treatment or placebo. Unfortunately, the RCT evidence in children is limited due to small number of studies, short duration of follow-up, and minimal data on significant outcomes – cirrhosis and HCC. Since cirrhosis and HCC development in childhood is rare, RCT's in children use intermediate outcomes (HBeAg seroconversion and viral suppression) to inform clinical decisions when treating children. Like in adults, the currently approved therapies for children are well tolerated. Care must be taken to determine the best regimens in order to minimize development of resistance and side effects. Caregiver and patient preferences and capabilities must also be considered when deciding the appropriate therapy and treatment course.

References

1. Terrault NA, Bzowej NH, Chang KM, Hwang JP, Jonas MM, Murad MH (2016) AASLD guidelines for treatment of chronic hepatitis B. Hepatology 63(10):261–283
2. World Health Organization (2015, March) Guidelines for the prevention, care and treatment of persons with chronic hepatitis B infection. http://www.who.int/hiv/pub/hepatitis/hepatitis-b-guidelines/en/
3. Sokal EM, Paganelli M, Wirth S, Socha P, Vajro P, Lacaille F et al (2013) Management of chronic hepatitis B in childhood: ESPGHAN clinical practice guidelines. J Hepatol 59:814–829
4. Jonas MM, Lok A, McMahon BJ, Brown RS, Wong JB, Ahmed AT et al (2016) Antiviral therapy in management of chronic hepatitis B viral infection in children: a systemic review and meta-analysis. Hepatology 63:307–318
5. Rijckborst V, Janssen HLA (2010) The role of interferon in hepatitis B therapy. Curr Hepat Rep 9(4):231–238
6. Bortolotti F, Jara P, Crivellaro C, Hierro L, Cadrobbi P, Frauca E et al (1998) Outcome of chronic hepatitis B in Caucasian children during a 20-year observation period. J Hepatol 29:184–190
7. Fujisawa T, Inui A, Sogo T, Komatsu H (2004) Long-term history of chronic hepatitis B virus infection in children. [Japanese]. Nippon rinsho. Jpn J Clin Med 62(Suppl 8):303–308.
8. Barbera C, Bortolotti F, Crivellaro C, Coscia A, Zancan L, Cadrobbi P et al (1994) Recombinant interferon-alpha 2a hastens the rate of HBeAg clearance in children with chronic hepatitis B. Hepatology 20:287–290
9. Utili R, Sagnelli E, Galanti B, Aprea L, Cesaro G, Digilio L et al (1991) Prolonged treatment of children with chronic hepatitis B with recombinant alpha 2a-interferon: a controlled, randomized study. Am J Gastroenterol 86:327–330
10. Sokal EM, Conjeevaram HS, Roberts EA, Alvarez F, Bern EM, Goyens P et al (1998) Interferon alfa therapy for chronic hepatitis B in children: a multinational randomized controlled trial. Gastroenterology 114:988–995
11. Gregorio GV, Jara P, Hierro L, Diaz C, de la Vega A, Vegnente A et al (1996) Lymphoblastoid interferon alfa with or without steroid pretreatment in children with chronic hepatitis B: a multicenter controlled trial. Hepatology 23:700–707
12. Ruiz-Moreno M, Rua MJ, Molina J, Moraleda G, Moreno A, Garcia-Aguado J, Carreno V (1991) Prospective, randomized controlled trial of interferon-alpha in children with chronic hepatitis B. Hepatology 13:1035–1039
13. Ruiz Moreno M, Jimenez J, Porres JC, Bartolome J, Moreno A, Carreno V (1990) A controlled trial of recombinant interferon-alpha in Caucasian children with chronic hepatitis B. Digestion 45:26–33
14. Vajro P, Tedesco M, Fontanella A, De Vincenzo A, Vecchione R, Ammendola R et al (1996) Prolonged and high dose recombinant interferon alpha-2b alone or after prednisone priming accelerates termination of active viral replication in children with chronic hepatitis B infection. Pediatr Infect Dis J 15:223–231
15. Lai CL, Lin HJ, Lau JN, Flok AS, Wu PC, Chung HT et al (1991) Effect of recombinant alpha 2 interferon with or without prednisone in Chinese HBsAg carrier children. Q J Med 78:155–163
16. De Clercq E, Ferir G, Kaptein S, Neyts J (2010) Antiviral treatment of chronic hepatitis B virus (HBV) infections. Viruses 2:1279–1305
17. Chang CN, Skalski V, Zhou JH, Cheng YC (1992) Biochemical pharmacology of (+) and (−)- 2′3′-dideoxy-3′thiacytidine as anti-hepatitis B virus agents. J Biol Chem 267:22414–22420
18. Lai CL, Yuen MF (2000) Profound suppression of hepatitis B virus replication with lamivudine. J Med Virol 61:367–373
19. Dienstag JL, Schiff ER, Wright TL, Perrillo RP, Hann HW, Goodman Z et al (1999) Lamivudine as initial

treatment for chronic hepatitis B in the United States. N Engl J Med 341:1256–1263
20. Lai CL, Chine RW, Leung NWY, Chang TT, Guan R, Tai DI et al (1998) A one year trial of lamivudine for chronic hepatitis B. N Engl J Med 339:61–68
21. Sokal EM, Kelly DA, Mizerski J, Badia IB, Arelas JA, Schwarz KB et al (2006) Long-term lamivudine therapy for children with HBeAg-positive chronic hepatitis B. Hepatology 43(2):225–232
22. Lok AS, Lai CL, Leung N, Yao GB, Cui ZY, Schiff ER et al (2003) Long-term safety of lamivudine treatment in patients with chronic hepatitis B. Gastroenterology 125:1714–1722
23. Pawlotsky JM, Dusheiko G, Hatzakis A, Lau D, Lau G, Lian TJ et al (2008) Virologic monitoring of hepatitis B virus therapy in clinical trials and practice: recommendations for a standardized approach. Gastroenterology 134:405–415
24. Jonas MM, Kelley DA, Mizersky J, Badia IB, Areias JA, Schwarz KB et al (2002) Clinical trial of lamivudine in children with chronic hepatitis B. N Engl J Med 346:1706–1713
25. Werle-Lapostolle B, Bowden S, Locarnini S, Wursthorn K, Petersen J, Lau G et al (2004) Persistence of cccDNA during the natural history of chronic hepatitis B and decline during adefovir dipivoxil therapy. Gastroenterology 126:1750–1758
26. Jonas MM, Kelly D, Pollack H, Mizerski J, Sorbel J, Frederick D et al (2012) Efficacy and safety of long-term adefovir dipivoxil therapy in children with chronic hepatitis B infection. Pediatr Infect Dis J 31:578–582
27. Gallego A, Sheldon J, Garcia-Samaniego J, Margall N, Romero M, Hornillos P et al (2008) Evaluation of initial virological response to adefovir and development of adefovir-resistant mutations in patients with chronic hepatitis B. J Viral Hepat 15:392–398
28. Zoulim F (2006) Entecavir: a new treatment option for chronic hepatitis B. J Clin Virol 36:8–12
29. Seifer M, Hamatake RK, Colonno RJ, Standring DN (1998) In vitro inhibition of hepadnavirus polymerases by the triphosphates of BMS-200475 and lobucavir. Antimicrob Agent Chemother 42:3200–3208
30. Jonas MM, Chang MH, Sokal E, Schwarz KB, Kelly D, Kim KM, et al (2015) Randomized Controlled Trial of Entecavir Versus Placebo in Children with HBeAg-positive Chronic Hepatitis B. Hepatology; published on-line July 2015. https://doi.org/10.1002/hep.28015
31. Delaney WE 4th, Ray AS, Yang H, Qi X, Xiong S, Zhu Y et al (2006) Intracellular metabolism and in vitro activity of tenofovir against hepatitis B virus. Antimicrob Agents Chemother 50:2471–2477
32. Delaney WE 4th, Borroto-Esoda K (2008) Therapy of chronic hepatitis B: trends and developments. Curr Opin Pharmacol 8:532–540
33. Murray KF, Szenborn L, Wysocki J, Rossi S, Corsa AC, Dinh P et al (2012) Randomized, placebo-controlled trial of tenofovir disoproxil fumarate in adolescents with chronic hepatitis B. Hepatology 56:2018–2026
34. Kitrinos KM, Corsa A, Liu Y, Flaherty J, Snow-Lampart A, Marcellin P et al (2014) No detectable resistance to tenofovir disoproxil fumarate (TDF) after 6 years of therapy with chronic hepatitis B. Hepatology 59(2):434–442
35. European Association For The Study of the Liver (2012) EASL clinical practice guidelines: management of chornic hepatitis B virus infection. J Hepatol 57(1):167–185
36. Comanor L, Minor J, Conjeevaram HS, Roberts EA, Alvarez F, Bern EM et al (2001) Impact of chronic hepatitis B and interferon-alpha therapy on growth of children. J Viral Hepat 8:139–147
37. Sokal EM, Kelly DA, Mizerski J, Badia IB, Areias JA, Schwarz KB et al (2006) Long-term lamivudine therapy for children with HBeAg-positive chronic hepatitis B. Hepatology 43:225–232
38. Fontana RJ (2009) Side effects of long-term antiviral therapy for hepatitis B. Hepatology 49:S185–S195

Natural History of Hepatitis C Virus Infection in Children

11

Nicole Green and Karen F. Murray

Abstract

Hepatitis C was first cloned and discovered to be a major cause of non-A, non-B hepatitis in 1989. Hepatitis C virus (HCV) is a RNA virus within the Flaviviridae family and comprises the genus *Hepacivirus*, of which there are six known genotypes. HCV is now known to be a leading cause of chronic liver disease in both industrialized and developing countries. Recent estimates suggest that over 200 million people worldwide have been infected with hepatitis C virus with an additional 3–4 million newly infected annually (El-Shabrawi MH, Kamal NM. World J Gastroenterol 19:7880, 2013). Eleven million of those globally infected with HCV are thought to be under 15 years of age (Gower E, Estes C, Blach S et al. J Hepatol 61:S45, 2014). Infection with HCV most commonly leads to persistent infection and can progress to chronic liver disease, cirrhosis, or hepatocellular carcinoma. While children account for a small proportion of the infected population, many of these children develop chronic hepatitis C and thus are at risk for its complications. The worldwide prevalence of HCV infection in children varies geographically, ranging from 0.05% to 0.36% in the USA (1.3% of children over the age of 6 (Mack CL, Gonzalez-Peralta RP, Gupta N et al. J Pediatr Gastroenterol Nutr 54:838, 2012)) and Europe to 1.8–5.8% in certain developing countries. The highest prevalence reported is in Egypt, sub-Saharan Africa, Amazon basin, and Mongolia (El-Shabrawi MH, Kamal NM. World J Gastroenterol 19:7880, 2013). Including individuals who were previously exposed but cleared the infection with those infected, the prevalence of HCV antibody positivity in North America is thought to approximate 0.2% of 6–11-year-olds and 0.4% of 12–19-year-olds (Mack CL, Gonzalez-Peralta RP, Gupta N et al. J Pediatr Gastroenterol Nutr 54:838, 2012). While a lot of what is known about hepatitis C comes from studying adults with the disease, children and adults demonstrate differences in modes of acquisition and transmission, rates of clearance and progression, and perhaps in response to treatment.

N. Green
Pediatric Gastroenterology, University of Washington School of Medicine, Seattle, WA, USA

K. F. Murray (✉)
Division of Gastroenterology and Hepatology, Department of Pediatrics, Seattle Children's and University of Washington, Seattle, WA, USA
e-mail: karen.murray@seattlechildrens.org

11.1 Transmission and Clearance

Transmission of HCV infection is through contaminated blood or other bodily fluids. Perinatal transmission represents the most common mode of acquisition of HCV in children, accounting for

M.-H. Chang, K. B. Schwarz (eds.), *Viral Hepatitis in Children*,
https://doi.org/10.1007/978-981-13-0050-9_11

3. Benova L, Mohamoud YA, Calvert C, Abu-Raddad LJ (2014) Vertical transmission of hepatitis C virus: systemic review and meta-analysis. Clin Infect Dis 59:765
4. Waasdorp HC, Golden-Mason L, Brocato M et al (2010) Innate immune function in placenta and cord blood of hepatitis C-seropositive mother-infant dyads. PLoS One 5:e12232
5. European Pediatric Hepatitis C Virus Network (2005) A significant sex-but note elective caesarean section-effect on mother to child transmission of hepatitis C virus infection. J Infect Dis 192:1872–1879
6. Mast EE, Hwang LY, Seto DS et al (2005) Risk factors for perinatal transmission of hepatitis C virus (HCV) and the natural history of HCV infection acquired in infancy. J Infect Dis 192:1880–1889
7. Maasoumy B, Wedemeyer H (2012) Natural history of acute and chronic hepatitis C. Best Pract Res Clin Gastroenterol 26:401–412
8. Ruiz-Extremera A, Munoz-Gamez JA, Salmeron-Ruiz MA et al (2011) Genetic variation in interleukin 28B with respect to vertical transmission of hepatitis C virus and spontaneous clearance in HCV-infected children. Hepatology 53:1830–1838
9. Mack CL, Gonzalez-Peralta RP, Gupta N et al (2012) NASPGHAN practice guidelines: diagnosis and management of hepatitis C infection in infants, children, and adolescents. J Pediatr Gastroenterol Nutr 54:838
10. Bortolotti F, Verucchi G, Camma C et al (2008) Long-term course of chronic hepatitis C in children: from viral clearance to end-stage liver disease. Gastroenterology 134:1900
11. Lehmann M, Meyer MF, Monazahian M et al (2004) High rate of spontaneous clearance of acute hepatitis C virus genotype 3 infection. J Med Virol 73:387–391
12. Jara P, Resti M, Hierro L et al (2003) Chronic hepatitis C virus infection in childhood: clinical patterns and evolution in 224 white children. Clin Infect Dis 36:275
13. Forton DM, Thomas HC, Murphy CA et al (2002) Hepatitis C and cognitive impairment in a cohort of patients with mild liver disease. Hepatology 35:433–439
14. Younossi Z, Kallman J, Kincaid J (2007) The effects of HCV infection and management of health-related quality of life. Hepatology 45:806–816
15. Nydegger A, Srivastava A, Wake M, Smith AL, Hardikar W (2008) Health-related quality of life in children with hepatitis C acquired in the first year of life. J Gastroenterol Hepatol 23(2):226–230
16. Rodrigue JR, Balistreri W, Haber B et al (2009) Impact of hepatitis C virus infection on children and their caregivers: quality of life, cognitive, and emotional outcomes. J Pediatr Gastroenterol Nutr 48:341
17. Goodman Z, Makhlouf H, Liu L et al (2008) Pathology of chronic hepatitis C in children: liver biopsy findings in Peds-C trial. Hepatology 47(3):836–843
18. European Paediatric Hepatitis C Virus Network (2005) Three broad modalities in the natural history of vertically acquired hepatitis C virus infection. Clin Infect Dis 41:45
19. Wilder J, Patel K (2014) A review of the natural history chronic hepatitis C infection. N Am J Med Sci 7(1):1–7
20. Badizadegan K, Jonas M, Ott M et al (1998) Histopathology of the liver in children with chronic hepatitis C viral infection. Hepatology 28:1416–1423
21. Schwarz KB, Gonzalez-Peralta RP, Murray KF et al (2011) The combination of ribavirin and peginterferon is superior to peginterferon and placebo for children and adolescents with chronic hepatitis C. Gasterterology 140:450
22. Mohan P, Colvin C, Glymph C et al (2007) Clinical spectrum of histopathologic features of chronic hepatitis C infection in children. J Pediatr 150:168
23. Gonzalez-Peralta RP, Langham MR Jr, Andres JM et al (2009) Hepatocellular carcinoma in 2 young adolescents with chronic hepatitis C. J Pediatr Gastroenterol Nutr 48:630
24. Kumar V, Kato N, Urabe Y et al (2011) Genome-wide association study identifies a susceptibility locus for HCV-induced hepatocellular carcinoma. Nat Genet 43(5):455–458

Management of Viral Hepatitis C in Children

12

Björn Fischler and Afrodite Psaros-Einberg

Abstract

Once hepatitis C virus (HCV) infection has infected a child, the risk of chronicity seems as high as in adults, i.e., 60–80%. Although symptomatic disease is rare and histological progression is in most cases slower than for adults, advanced fibrosis or in fact cirrhosis is noted in 2–5% by adolescence (Bortolotti F, Verucchi G, Cammà C, Cabibbo G, Zancan L, Indolfi G et al. Gastroenterology 134:1900–1907, 2008; Guido M, Bortolotti F, Leandro G, Jara P, Hierro L, Larrauri J et al. Am J Gastroenterol 98:660–663, 2003; Goodman ZD, Makhlouf HR, Liu L, Balistreri W, Gonzalez-Peralta RP, Haber B et al. Hepatology 47:836–843, 2008; Jara P, Resti M, Hierro L, Giacchino R, Barbera C, Zancan L et al. Clin Infect Dis 36:275–280, 2003). This would suggest that antiviral treatment during childhood or adolescence can be beneficial. Furthermore, if such treatment is successful, i.e., eradicates the infection, the future risks of transmitting the infection to sexual partners or offspring are eliminated. Additionally, there is usually no need for further follow-up after successful treatment with the achievement of sustained viral response (SVR) 12–24 weeks after cessation. The one exception is the continuous need for screening for hepatocellular carcinoma if cirrhosis was detected before treatment (Gonzalez-Peralta RP, Langham MR, Andres JM et al. J Pediatr Gastroenterol Nutr 48:630–635, 2009).

So far, all treatment modalities have first been tried in adults and thereafter in children. This is true for interferon (IFN) monotherapy, combination therapy with IFN (conventional or pegylated (PEG)) and ribavirin (RBV), as well as for the recently available IFN-free combinations of direct-acting antiviral (DAA) agents without or with RBV. For each new treatment modality, improved SVR rates have been reported, and results for children have often been slightly better than for adults. This might be attributed to shorter duration of infection, lower viral loads, and relatively fewer concomitant diseases in children.

B. Fischler (✉) · A. Psaros-Einberg
Department of Pediatrics, Karolinska University Hospital, CLINTEC, Karolinska Institutet, Stockholm, Sweden
e-mail: bjorn.fischler@sll.se; bjorn.fischler@karolinska.se

12.1 Interferon-Based Therapies

Small, non-randomized studies from the 1990s indicated moderate success for treatment with IFN monotherapy in infected children. In an analysis of published trials and abstracts, SVR was 27% for genotype 1 and 70% for all other genotypes combined [1]. For comparison 5% of untreated controls cleared the virus spontaneously.

M.-H. Chang, K. B. Schwarz (eds.), *Viral Hepatitis in Children*,
https://doi.org/10.1007/978-981-13-0050-9_12

Table 12.1 Results from pediatric studies with combination therapy consisting of pegylated interferon and ribavirin

Patient number and ages (reference)	Treatment type and doses	SVR genotype 1 (%)	SVR non-genotype 1 (%)	Side effects
n = 107, 3–17 years (ref. [2])	PEG-IFN alfa-2b (60 μg/m2/week) + RBV (15 mg/kg/day)[a]	53	93	1% discontinuation 5% thyroid problem
n = 65, 6–17 years (ref. [3])	PEG-IFN alfa-2a (100 μg/m2, maximum 180 μg) + RBV 15 mg/kg/day[b]	57	89	3% discontinuation 11% thyroid problem
n = 55[c], 5–17 years (ref. [4])	PEG-IFN alfa-2a (180 μg/1.73 m2) + RBV (15 mg/kg/day)	47	80	7% discontinuation 4% thyroid problem

[a]24 weeks for genotype (gt) 2 and 3 patients with low viral load (<600,000 IU/ml) and 48 weeks for gt1, gt4, and gt3 with high viral load

[b]24 weeks for gt 2 and 3, 48 weeks for gt 1,4,5,6

[c]Patients were randomized to receive PEG-INF in combination with placebo or with RBV. Only the latter group is described here

The addition of RBV and the subsequent change from conventional to PEG-IFN resulted in improved SVR rates. The three largest pediatric multicenter studies with this combination treatment with PEG-IFN and RBV are depicted in Table 12.1 [2–4]. In essence, the SVR rates were increased to 50–55% for genotype 1 and 80–90% for non-genotype 1 in these studies (Table 12.1). However, the rate of side effects was high. This included symptomatic side effects, such as flu-like symptoms, fatigue, loss of appetite, and depression, but also laboratory abnormalities, particularly related to bone marrow depression. The latter necessitated dose reduction in a considerable portion of patients. While these negative effects were reversible when treatment was stopped, this was not the case for the 5–10% of patients who developed thyroid abnormalities, most often hypothyroidism, during treatment. A majority of this subgroup were reported to be on daily thyroid hormone treatment and also after cessation of antiviral treatment.

Another concern was the effect on height during and after treatment. Growth velocity was clearly decreased during the actual treatment, and this was more evident in patients treated for 12 months than in those treated for 6 months [2]. A certain catch-up in growth was suggested after treatment cessation. Thus, in the study of 107 patients treated with PEG-IFN alfa-2b (60 μg/m2/week) in combination with RBV (15 mg/kg/day), the growth velocity was doubled during the follow-up period (5.73 ± 4.1 cm/year) compared to the low level during the treatment period (2.47 ± 2.22 cm/year) [2]. Still, at the end of the follow-up period of 24 weeks, the mean height percentile (44.3) remained slightly below the median and also below the mean baseline height percentile (50.9). Recently, long-term follow-up (median 5.5 years) data from this study were published [5]. Among patients treated for 24 weeks, full recovery of height z-scores to baseline was observed by 1 year of follow-up, whereas only partial recovery was observed during 5 years of follow-up in patients treated for 48 weeks. In fact, 12 of 30 (40%) girls and 7 of 18 (39%) boys who received 48 weeks of treatment had a > 15 percentile-point decrease in height from baseline to the end of follow-up.

One of the two multicenter studies combining RBV with PEG-IFN alfa-2a instead of PEG-IFN alfa-2b in 65 patients suggested no difference in z-score for height at baseline compared to end of treatment, but no long-term follow-up data have been published from this study [3]. For comparison, in the other multicenter study with this combination, subnormal z-scores for height both at end of treatment and 2-year follow-up were noted in a large proportion of patients [6].

In summary, despite possible differences between combinations using PEG-IFN alfa-2a or IFN alfa-2b, decreased growth velocity during treatment should be expected, and lack of normalization of z-scores for height can be anticipated in a proportion of patients treated for 48 weeks.

12.2 First-Generation Protease Inhibitors

The suboptimal results of "standard of care" (SOC) combination treatment with PEG-IFN and ribavirin for genotype 1 patients spurred the development of new drugs directed against HCV. The first improvement came with the addition of either one of the two protease inhibitors boceprevir and telaprevir to SOC treatment, which resulted in improvements in SVR from below 50% for genotype 1 to around 70% in adults [7, 8]. However, new side effects were added to those already seen for SOC, and although pediatric studies were initiated, they were never fulfilled and so far have not resulted in any publications [9, 10].

In a single case report of an adolescent who had been liver transplanted for hepatitis C-related hepatocellular carcinoma, successful treatment with PEG-IFN, RBV, and boceprevir was described [11].

12.3 Treatment with Oral, Interferon-Free Combinations of Direct-Acting Antiviral Agents

Within a few years, it became evident that the development of newer direct-acting antivirals (DAA) would result in IFN-free combination treatments with further increase in SVR. By 2014, large adult studies showed remarkable improvements in the outcome for genotype 1 patients, bringing SVR above 90%, both in treatment-naïve and treatment-experienced patients [12–14]. Furthermore, patients with compensated cirrhosis had equally good outcome, and patients with decompensated cirrhosis could also be treated. Additionally, patients on the waiting list for liver transplantation could be treated to achieve SVR before transplantation and thereby avoid reinfection, and already liver-transplanted, reinfected patients could also be treated with very good results. Compared to SOC treatment, the DAA combinations had very mild side effects, mostly related to the concomitant use of ribavirin.

By early 2017, further development of new drugs has resulted in several possible combinations for adults and reduced the need to add ribavirin (Table 12.2). The duration of treatment is commonly 12 weeks, but a proportion of genotype 1 patients need only 8 weeks. Furthermore, very effective interferon-free combinations are now available for all genotypes [15, 16]. Guidelines for adult chronic HCV infection today recommend such treatment for all patients, with the priority of those with moderate to severe fibrosis and/or patients in transplant settings or with other immunosuppressive treatments [17–19].

It has been suggested that treatment in children should be deferred until results of pediatric controlled studies on interferon-free DAA combinations are available [5]. However, for high-risk patients such delay may not be feasible or advisable. Thus, off-label use of the new DAA combinations has been described in some pediatric case reports (Table 12.3). Notably, very sick children and adolescents have been successfully treated, the youngest being only 1 year of age [20–23]. Adolescents were given adult doses, while smaller children received 25 or 50% of adult doses. In one of these reports, we described a stem cell-transplanted teenager with a complicated history who was successfully treated with sofosbuvir and simeprevir for 12 weeks but experienced severe peripheral edema clearly connected to the treatment [21]. It was suggested that drug interaction between simeprevir and nifedipine within the cytochrome P450 system could have precipitated this side effect. We have since then treated three other children (one after liver transplantation, one in conjunction with treatment for Ewing's sarcoma, and one with advanced fibrosis), aged 9–17 years with the fixed combination of sofosbuvir and ledipasvir (Harvoni^R) in adult doses for 12 weeks. All three had SVR and no side effects (unpublished observation Psaros Einberg A, Fischler B).

Very recently the results of a controlled study on the use of Harvoni^R for 12 weeks with adult

Table 12.2 Direct-acting antiviral drugs currently licensed for adults

Substance class	Substance	Drug name	Genotype
NS5B polymerase inhibitor (nucleotide analogue)	Sofosbuvir	Sovaldi	All genotypes, but Harvoni not for genotypes 2 and 3
		Harvoni[a]	
		Epclusa[b]	
NS5B polymerase inhibitor (non- nucleotide analogue)	Dasabuvir	Exviera	Combination with Viekirax for genotype 1
NS/4A protease inhibitor	Simeprevir	Olysio	1 and 4
	Paritaprevir	Viekirax	1 and 4[c]
	Grazoprevir	Zepatier	1 and 4[d]
NS5A inhibitor	Daklatasvir	Daklinza	1, 3, and 4
	Ledipasvir	Harvoni[a]	1, 4, 5, and 6
	Ombitasvir	Viekirax[c]	1 and 4
	Elbasvir	Zepatier[d]	1and 4
	Velpatasvir	Epclusa[b]	All genotypes

[a]Harvoni: Fixed combination of sofosbuvir and ledipasvir
[b]Epclusa: Fixed combination of sofosbuvir and velpatasvir
[c]Viekirax: Fixed combination of ombitasvir, paritaprevir, and ritonavir (ritonavir inhibits CYP3A resulting in an increased systemic exposure to paritaprevir)
[d]Zepatier: Fixed combination of grazoprevir and elbasvir

doses for HCV-infected patients with genotype 1 aged 12–17 years were published [24]. This fixed combination resulted in SVR at 12 weeks after cessation in an impressive 98 out of 100 patients (98%), including 1 with cirrhosis. The two without SVR were lost to follow-up. The three most commonly reported adverse events were headache (27% of patients), diarrhea (14%), and fatigue (13%). No severe adverse events were reported. Further studies, including pharmacokinetic investigations with this and other combinations, in younger children are ongoing [25, 26].

12.4 Summary

For the near future, it is suggested that all pediatric patients with chronic HCV infection where spontaneous recovery is unlikely should be considered for treatment with interferon-free combinations at some point before adulthood. With the strong data from adult studies as well as the abovementioned published study on the use of fixed combination sofosbuvir and ledipasvir for adolescents, this treatment can be readily used for not only genotype 1 but also for genotype 4 for patients 12 years or older [17–19, 24]. For pediatric patients with genotypes 2 and 3, there are available combinations with high efficacy and low toxicity proven in adults (Table 12.1) which could be considered at least for adolescents in need of prompt treatment [16]. For patients below 12 years of age with urgent need of treatment, the use of reduced doses as described in Table 12.3 could be suggested [20, 23]. Finally, the use of interferon-based regimens for pediatric patients with chronic HCV infection should be discouraged.

Table 12.3 Published case reports on children treated with interferon-free combinations of direct-acting antiviral agents

Age (reference)	Setting	Treatment	Outcome	Side effects
4 years (ref. [20])	3 months post umbilical cord blood transplantation for acute lymphoblastic leukemia, genotype 1a	Sofosbuvir 200 mg + simeprevir 75 mg (i.e., 50% of adult doses), 24 weeks	SVR 24 weeks after treatment cessation	Not reported
15 years (ref. [21])	1 year post stem cell transplantation for sickle cell disease, genotype 4c	Sofosbuvir 400 mg + simeprevir 150 mg, 12 weeks	SVR 21 weeks after treatment cessation	Severe peripheral edema, reversible after treatment cessation
14 years (ref. [22])	Decompensated cirrhosis due to chronic hepatitis C, genotype 1a. Listed for liver transplantation	Sofosbuvir 400 mg + ledipasvir 90 mg, fixed combination, 12 weeks	SVR 4 weeks after treatment cessation	None
1 year (ref. [23])	Pre- and post- liver transplantation for biliary atresia, genotype 1b	Sofosbuvir 100 mg + ledipasvir 22.5 mg (i.e., 25% of adult doses), fixed combination + RBV 15 mg/kg/d, 12 weeks	SVR 12 weeks after treatment cessation	None
16 years (ref. [23])	Post-liver transplantation for Budd-Chiari syndrome and cirrhosis, genotype 1 b	Sofosbuvir 400 mg + ledipasvir 90 mg, fixed combination + RBV 15 mg/kg/d, 12 weeks	SVR 12 weeks after treatment cessation	None

References

1. Jacobson KR, Murray K, Zellos A, Schwarz KB (2002) An analysis of published trials of interferon monotherapy in children with chronic hepatitis C. J Pediatr Gastroenterol Nutr 34:52–58
2. Wirth S, Ribes-Koninckx C, Calzado MA, Bortolotti F, Zancan L, Jara P et al (2010) High sustained virologic response rates in children with chronic hepatitis C receiving peginterferon alfa-2b plus ribavirin. J Hepatol 52:501–507
3. Sokal EM, Bourgois A, Stephenne X, Silveira T, Porta G, Gardovska D, Fischler B, Kelly DA (2010) Peginterferon alfa-2a plus ribavirin for chronic hepatitis C virus infection in children and adolescents. J Hepatol 52:827–831
4. Schwarz KB, Gonzalez-Peralta RP, Murray KF, Molleston JP, Haber BA, Jonas MM et al (2011) The combination of ribavirin and peginterferon is superior to peginterferon and placebo for children and adolescents with chronic hepatitis C. Gastroenterology 140:450–458
5. Haber B, Alonso E, Pedreira A, Rodriguez-Baez N, Ciocca M, Lacaille F, Lang T, Gonzalez T, Goodman Z, Yang Z, Jackson B, Noviello S, Albrecht JK (2017) Long-term follow-up of children treated with peginterferon and ribavirin for hepatitis c virus infection. J Pediatr Gastroenterol Nutr 64:89–94
6. Jonas MM, Balistreri W, Gonzalez-Peralta RP, Haber B, Lobritto S, Mohan P, Molleston JP, Murray KF, Narkewicz MR, Rosenthal P, Schwarz KB, Barton BA, Shepherd JA, Mitchell PD, Duggan C (2012) Pegylated interferon for chronic hepatitis C in children affects growth and body composition: results from the pediatric study of hepatitis C (PEDS-C) trial. Hepatology 56(2):523–531
7. Jacobson IM, McHutchison JG, Dusheiko G, Di Bisceglie AM, Reddy KR, Bzowej NH, Marcellin P, Muir AJ, Ferenci P, Flisiak R, George J, Rizzetto M, Shouval D, Sola R, Terg RA, Yoshida EM, Adda N, Bengtsson L, Sankoh AJ, Kieffer TL, George S, Kauffman RS, Zeuzem S, ADVANCE Study Team (2011) Telaprevir for previously untreated chronic hepatitis C virus infection. N Engl J Med 364(25):2405–2416
8. Poordad F, McCone J Jr, Bacon BR, Bruno S, Manns MP, Sulkowski MS, Jacobson IM, Reddy KR, Goodman ZD, Boparai N, DiNubile MJ, Sniukiene V, Brass CA, Albrecht JK, Bronowicki JP, SPRINT-2 (2011) Investigators Boceprevir for untreated chronic HCV genotype 1 infection. N Engl J Med 364(13):1195–1206
9. Available at https://clinicaltrials.gov/ct2/show/NCT01701063?term=telaprevir+and+children&rank=2

10. Available at: https://clinicaltrials.gov/ct2/show/NCT01590225?term=boceprevir+and+children&rank=2
11. Malik S, Dekio F, Wen JW (2014) Liver transplantation in a child with multifocal hepatocellular carcinoma hepatitis C and management of post-transplant viral recurrence using boceprevir. Pediatr Transplant 18(2):E64–E68
12. Feld JJ, Kowdley KV, Coakley E et al (2014) Treatment of HCV with ABT-450/r-ombitasvir and dasabuvir with ribavirin. N Engl J Med 370:1594–1603
13. Sulkowski MS, Gardiner DF, Rodriguez-Torres M et al (2014) Daclatasvir plus sofosbuvir for previously treated or untreated chronic HCV infection. N Engl J Med 370:211–221
14. Lawitz E, Poordad FF, Pang PS et al (2014) Sofosbuvir and ledipasvir fixed dose combination with and without ribavirin in treatment-naive and previously treated patients with genotype 1 hepatitis C virus infection (LONESTAR): an open-label, randomised, phase 2 trial. Lancet 383:515–523
15. Lawitz E, Gane E, Pearlman B et al (2015) Efficacy and safety of 12 weeks versus 18 weeks of treatment with grazoprevir (MK-5172) and elbasvir (MK-8742) with or without ribavirin for hepatitis C virus genotype 1 infection in previously untreated patients with cirrhosis and patients with previous null response with or without cirrhosis (CWORTHY): a randomised, open-label phase 2 trial. Lancet 385:1075–1086
16. Foster GR, Afdhal N, Roberts SK, Bräu N, Gane EJ, Pianko S, Lawitz E, Thompson A, Shiffman ML, Cooper C, Towner WJ, Conway B, Ruane P, Bourlière M, Asselah T, Berg T, Zeuzem S, Rosenberg W, Agarwal K, Stedman CA, Mo H, Dvory-Sobol H, Han L, Wang J, McNally J, Osinusi A, Brainard DM, JG MH, Mazzotta F, Tran TT, Gordon SC, Patel K, Reau N, Mangia A, Sulkowski M, ASTRAL-2 Investigators, ASTRAL-3 Investigators (2015, Dec 31) Sofosbuvir and Velpatasvir for HCV Genotype 2 and 3 Infection. N Engl J Med 373(27):2608–2617
17. Lagging M, Wejstål R, Norkrans G, Karlström O, Aleman S, Weiland O, Castedal M, Westin J, the Swedish Consensus Group (2017) Treatment of hepatitis C virus infection: updated Sweish guidelines 2016. Infect Dis 49(8):561–575
18. European Association for the Study of the Liver (2017) EASL recommendations on treatment of hepatitis C 2016. J Hepatol 66:153–194
19. American Association for the Study of Liver Diseases and Infectious Diseases Society of America. Recommendations for testing, managing, and treating hepatitis C. Available at: http://www.hcvguidelines.org/
20. Thomas P, Santiago T, Dallas MH (2016) Treatment of hepatitis C in a pediatric patient using simeprevir and sofosbuvir immediately after an umbilical cord blood transplantation. Bone Marrow Transplant 51:735–737
21. Fischler B, Priftakis P, Sundin M (2016) Sofosbuvir and Simeprevir treatment of a stem cell transplanted teenager with chronic hepatitis C infection. Pediatr Infect Dis J 35:708–710
22. Smith SK, Rosenthal P (2016) Clearance of hepatitis C virus after fixed-dose combination Ledipasvir/Sofosbuvir in an adolescent female with decompensated cirrhosis. J Pediatr Gastroenterol Nutr 63(5):516–517
23. Huysentruyt K, Stephenne X, Varma S, Scheers I, Leclercq G, Smets F, Sokal E (2017) Sofosbuvir/ledipasvir and ribavirin tolerability and efficacy in pediatric liver transplant recipients. Liver Transpl 23(4):552–553
24. Balistreri WF, Murray KF, Rosenthal P, Bansal S, Chuan-Hao L, Kersey K, Massetto B, Zhu Y, Kanwar B, German P, Svarovskaia E, Brainard DM, Wen J, Gonzalez-Peralta RP, Jonas MM, Schwarz K (2017) The safety and effectiveness of Ledipasvir-Sofosbuvir in adolescents 12 to 17 years old with hepatitis C virus genotype 1 infection. Hepatology 66(2):371–378
25. Available at: https://clinicaltrials.gov/ct2/show/NCT02249182?term=harvoni+and+children&rank=1
26. Available at: https://clinicaltrials.gov/ct2/show/NCT02486406?term=paritaprevir+and+children&rank=1

13 Hepatitis D

Keisha R. Barton and Daniel H. Leung

Abstract

Hepatitis D virus (HDV), or delta virus, is a single-stranded circular RNA virus that is dependent on hepatitis B virus (HBV) surface antigen (HBsAg) for transmission. It is highly pathogenic with a high incidence of progression to cirrhosis and other long-term complications including death. It affects 15–20 million people worldwide despite universal HBV vaccination and due to lack of testing and under-recognition. The standard therapy for treatment is suboptimal in adults, and there are no currently approved treatment modalities for children. Novel research-based therapies including prenylation inhibitors, viral entry inhibitors, and nucleic acid inhibitors have potential to reduce disease morbidity and mortality.

13.1 Introduction/Historical Context

Hepatitis D virus (HDV), or delta virus, is a single-stranded circular RNA virus that is dependent on hepatitis B virus (HBV) surface antigen (HBsAg) for transmission [1]. It is also the smallest known virus to infect humans. Despite this, it remains highly pathogenic with a high incidence of long-term complications and sequelae, most importantly evolution to cirrhosis [2]. As its prevalence in the United States remains relatively low, HDV continues to raise therapeutic perplexities given the lack of recognition and testing which often leads to a delay in treatment initiation. HDV in children is even more of a challenge as there have been few studies/trials to date on the efficacy of current therapies in the pediatric population. Our goals in this chapter will be to review the diagnosis and prevention of significant disease in children, discuss the newly developing therapies for HDV, and examine some future directions for pediatric HDV.

The "incidental" discovery of HDV was made by an Italian physician Dr. Mario Rizzetto in 1977. While he was examining liver biopsies of HBsAg-positive patients, Dr. Rizzetto found a unique antigen that was distinct from surface or core antigens [1]. Specifically, under electron microscopy, this new antigen was found exclusively in the hepatic nuclei of the liver biopsies from HBsAg-positive patients who strangely lacked any ultrastructural evidence of HB core particles. This novel antigen was consistently absent in patients with HBsAg seronegativity, with inactive chronic carriers, and with acute self-limiting hepatitis or those who were asymptomatic. Further, it was most prevalent in patients

K. R. Barton · D. H. Leung (✉)
Division of Pediatric Gastroenterology, Hepatology, and Nutrition, Texas Children's Hospital, Department of Pediatrics, Baylor College of Medicine, Houston, TX, USA
e-mail: dhleung@texaschildrens.org

M.-H. Chang, K. B. Schwarz (eds.), *Viral Hepatitis in Children*,
https://doi.org/10.1007/978-981-13-0050-9_13

who were immunosuppressed (i.e., receiving medications such as steroids or azathioprine) and/or had a more disrupted histological liver architecture. This prompted the consideration of what is now known as HDV as a virus dependent on HBsAg and specifically more common in patients with chronic persistent hepatitis or inactive cirrhosis [1]. At that time, Rizzetto described the "nature of the new antigen [as] obscure" and although there have been some advances; this statement still rings true today, particularly in the pediatric population.

13.2 Epidemiology

Since its discovery in the late 1970s, it has been well established that the highest prevalence of HDV is in regions of lower socioeconomic status in countries on the continents of Africa and South America, Turkey, Italy, and Russia (Fig. 13.1) [2]. In the first decade after its reporting (1980s), there was a worldwide prevalence of chronic HDV in 15–20 million individuals (equates to roughly 5% of the estimated 350 million chronic HBV carriers). Although the prevalence of chronic HBV infection is high in Southeast Asia (specifically China), the previously reported rate of HDV is low ~0.8–1.2% [small-scale study of only ~1500 patients] [3]. The true prevalence is actually unknown and even underestimated as it is confounded by limited testing for HDV in China and lack of large-scale studies. The lack of testing appears to have stemmed from a misguided belief that HDV was unlikely to be relevant [4]. In a retrospective study of nearly 11,000 patients who were HBsAg positive for 6 months in Guangdong, China, 30% did not undergo testing for HDV [4]. Of the remaining 8151 treatment-naïve patients who were screened with anti-HDV IgM, the reported prevalence rate was 6.5% (nearly 6x the prevalence rate of the previous study). Further large-scale studies are necessary to evaluate the true prevalence of HDV infection in China and Southeast Asia.

In the United States, the reported prevalence of HDV greatly varies based on risk factors, ranging from 3.8% of blood donors, 15% of those who are HIV coinfected, 30% of developmentally disabled individuals with chronic HBV, and

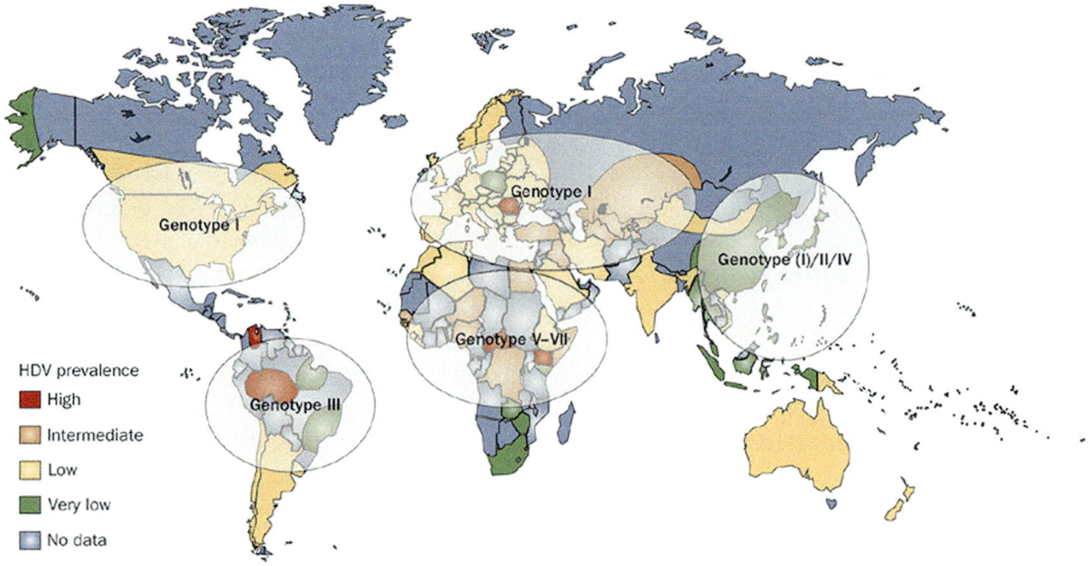

Fig. 13.1 Global epidemiology of HDV infection according to viral genotype. HDV genotype 1 is the most frequent genotype and is distributed throughout the world, especially in Europe, the Middle East, North America, and North Africa. By contrast, HDV genotype 2 is observed in the Far East, and HDV genotype 3 is seen exclusively in the northern part of South America. Abbreviation: *HDV* hepatitis D virus. (Reproduced with permission from Ref. [5])

Springer Nature remains neutral with regard to jurisdictional claims in published maps and institutional affiliations

67% of injection drug users [5, 6]. While hepatitis B vaccine was licensed for use in the United States in 1982, use of the HBV vaccine initially had little impact on HBV incidence, which actually increased in the early 1980s. In June 1982, the Advisory Committee on Immunization Practices (ACIP) made initial vaccination recommendations only for high-risk groups (i.e., men who have sex with men, injection drug users, and heterosexual individuals with multiple partners). Unfortunately, there were low vaccination rates in these groups for multiple reasons, including affordability and both patient and provider naiveté in identifying high-risk behavior [7]. However, in the late 1980s, there was a discrete reduction in the United States when fewer cases were reported specifically among the aforementioned high-risk groups. In these groups, the decline in incidence was likely related to behavioral changes including use of disposable needles, a successful campaign for protection against sexually transmitted diseases, and improved safety procedures against blood-borne illnesses [6]. This was partially in response to the very public epidemic of acquired immunodeficiency syndrome (AIDS) rather than vaccine use. By the 1990s, what followed were anecdotal reports of decreased prevalence of HDV infection [8], most likely due to the widespread use of HBV vaccine in response to regulations issued by the Occupational Safety and Health Administration (OSHA). However this is limited by little to no epidemiologic studies of HDV prevalence in the United States as there have not been validated Centers for Disease Control and Prevention (CDC) or World Health Organization (WHO) reports to substantiate. The implementation of routine screening of HBsAg in pregnant mothers in 1988, routine infant and childhood catch-up HBV vaccination in 1991, and CDC recommendations for adolescent HBV vaccination in 1997 [9] further amplified the reduction of HBV infection and inherently HDV as well. This subsequently led to a decrease in evaluation and vigilance for the presence of HDV and promoted a false sense of security that the virus was near eradication [10].

13.3 Viral Characteristics

The HDV virion contains the smallest genetic material of any animal virus, 1.7 kilobase (kb) pairs compared to 3.2 kb and 9.6 kb in HBV and HCV, respectively. However, it is still considered a large particle (36 nanometers) [9–11] and is comprised of HDV antigen (HDAg) and HDV RNA. Currently, there are two known types of HDV antigens—small and large. The function of the small HDAg (S-HDAg) "promotes" HDV RNA synthesis, while in contrast, the large HDAg (L-HDAg) "inhibits" HDV RNA synthesis but remains essential for the assembly of new viral particles [10]. S-HDAg and L-HDAg have different posttranslational modification processes. S-HDAg undergoes phosphorylation at both the serine and threonine residues, while L-HDAg only undergoes phosphorylation at the serine residue. Hong and Chen found that phosphorylation at serine −177 on S-HDAg is critical for its interaction with RNA polymerase and the promotion of RNA synthesis [12]. Meanwhile, L-HDAg undergoes isoprenylation (addition of a hydrophobic isoprenoid group to a protein to facilitate attachment to cell membranes) which results in farnesylation (a process by which a cysteine residue in the C-terminal region of a protein is post-translationally modified with an isoprenoid lipid, resulting in increased affinity of the protein for the membrane) of cysteine-211. This modification inhibits replication but importantly facilitates assembly by directly enforcing binding between L-HDAg and HBV exterior proteins [13]. The sodium taurocholate cotransporting polypeptide (NCTP) receptor is the first door of entry for HDV into the hepatocyte. HDV (enveloped by HBV) acts as a ligand to the NCTP receptor and endocytosis occurs. HDV itself does not have its own enzymes (i.e., polymerases or proteases) that aid in viral replication, and therefore it relies solely on host polymerases.

There are at least eight genotypes of HDV (no known subtypes), and they have a geographic-specific predilection (Fig. 13.1). Genotype 1 is the most prevalent worldwide and also the most common HDV genotype found in the United

States. It is also the most highly pathogenic. In a prospective Taiwanese study, those with HDV genotype 1 superinfection had a lower biochemical remission rate and increased negative outcomes including higher rate of progression to cirrhosis, development of hepatocellular carcinoma, and increased mortality [10]. Genotype 2 is seen more commonly in Southeast Asia, whereas genotype 3 is exclusively reported in the northern aspect of South America [14]. The remaining genotypes, 4–8, are primarily found in patients living in Africa.

13.4 Pathogenesis

There are two forms of interaction between HBV and HDV—coinfection and superinfection. It is critical to distinguish between these two as both the management and prognosis differ significantly.

Coinfection signifies an acute HBV infection and an acute HDV infection that occur simultaneously (Fig. 13.2). Appearance of both serum HBsAg and HDAg is accompanied by a rise in alanine aminotransferase (ALT) followed

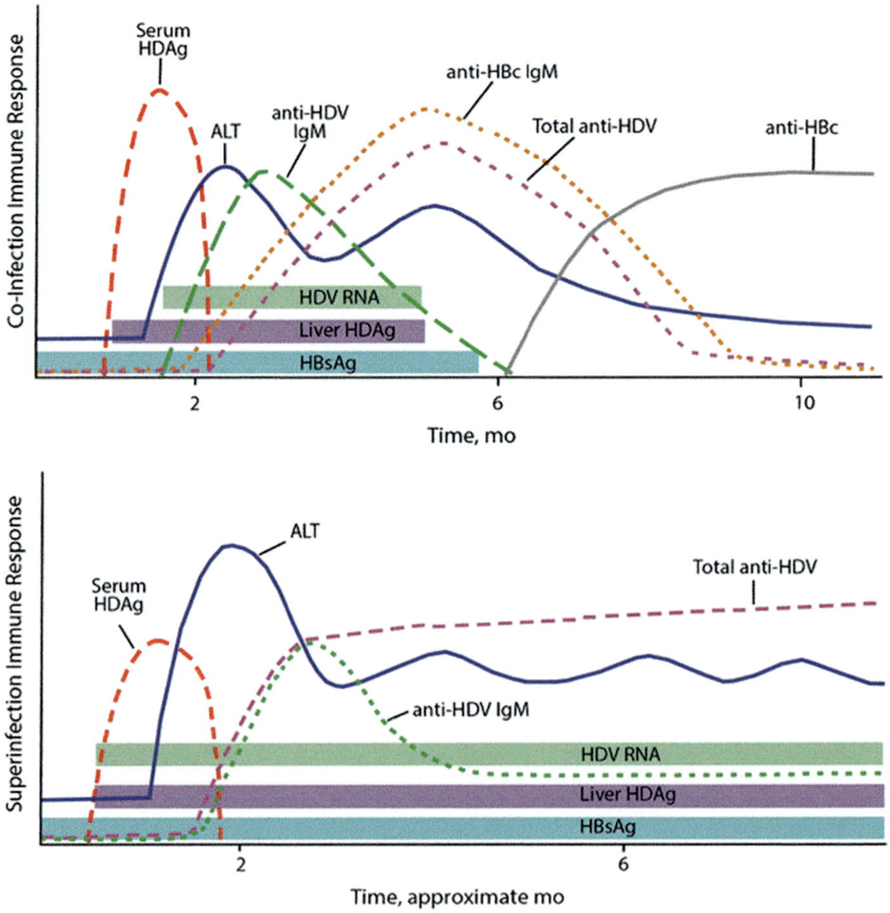

Fig. 13.2 Typical serological course of HBV-HDV coinfection (top) and HBV-HDV superinfection (bottom). *ALT* alanine transaminase, *anti-HDV* HDV antibody, *HBc* hepatitis B core antibody, *HBsAg* hepatitis B virus surface antigen, *HBV* hepatitis B virus, *HDV* hepatitis D virus, *HDAg* hepatitis delta antigen, *IgM* immunoglobulin M. (Reproduced with permission from Ref. [14])

by HDV viremia. There is classically a double peak in ALT rise, initially due to HBV replication and secondarily triggered by HDV replication [6]. Anti-HDV IgM (marker of disease activity) quickly appears. Detection of anti-HDV IgM is often short-lived, and subsequent seroconversion to anti-HDV IgG occurs over time and remains positive in serum long after the acute infection has cleared [15]. HBV infection is detected with anti-HBc IgM and HBV viremia [6]. In late stages of coinfection, HBV replication is suppressed (in contrast to HBV monoinfection); however significant liver disease (compensated cirrhosis, chronic active liver disease) may still progress. This suggests that HDV is actively involved in the advancement of liver disease [15]. In adults, HBV/HDV coinfection generally has a benign, self-limited course though it rarely can be associated with a severe acute hepatitis leading to fulminant hepatitis [15]. About 20% of patients with coinfection have progression to cirrhosis [16]. It is important to note that HBV/HDV coinfection presents similarly to acute HBV infection and a high index of suspicion is necessary to make an accurate diagnosis.

In contrast, superinfection occurs in patients with established chronic HBV who subsequently become infected with HDV. Superinfection is the more common avenue of acquiring HDV. Similar to coinfection, serologies from superinfected patients also demonstrate anti-HDV IgM but have anti-HBc IgG only, not IgM [8] (Fig. 13.2). Unfortunately, there are no differentiating risk factors between superinfection and coinfection. In a 12-year case-control Italian study conducted by Mele et al., independent risk factors for HDV infection were elucidated. A total of 344 patients were diagnosed with acute HDV infection with the majority being coinfection (63%) despite universal HBV vaccination [17]. Independent risk factors including intravenous drug use, hospitalization, receipt of beauty treatments (i.e., tattooing, piercings, manicures, and barber shop shavings), dental therapy, two or more sexual partners in the past year, and cohabitation with an intravenous drug user were shown to have odds ratios greater than 1 [compared to HAV controls] [17]. There was no significant association with gender or age. In a study evaluating HIV-/HBV-coinfected patients in Iran, differing risk factors were identified. Of the 178 HIV-/HBV-coinfected patients, 19% were found to be HDV Ab positive. Prior history of blood transfusion and prison history represented the most significant risk factors in this group. There was no association with unsafe sexual practice, injection drug abuse, age, or marital status. These two studies illustrate that risk factors can be geographically and population dependent and that additional studies need to be conducted in order to assess risk factors by region/country [18].

There is limited understanding about the exact pathogenesis of HBV/HDV infection, let alone the histologic and immunologic differences between superinfection and coinfection. Although HDV was initially thought to be directly toxic to hepatocytes based on in vitro [19] and human studies [20], it is now known that majority of the damage from HDV is secondary to cytotoxic T lymphocytes [21]. Theories regarding the much more severe course of superinfection as compared to coinfection are postulated to have a correlation with the host immune system. In superinfection, an immunotolerant host or HBV carrier may not functionally be able to recognize or clear their infection, whereas in HDV coinfection, a theoretically normal host with preserved immunologic function can successfully clear the virus [22]. Another theory is the presence of perforin-positive CD4 T cells implicated to play a role in the severity of HIV-infected patients. CD4 T cells are vital to the immune response and integral in stimulating antigen- presenting cells (APC) and cytokine release. Recent studies have shown there are increased numbers of perforin-positive CD4 T cells in patients with HDV compared with HBV or HCV alone [23]. It is clear that further studies regarding the immunology (both innate and adaptive immune systems) of HDV are highly necessary to further elucidate this topic.

Fulminant liver failure, often with massive necrosis, occurs in 5% of superinfected individuals compared to only ~1% of coinfected patients [13]. Superinfection also leads to chronic HDV infection at a significantly high rate. In fact,

90% of patients with HBV/HDV superinfection result in chronic HDV, and unfortunately, 70% proceed to cirrhosis within 5–10 years of diagnosis [24] and experience earlier decompensation, hepatocellular carcinoma (HCC), and a lower 5-year survival rate [14, 25, 26]. In a natural history study of compensated cirrhosis secondary to HDV superinfection in 166 Romanian patients [27], the median time to first decompensation (ascites, jaundice, portal hypertension, gastrointestinal bleeding, HCC, etc.) after diagnosis of compensated cirrhosis was less than 2 years (21 ± 19 months). Further, the median survival was less than 5 years (58.3 months). A multicenter European study similarly inquired about the morbidity and mortality of HDV in compensated cirrhosis. In this study, there was a threefold increase in HCC and a twofold increase in mortality relative to cirrhotics that were HDV negative [28]. In a multicenter Italian natural history study, the estimated liver transplant-free survival rate was 49% at 5 years and 40% at 10 years for patients with HBV/HDV-related cirrhosis ($p < 0.01$) [29]. These examples illustrate the aggressive nature of HDV infection with regard to decompensation, morbidity, and mortality. With regard to HCC risk, Abbas et al. identified features such as decreased liver size, more severe portal hypertension, and earlier TNM classification (global system for classifying the extent of spread of cancer) were more common with HDV infection-associated cirrhosis compared to HBV alone. This may suggest independent risk factors for HCC with HDV infection compared to HBV monoinfection [30].

13.5 Diagnosis, Screening, and Prevention

13.5.1 Diagnosis

It is strongly recommended that all adult patients with chronic HBV undergo routine screening for HDV given its propensity to be very aggressive [14]. Common risk factors for HDV in adults include intravenous drug use or shared needles, living in an endemic area, men who have sex with men, and patients that undergo hemodialysis [8]. These risk factors, notably IV exposure, have implications in HDV among children and adolescents. In Pakistani children, frequent use of intravenous drips for therapeutic purposes at hospitals was observed more in the HDV group than HBV monoinfected [31]. There is limited literature on perinatal or vertical HDV transmission. A study of 185 Saudi pregnant women who were HBsAg carriers found that 9.7% were also anti-HDV positive. However, follow-up of 17 infants born to anti-HDV-positive mothers revealed that none developed HDV infection [32]. This suggests that vertical transmission is relatively uncommon, which is important to note in the pediatric population.

Similar to other hepatitides, the diagnosis of HDV is made serologically with the presence of HDV antigen and anti-HDV antibodies in combination with HBV serologies +/− HDV RNA quantitative PCR [25] (Table 13.1). Within 2 months following HDV infection, >90% of patients will develop HDV antibodies [14]. In the United States, antibody (anti-HDV IgM and IgG) and HDV RNA qualitative PCR testing are the major diagnostic tests, although HDV RNA quantitative PCR testing has recently become available (ARUP Laboratories, FDA approval not required), though not as mainstream as in Europe. Specimens can also be sent to the Centers for Disease Control and Prevention if there is a high suspicion for HDV [14].

Recently a one-step real-time PCR for HDV RNA for all eight genotypes was developed [33]. This advancement may be most helpful for disease monitoring with treatment because serum viral load does not appear to correlate to disease activity or severity [34]. In addition, given variability of the genome sequence, the HDV RNA PCR may be negative if inadequate primers are used [14]. Therefore HDV IgM should always be tested in patients with chronic HBV even if the HDV viral load is negative. Genotyping is not widely available, but considering there are prognostic implications depending on genotype, this may be a future consideration for routine testing.

After HDV infection is confirmed in adults, liver biopsy is routinely recommended to assess

Table 13.1 Interpretation of HepB and HepD serologic and nucleic acid testing

HBV									
HBsAg	Presence indicates that an individual has HBV infection and is infectious. Loss suggests cure of HBV								
Anti-HBc, total	Presence indicates past or present HBV infection								
Anti-HBc, IgM	Presence usually indicates HBV infection within the preceding 4–6 months (acute infection)								
HBeAg	Presence indicates active viral replication and high infectivity. Absence may indicate prior or pending seroconversion. However loss of HBeAg in the setting of detectable virus indicates a mutation in the precore or core promotor regions								
Anti-HBe	Presence indicates resolving infection (seroconversion) or response to therapy								
Anti-HBs	Presence indicates recovery and immunity against HBV infection or history of immunization								
HBV DNA	Presence indicates HBV infection								
HDV									
Anti-HDV, total	Presence coincident with HBsAg indicates past or present HBV/HDV coinfection (eventual loss) or superinfection (persistence)								
Anti-HDV IgM	Presence coincident with HBsAg indicates past or present HBV/HDV coinfection or superinfection. Negative amidst anti-HDV total indicates resolved infection								
HDV RNA	Presence indicates active infection								
Hepatitis virus	Anti-HAV IgM	HBsAg	HBV DNA	Anti-HBc IgM	Anti-HBc total	Total HCV ab	HCV RNA	Anti-HDV total	HDV RNA
Acute HBV	–	+	+	+	–	–	–	–	–
Acute HBV with HDV coinfection	–	+	+	+	–	–	–	+	+
Acute HBV with HDV superinfection	–	+	+	–	–	–	–	+	+

Reproduced with permission from Ref. [14]

HAV hepatitis A virus, *HBc* hepatitis B core, *anti-HBc* hepatitis B core antibody, *anti-HBe* hepatitis B e antibody, *anti-HBs* hepatitis B surface antibody, *HBsAg* hepatitis B virus surface antigen, *HBV* hepatitis B virus, *HCV* hepatitis C virus, *HDV* hepatitis D virus, *IgM* immunoglobulin M (Adapted from Leung et al. 2015).

for degree of inflammation and fibrosis. As previously mentioned, this recommendation stems from literature illustrating that HDV- infected patients progress to cirrhosis more rapidly [35]. There are no current pediatric series to offer recommendations for liver biopsy timing. In a pediatric patient with known HBV/HDV infection with a persistently elevated ALT>100 U/L for 6 months and with low HBV DNA (<2000 IU/mL = inactive chronic carrier), strong consideration for liver biopsy should be made to guide clinical management (i.e., aggressive HBV therapy, primary HDV treatment, or liver transplant).

13.5.2 Screening for Other Diseases

Routine screening for hepatitis C virus (HCV) and human immunodeficiency virus (HIV) is recommended because of the parallel routes of transmission (i.e., intravenous drug use and high-risk sexual activity). Interestingly, this also parallels the geographic risk of transmission. A study in Central Europe showed that approximately one-third of the HDV-infected patients tested positively for HCV [36]. In studies in Spain, 5% of HIV-infected patients had multiple hepatitides with hepatitis B, C, and D being the most common, respectively, in that order [37]. In addition, HIV is an independent risk factor for liver disease for a variety of reasons. As discussed by Castellares et al. in a large cohort of >2000 HIV+ patients, there is a higher incidence of liver fibrosis as measured by transient elastometry (Fibroscan®). Potential etiologies of liver fibrosis other than caused by hepatitides included antiretroviral therapy toxicity and higher incidence of alcohol abuse in patients with chronic hepatitis [38]. It has been proposed that the mitochondrial toxicity of nucleoside analogue and glucose or lipid abnormalities associated with protease inhibitors may produce and/or enhance fibrosis [38].

An association with autoimmunity has been described with chronic HDV. In particular, an elevation of LKM-3 autoantibodies (liver/kidney/muscle 3), a marker suggestive of autoimmune hepatitis (AIH), has been shown. In an Italian study, 13% of patients with chronic HDV were positive for LKM-3 autoantibodies, whereas there was no evidence of autoantibodies in HBV-monoinfected patients [39]. This suggests that HDV itself may be antigenic creating an antibody response. It is difficult to assess whether this antibody response is secondary to autoimmunity or a response to viral infection. Of note, the majority of patients in this multicenter study were male, arguing against autoimmunity given that AIH usually have a female predominance. In a subsequent study by Strassburg et al., a difference in LKM-3 titers was found in German patients with chronic HDV and AIH. Patients with AIH had higher titers than patients with chronic HDV [40]. A Grecian study aimed to study the characteristics with concomitant viral hepatitis (HBV, HBV/HBD, or HCV) and autoimmune hepatitis. The diagnosis of autoimmune hepatitis was based on the 2008 criteria of the International Autoimmune Hepatitis Group (IAIHG) [41]. Their conclusions were that combined viral hepatitis and autoimmune disease were difficult to recognize (similar clinical features and histology) and treatment modalities were confounding. Patients with viral hepatitis were often treated with interferon which could induce autoimmune hepatitis, and those with autoimmune hepatitis were often treated with immunosuppression which could enhance viral replication in patients with viral hepatitis [42]. Further studies need to be implemented to determine clinical significance and whether disease severity is intensified in patients with a potential HDV/AIH overlap syndrome or if therapies including azathioprine, mycophenolate, or steroids are beneficial.

13.5.3 Prevention

Vaccination against hepatitis B is an effective way to prevent hepatitis D infection as hepatitis B surface antigen represents the critical component required for the entry of hepatitis D into hepatocytes. By virtue of its seroprotection against HBV, hepatitis B immunization can only prevent hepatitis D coinfection, but not superinfection. HDV superinfection requires a host with established chronic HBV infection, so vaccination against HBV would be futile. In the last decade, there have been numerous yet unsuccessful attempts to develop a much needed hepatitis D vaccine. The woodchuck has been used a model for testing as it can be chronically infected with woodchuck hepatitis virus (WHV) and then superinfected with HDV. The clinical course is similar to patients with HBV/HDV superinfection. The specific HDV proteins, small [HDAg p24] and large [HDAg p27], have been investigated to develop a vaccine. In initial studies, there was an antibody response but yet no protection from superinfection [43]. This is largely due to the inability to develop a specific and sustained CD8 T cell response to HDV [44]. New strategies for vaccine development must be proposed and tested.

13.6 Treatment

Treatment, specifically eradication of HDV, has proven to be challenging over the years. The primary outcome of treatment is complete suppression of HDV RNA replication. This clinical remission is generally associated with normalization of aminotransferases and histologic recovery [45]. Ideally, eradication of hepatitis B with antiviral therapies directed at this virus would eliminate hepatitis D. However, eradication of hepatitis B from the reservoir of HBV cccDNA (covalently closed circular DNA) has proven to be challenging and may also not resolve a superinfection. Directed hepatitis D therapies must be explored.

Standard of care in the 1980s and 1990s was recombinant or natural interferon-alpha (IFNα) given thrice weekly for 48 weeks. The mechanism of action of IFN is unclear although it is theorized that it initiates an inhibitory effect on HBV and/or has immune system modulating effects [46]. These treatments ameliorated elevated alanine aminotransferases (ALT) in less than half of cases (~20–50%), but unfortunately even these effects were generally transient [45]. In an Italian study, a cohort of 61 HDV patients that were randomized to either interferon-alpha treatment or no treatment for 12 months, there was histologic improvement in patients that received IFN with decreased portal inflammation (57% vs 36%) and declining ALT levels in the treatment group. However, relapse occurred in 87.5% of patients after cessation of therapy [47].

Given these mediocre results, further studies were conducted to illuminate the possibility of improved outcomes with higher dosing and duration of therapy. In a small cohort of 36 patients, there was a suggestion that higher doses (i.e., nine million units vs three million) were beneficial and resulted in improved long-term outcomes, including long-term survival, ALT normalization (71% vs 29%), undetectable HDV (50% vs 21%), and improvement in hepatic fibrosis score [48, 49]. Unfortunately, nearly all patients with detectable HDV RNA rebounded after cessation of treatment.

13.6.1 Pegylated Interferon-Alpha

Currently, the first line of treatment against HDV is pegylated interferon (PEG-IFNα). Its use leads to undetectable serum HDV RNA in only 25–40% of cases after 48 weeks of treatment [50]. Standard IFN has a relatively short half-life (4–5 h) which requires thrice weekly dosing. Pegylation is a modification process that covalently conjugates polyethylene glycol (PEG), a non-immunogenic polymer, to a specific molecule (i.e., drug, protein, etc.). This process changes the innate properties of the molecule resulting in improved drug solubility and decreased immunogenicity [51]. There are two forms of PEG-IFNα, 2a and 2b. Although in vitro studies revealed greater potency of 2b compared to 2a, in vivo studies show no difference in activity [51].

PEG-IFNα is now the preferred treatment in comparison to natural IFNα because of a longer half-life, which allows for weekly dosing. The standard of care for chronic HDV treatment in adults is subcutaneous PEG-IFNα weekly at a dose of 1.5 MU/kg. As with previous studies using natural IFNα, there is also suggestion that longer PEG-IFNα therapy may be superior. In a study conducted by Niro et al. using PEG-IFNα-2b in a small cohort of 38 patients, longer courses of treatment (72 weeks) resulted in sustained HDV negativity in 20% of patients with chronic HDV [52]. In addition, there was a study arm that concomitantly used ribavirin with no effected on sustained viral response.

PEG-IFNα therapy is not currently FDA approved for use in children. Data for length of therapy and efficacy are lacking in pediatric cases. In addition there is no consensus recommendation for indications for HDV treatment, dosing or timing of treatment. Our center's current practice is finite treatment for 48 weeks [14]. Through literature review and site-specific indications, we recommend treatment if there is significant fibrosis on liver biopsy (≥F2 Metavir) or notable portal inflammation accompanied with liver transaminases >250 U/L despite successful suppression of HBV viral load. Although there are not targeted studies, in our opinion, patients with persistent HDV RNA serum positivity, elevated ALT, and anti-HDV IgM are unlikely to respond to further treatment up to 72 weeks or will relapse following cessation of treatment.

13.6.2 HBV Polymerase Inhibitors

Hepatitis B polymerase inhibitors, or nucleos(t)ide analogs (NA), such as adefovir, lamivudine, tenofovir, and entecavir target HBV replication. However, for long-term consideration, tenofovir and entecavir have the lowest resistance rates at 0% and 1.6% [53, 54]. In patients infected with HDV in conjunction with advanced liver disease,

NA are often used to suppress HBV replication [55]. Given their inability to completely eradicate HBV, it is not surprising that have no significant impact on HDV RNA although they may have theoretical benefit. In the Hep-Net International Delta Hepatitis Interventional Trial (HIDIT-1), 90 adult HDV patients were randomized to receive either 180 mcg of PEG-IFNα2a weekly plus either 10 mg of adefovir or placebo daily or 10 mg of adefovir dipivoxil alone for 48 weeks. Combination therapy had no advantages of reducing serum HBV DNA or HDV RNA [56]. One 2016 opinion paper by Wranke and Wedemeyer proposes that anti-HBV therapy be initiated if HBV DNA levels are persistently >2000 IU/ml [57] suggestive of either HBV reactivation or immune clearance.

13.7 Novel Treatments/Future Therapies

New therapies for HDV eradication are on the horizon including drugs that work to directly inhibit the viral lifecycle. As described previously, the sodium taurocholate cotransporting polypeptide (NCTP) receptor is the first door of entry for HDV into the hepatocyte and is a therapeutic target. Host RNA polymerases replicate HDV RNA that subsequently encodes the large protein L-HDAg (large hepatitis D antigen). Viral assembly requires the critical interaction between L-HDAg and HBsAg [58]. In this step, there is lipid modification of the L-HDAg, which is required for particle formulation, and this step is known as prenylation. Prenylation involves a prenyl lipid (farnesyl or geranyl) that is covalently bonded to a cysteine within a specific motif encoded within the carboxyl terminus [59]. Interestingly, L-HDAg directs the addition of farnesyl, which represents another site for viral disruption. Innovative therapies for HDV have been constructed to inhibit many of these critical steps in viral assembly and are summarized below.

13.7.1 Entry Inhibitors

Myrcludex B is a new drug that can block the uptake of HDV at the level of the sodium taurocholate cotransporting polypeptide (NTCP) liver receptor [60, 61]. Work using both in vitro and in vivo models (mouse) has validated this mechanism by demonstrating reduced HBV and HDV virus uptake into hepatocytes after administration of the drug [62]. Myrcludex B is derived from the N-terminal domain of the large HBV surface protein (myristoylated lipopeptide contains 47 amino acids of the pre-S1 domain of L-HBsAg). Its mechanism of antiviral action is via specific inactivation via binding of the myristoylated domain to NTCP. This synthetic homologous peptide competes for the binding with the natural HBsAg and results in the restriction of virion uptake in the cell [63]. Phase II clinical trials are ongoing regarding the potential from Myrcludex B in combination with PEG-IFNα [64]. Preliminary results revealed negative HDV RNA after 24 weeks in five out of seven patients, but a rebound of virus was detected after Myrcludex B was discontinued [64]. There are ongoing studies evaluating the potential user of higher doses of Myrcludex B in addition to longer combinations with PEG-IFNα.

13.7.2 Prenylation Inhibitors

Farnesylation inhibitors prevent the protein farnesyltransferase which is vital in the prenylation process. If prenylation does not occur, then viral assembly and secretion are halted. Prenylation inhibitors have also been confirmed in in vitro and in vivo studies [65]. A recent National Institute of Health (NIH) phase IIa double-blinded randomized control trial studied the effectiveness of lonafarnib, an oral farnesyltransferase inhibitor. This was the first study investigating a prenylation inhibitor in HDV infection. There were three groups: [1] subjects receiving lonafarnib 100 mg twice daily, [2] subjects receiving lonafarnib 200 mg twice daily, and [3] subjects receiving placebo [66]. HDV RNA was decreased in both treatment groups and was associated with the plasma concentration of lonafarnib. HBV DNA increased with HDV RNA decrease. HDV RNA returned to baseline when treatment was discontinued.

13.7.3 Nucleic Acid Polymers

Nucleic acid polymer (NAP) is a potential therapy that aims to block the release of HBsAg particles. The NAPs REP 2055 and REP 2139-Ca showed a decline in HBsAg and HBV DNA and the development of anti-HBs antibodies when administered to patients with solitary HBV infection [67]. Increased HDV load was noted in all patients after discontinuation of the NAP. In a recent oral presentation by Bazinet et al. presented at the 50th Annual Meeting of the European Association for the Study of the Liver, HDV RNA was reduced in all patients after 15 weeks of treatment with a NAP. The long-term follow-up with REP 2139-Ca/PEG-IFNa-2a combination therapy is still under study [68].

13.7.4 Role of Transplantation

In cases of decompensated liver failure and failed medical therapy, liver transplantation becomes the only form of therapy and is lifesaving. Given the aggressive and rapid progression of HDV disease, it may be prudent to evaluate patients for liver transplant during early stages of disease. Following transplantation, vaccination against HBV is warranted for those HBV negative to prevent reinfection. The transplanted liver is exposed to HDV during the time of transplantation, and this can affect the hepatocytes. It is purported that HDAg is detectable in the allograft months to years after transplantation [69]. In a prospective European study involving the long-term clinical outcomes following liver transplantation for hepatitis D, the 5-year survival rate was estimated at88%, much greater than for hepatitis B alone [70]. Successful liver transplantation for HDV is promising if HBV/HDV reinfection does not occur [69]. In patients who received continuous passive anti-HB immunoprophylaxis (all but 4), 89.7% remained HBV negative [70].

13.8 Summary

Hepatitis delta virus is a small but deadly RNA virus dependent on hepatitis B for transmission and entry into hepatocytes. It remains extraordinarily pathogenic, but outcomes are vastly different depending on whether there is HBV/HDV coinfection or HDV superinfection in chronically infected HBV patients. Early testing for HDV is strongly recommended in patients from endemic areas along with prevention of HBV with vaccination and consideration of liver biopsy in severe cases. Genotype 1 is the most common worldwide and unfortunately also the most pathogenic. Pegylated interferon-alpha remains the only current therapy (yet not approved in children) for HDV infection but benefits <1/3 of patients. Further studies of new therapies (viral entry inhibitors, prenylation inhibitors, and nucleic acid polymers) are beginning to come onto the horizon as potential future therapies.

References

1. Rizzetto M, Canese M, Arico S (1977) Immunofluorescence detection of a new antigen antibody system (anti-) associated to hepatitis B virus in liver and serum of HBsAg carriers. Gut 18:997–1003
2. Rizzetto M, Ponzetto A, Forzani I (1990) Hepatitis delta virus as a global health problem. Vaccine 8(Suppl):S10–S14
3. Shen L, Gu Y, Sun L et al (2012) Development of a hepatitis delta virus antibody assay for study of the prevalence of HDV among individuals infected with hepatitis B virus in China. J Med Virol 84(3):445–449. https://doi.org/10.1002/jmv.23212
4. Liao B, Zhang F, Lin S et al (2014) Epidemiological, clini- cal and histological characteristics of HBV/HDV co-infection: a retrospective cross-sectional study in Guangdong, China. PLoS One 9(12):e115888. https://doi.org/10.1371/journal.pone.0115888

disease that is indistinguishable from other viruses such as HAV, although in contrast to hepatitis A virus, most HEV infections occur in late childhood or early adulthood [37]. In addition, direct person-to-person transmission of HEV does not appear to be common [34, 35, 38]. HEV seroprevalence ranges from 7.8 to 45% in endemic areas to nearly 100% in some developing countries [33, 39]. Symptomatic HEV attack rates are highest among young adults during epidemics ranging from 3 to 30% and lowest among children at 0.2–10% [40, 41]. Overall HEV prevalence in a community is closely related to socioeconomic level and access to safe drinking water and sanitation [33, 39]. In one report, HEV seroprevalence rate reaches more than 95% in children living in endemic areas by the age of 10 years [42]. HEV is responsible for sporadic cases and epidemic outbreaks of acute hepatitis related to poor hygiene and sanitation in many Asian and African countries [4]. Sporadic cases of HEV infection in industrialized countries are often reported in individuals with a travel history to endemic areas whom are infected by indigenous HEV strains (genotype 1 or 2).

HEV-infected pregnant women are at an increased risk for acute or fulminant liver failure (FHF) and death [40, 41], compared to pregnant women without HEV infection [43]. This clinical predisposition was first reported during HEV genotype 1 outbreaks on the Indian subcontinent and Africa [42, 44]. In contrast, little or no increased morbidity has been reported among pregnant HEV-infected women in other HEV-endemic countries, such as Egypt [36, 43, 45]. That said, a large prospective study from Northern India found that up to 60% of viral hepatitis cases in pregnant women were attributed to HEV infection, with mortality and FHF higher among HEV-infected pregnant mothers (41%) than non-HEV-infected mothers (7%) [43].

Among pregnant women, infection contracted during the third trimester is associated with severe disease, resulting in a mortality rate of 15–25%. Maternal-to-fetal HEV transmission has also been demonstrated, with rates ranging from 23.3% to 50%. In a large prenatal study in India, 28 of 469 pregnant women were positive for HEV RNA; 12 of these women had acute liver disease, and 2 died undelivered. The remaining 16 women had mild disease with full recovery. Of 26 infants born, all were positive for HEV RNA and developed acute infection. The high risk of vertical transmission of HEV infection from mother to infant was investigated and transmission rates of up to 100% were reported. This high transmission rate is not the only important factor for neonatal outcome, and there could have been a selection bias in the study. While many cases with vertical transmission result in high neonatal mortality, in this study those newborn infants who survived had self-limiting disease with short-lasting viremia [42].

In recent years, increasing attention has been directed to cases of HEV infection among individuals in Europe, New Zealand, North America, Japan, and South America with no history of travel to regions endemic for HEV, such as the Indian subcontinent and Africa. These cases have been characterized by genetically distinct subtypes of HEV (genotypes 3 or 4) and considered autochthonous or locally acquired [46–50]. In the absence of fecal-water contamination or epidemic spread, autochthonous infections challenged initial theories regarding HEV transmission, particularly in industrialized settings [51, 52]. Zoonotic reservoirs, particularly swine, were ultimately identified as potential sources of autochthonous infection and the direct zoonotic transmission of HEV through contaminated meat demonstrated in Japan in 2003 [16, 53]. Since that time, HEV genotypes 3 and 4 have been isolated from multiple meat products, including pig liver, deer meat, and pork, with human infections documented secondary to the consumption of insufficiently cooked, HEV-infected foods [52–58].

HEV seroprevalence estimates among industrialized western countries in Europe and North America range from 6% to 21%, with pediatric estimates ranging from 0% to 4.6% [59, 60–62]. In the United States, data from the National Health and Nutrition Evaluation Survey (NHANES, 1998–2004) demonstrated a pediatric HEV seroprevalence of 0.8% among males and 1.1% among females, ages 6–19 years [60]. While most studies to date have focused primarily on adult populations, an increasing number of recent reports have approached the pediatric burden of autochthonous HEV, especially among immunocompromised hosts [59, 63]. This growing recognition of the role of HEV infection among children suggests that autochthonous HEV remains an emerging pathogen in this population.

Globally, HEV genotypes 1 and 3 have also been reported to circulate in the Indian subcontinent and Africa. A recent study in China reported a 15% HEV seroprevalence among children; however, in this region most infections were due to HEV genotypes 1 and 4 [64–66]. Like HAV, the majority of HEV infections in children are asymptomatic [67], and it is likely that this high seroprevalence also represents autochthonous HEV, as opposed to travel-related, or epidemic, infection.

Nosocomial spread has been reported in the pediatric population [68]. Perinatal (including breastfeeding) and parenteral transmission have been rarely reported. Transfusion of blood or blood products has recently been recognized as a mode of transmission for HEV [69, 70]. HEV transfusion-associated transmission was reported in a HEV PCR-positive child following erythrocyte transfusion along with other HEV-infected recipients from an asymptomatic donor [71].

Pediatric solid organ transplant (SOT) recipients are at increased risk for HEV infection, chronic hepatitis, and fulminant liver failure. Among pediatric Canadian liver transplant recipients, HEV seroprevalence was reported to be 15% among those with normal hepatitis tests, compared to 86% for those with abnormal liver enzymes. One case of chronic hepatitis E virus infection was identified within this cohort [72]. In a similar German pediatric serologic study among liver and/or kidney transplants, a lower HEV seroprevalence was reported overall (3.2% in transplant patients versus 7.4% among immunocompetent patients), with 1 case of chronic hepatitis identified among 124 SOT recipients [73].

14.5 Clinical Manifestations of HEV

Among most previously healthy individuals, HEV manifests as a self-limiting, acute, icteric hepatitis with symptoms including jaundice, malaise, anorexia, fever, abdominal pain, hepatomegaly, and arthralgia. The clinical course of HEV is indistinguishable from that of HAV, with the incubation period ranging from 2 to 9 weeks or 15 to 60 days, with a mean of 40 days [9, 59, 74].

Clinical disease is more common among adults than children [9, 59, 74]. The incidence of acute hepatitis with jaundice increases with age. While pregnant women and individuals with chronic liver disease are at increased risk for FHF and death, overall mortality rates associated with HEV are low in the general population, with case fatality rates ranging from 0.1 to 3.0% [75]. Among western industrialized countries, autochthonous HEV infection predominately affects immunocompromised individuals but is clinically indistinguishable from endemic HEV. That said, overall morbidity and mortality are higher, with 8–11% of infected individuals developing fulminant hepatitis and liver failure [43].

Due to mechanisms which remain unclear, infection with HEV genotype 1 results in a high disease attack rate among pregnant women, leading to increased morbidity and fatality rates. The risks of these adverse events escalate with each trimester of pregnancy [18]. This type of HEV infection may lead to FHF, hepatic encephalopathy, disseminated intravascular coagulation, fetal distress, premature deliveries, and death of both the mother and fetus with estimated mortality rates ranging from 30 to 100% [18, 76–78].

Two large reports from India showed HEV or HAV/HEV coinfection to be leading causes of acute liver failure (ALF) and acute on chronic liver disease [79, 80]. However, the prevalence of ALF from HEV infection in children remains unknown in the United States and Europe. The Pediatric ALF (PALF) consortium does not routinely test for evidence of HEV infection in the absence of a travel history to endemic countries. However, locally acquired HEV genotype 3 infection has been demonstrated to be a potential etiology for ALF among both children and adults in other developed countries such as Argentina [74, 81, 82]. Children who develop ALF often have underlying chronic liver disease [79, 80, 83, 84]. While sporadic cases of hepatitis E have been associated with FHF in Japan, HEV remains a rare cause of acute liver failure in Japanese children [85].

Children receiving immunosuppressive therapy following solid organ transplantation or bone marrow transplantation, or for conditions such as rheumatologic disease, nephrotic syndrome, and inflammatory bowel disease, are also at risk for chronic HEV infection and chronic liver disease. The overall prevalence of acute or chronic HEV infection in such immunocompromised children is unknown. HEV genotype 3 infection has been described in patients with hematological disease and in HIV-positive patients with low CD4 counts [86].

Individuals with underlying chronic liver disease can have a poor outcome with mortality approaching 70% [27, 50]. Children receiving immunosuppressive therapy after organ transplantation are at risk for chronic HEV infection [87]. Chronic HEV infection can result in progressive liver fibrosis, cirrhosis, and subsequent liver failure, which occasionally requires liver transplantation [86, 88, 89]. Two children with chronic HEV infection after kidney transplantation were able to clear the virus after reduction in immunosuppressive therapy; otherwise liver cirrhosis could develop as reported in adult cases [90]. Extrahepatic manifestations such as neurological disorders (e.g., Guillain-Barre), acute pancreatitis, severe thrombocytopenia, hemolytic anemia, and hemophagocytic lymphohistiocytosis have been associated with locally acquired acute and chronic HEV genotype 3 infection both in adults and children [91, 92]. Neurologic manifestations or kidney disease such as HEV-related Guillain-Barre syndrome, membranoproliferative glomerulonephritis, membranous glomerulonephritis, or nephrotic syndrome in kidney or liver transplant patients with chronic HEV genotype 3 infection have not yet been reported in immunosuppressed children [74, 93]. Interestingly, proteinuria decreased or disappeared in these patients after HEV clearance. Chronic HEV infection has also been documented after stem cell transplantation in an adolescent who later developed cirrhosis and portal hypertension [72].

If liver transplantation is required once chronic infection is established, it is likely that chronic hepatitis E will recur in the liver graft [87]. Risk factors independently associated with chronic infection include heavy immunosuppression, reflected by a shorter time from transplantation to infection; lower CD2, CD3, CD4, and total lymphocyte counts; and use of tacrolimus-based rather than cyclosporine-based regimen [88].

Unless HEV screening is routine, the diagnosis can easily be missed because the clinical features of acute and chronic HEV infection are often nonspecific [94]. Most patients have no symptoms, subtle biological abnormalities, and very few present with jaundice.

Hepatitis E is frequently misdiagnosed as drug-induced liver injury or hepatitis of unknown etiology. HEV infection has a poor prognosis in patients with preexisting chronic liver disease and pregnant women in their third trimester. Patients with unexplained hepatitis should be tested for HEV, regardless of their age, demographics, or travel history.

14.6 Diagnosis of HEV Infection

The diagnosis of hepatitis E virus (HEV) infection relies primarily upon serologic and molecular markers of active and past infection (Fig. 14.1) [95]. Tissue immune-histochemical stain for HEV has been recently developed and is commercially available, although of questionable clinical utility given the infrequency of tissue biopsy in the setting of active disease [95, 96]. It is of note that no tests, to date, have been approved by the Food and Drug Administration (FDA) for the diagnosis of HEV infection in the United States.

14.6.1 Serologic Diagnosis

The adaptive immune response to HEV provides the basis for the serologic diagnosis of HEV infection. Clinical symptoms of HEV infection typically present 6–8 weeks following initial exposure, at which time anti-HEV IgM Ab becomes detectable in approximately 90% of patients [97, 98]. This antibody can persist from weeks to months following infection, after which time the patient is typically asymptomatic, with no further evidence of disease. Anti-HEV IgG

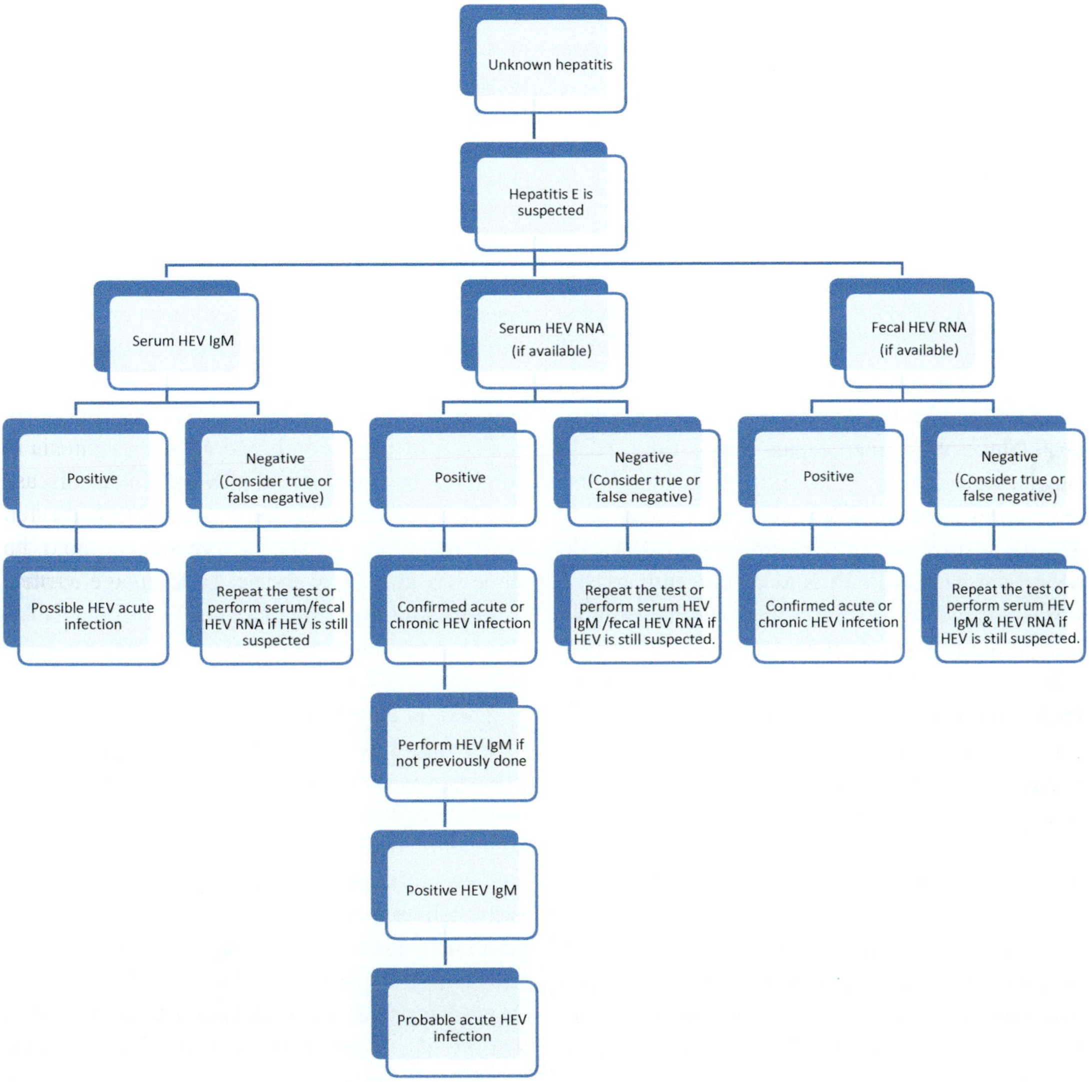

Fig. 14.1 Proposed diagram for serologic investigation for hepatitis E virus infection

appears shortly thereafter, at about 8–10 weeks following infection, and can persist for several years. The presence of anti-HEV IgG is generally considered seroprotective against all four genotypes of HEV.

The serologic diagnosis of HEV is made through the use of in-house or commercially available anti-HEV IgM and IgG test kits. Although HEV exists as four distinct genotypes, there is one serotype, allowing for HEV serologic assays to employ recombinant-based HEV antigen to capture evidence of anti-HEV IgG or IgM. While such serologic assays have historically demonstrated a variable range of sensitivity and specificity, from 52 to 98% and 84 to 99%, respectively, more recent second- and third-generation assays have demonstrated increasingly reliable performance [99, 100]. Limits to serologic testing, particularly in the immunocompromised population, include a lack of sensitivity among individuals who may have been treated with rituximab or other anti-B-lymphocyte agents at the time of infection, as well as decreased specificity among those treated with IVIG, given the well-recognized HEV seroprevalence in the general population. As a result, despite ongoing improvement, testing for HEV markers can be difficult to interpret and may pose problems in the diagnosis of infection [99].

14.6.2 HEV RNA Polymerase Chain Reaction

The use of RNA polymerase chain reaction for the diagnosis of HEV offers a number of advantages, particularly in the immunocompromised host [95]. While these assays have also yet to be approved by the FDA and are not commercially available in the United States at this time, HEV can be detected by PCR from both blood and stool up to 2 weeks prior to the onset of hepatitis and for several weeks after infection [1]. While no standardized HEV PCR assay currently exists, a WHO standard was developed and is available for laboratory use. HEV RNA assays target ORF2/3, responsible for structural proteins of HEV, and have been demonstrated to be highly sensitive and specific in a number of clinical studies [95].

14.7 Treatment of HEV

HEV is generally a self-limiting disease in healthy or immunocompetent individuals, evolving over a few weeks to months. Some patients might require supportive treatment of symptoms, but almost all are able to clear the HEV infection spontaneously. Fulminant hepatitis may occur in genotype 1 HEV infection and other genotypes infecting a child with underlying liver disease. Immunocompromised children and those with underlying liver disease should be considered at increased risk for morbidity, as HEV infection can progress to fulminant hepatic failure (FHF) or acute or chronic liver failure in this setting. Administration of immunoglobulin has not been helpful in preventing the disease in HEV-endemic areas [101, 102].

The treatment goal for chronic HEV infection is complete eradication of the virus. Although systematic guidelines do not yet exist, reduction of immunosuppressive therapy targeting T cells (particularly calcineurin inhibitors) is clinically recommended among individuals on immunosuppressive medications (e.g., solid organ transplant recipients) to resolve chronic HEV infection. Figure 14.2 demonstrates a proposed algorithm for the management of hepatitis E infection in children following solid organ transplantation [86, 89, 103–105]. This approach may allow spontaneous HEV clearance in 30% of cases [103, 106]. When the approach fails or leads to acute rejection, antiviral therapy is widely considered in order to avoid liver cirrhosis and liver graft loss. A 2–3-month course of monotherapy with pegylated interferon-α-2a (PEG-IFN-α-2a), PEG-IFN-α-2b, or ribavirin (or a combination of these medications) has been proposed, although interferon use may be a potential risk factor for acute rejection in SOT recipients [107]. Alternatively, ribavirin alone has also been shown to produce complete recovery and avoid the need for liver transplantation in case reports and small series [86, 89, 103–105, 108].

There is currently no consensus as to how to treat patients with HEV infection in pregnancy. Ribavirin is potentially teratogenic, and the use of pegylated interferon is generally avoided in pregnancy due to fetal concerns. In pregnant women with a near-term fetus, it is logical that early delivery of the viable fetus could be suggested to prevent maternal mortality. Therapeutic termination of pregnancy has not been reported in mothers with HEV infection as a beneficial therapy like in pregnancy-related disorders such as HELLP syndrome and acute fatty liver of pregnancy [109].

14.8 Prevention of HEV

Infants born to asymptomatic anti-HEV-positive mothers are at low risk for HEV infection. No data suggest cesarean section prevents HEV transmission. Given the low amount of HEV in colostrum (low infectivity), breastfeeding, an important nutrition source in endemic areas, should not be discouraged [110]. However, mothers with symptomatic or severe HEV infection with high viral loads should be advised not to breastfeed, due to potential risk of transmission.

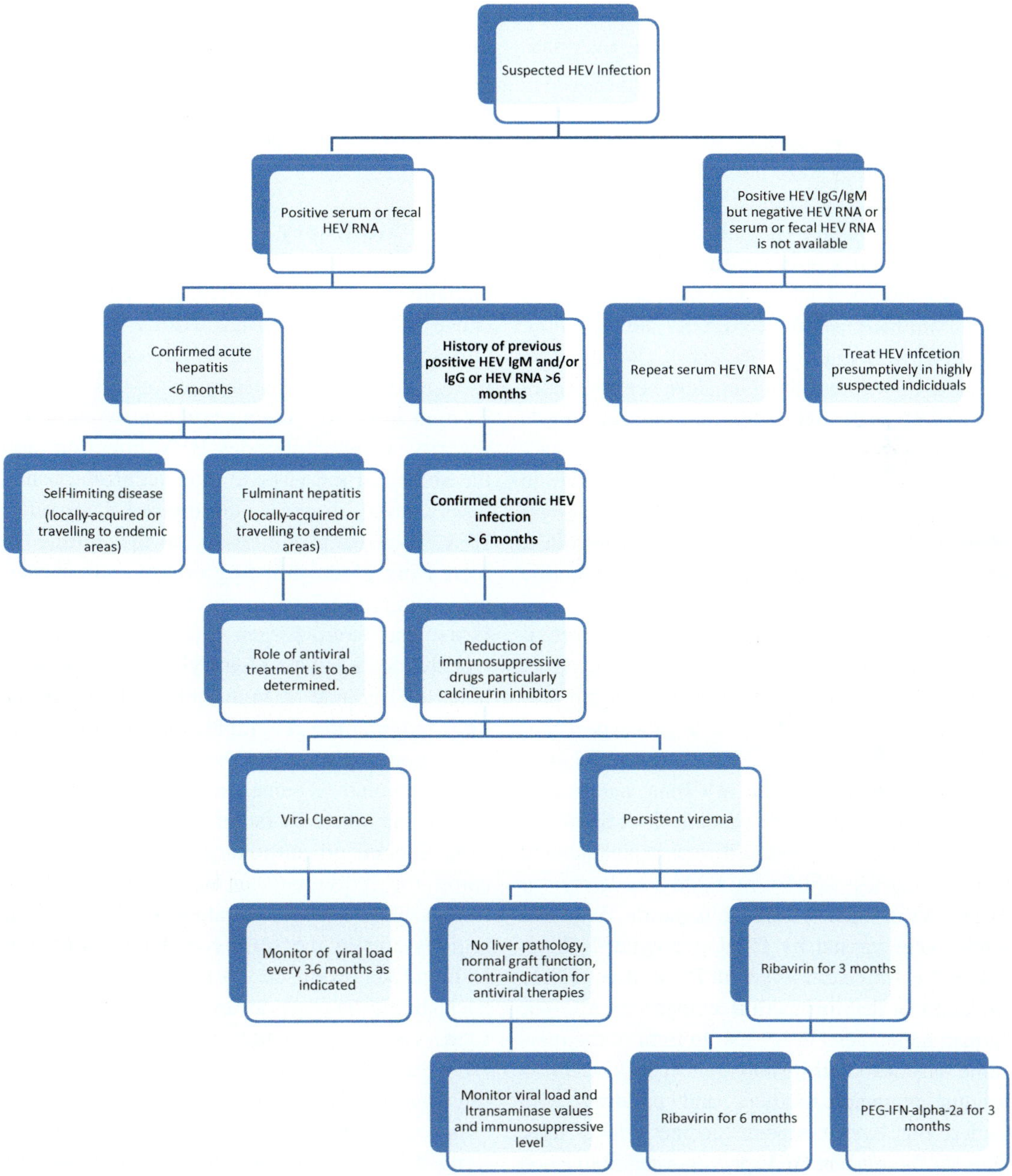

Fig. 14.2 Proposed algorithm for management of hepatitis E virus infection in children following solid organ transplantation

Appropriate prophylactic strategies and measures should be exercised to reduce the risk of exposure to the virus. High-risk groups include pregnant teens, children who are immunosuppressed, and solid organ transplant recipients. Special care should be taken by pregnant mothers to avoid potentially contaminated water sources in HEV-endemic regions, particularly during outbreaks and monsoon season. In addition, immunocompromised hosts (e.g., solid organ transplant recipients, oncology patients) should be cautioned regarding the risk of autochthonous HEV transmission and infection through undercooked meat products, including smoked pig liver sausage, venison, and pork [54, 57, 58].

Anti-HEV antibodies can also be induced by vaccination. HEV vaccines were reported to be effective, but they have not yet been used in the clinical setting. Currently there is no FDA-approved vaccine for HEV. To date, two types of recombinant HEV vaccine have been developed and are genotype 1-based. The first, developed by GlaxoSmithKline (Brentford, UK) and the Walter Reed Army Institute of Research (Washington, DC, USA), was tested in Nepalese healthy males (n = 1900) with high safety and efficacy levels after the third dose [111]. Unfortunately this vaccine has not been further developed [111]. In 2007, a second HEV vaccine (HEV 239) was studied in a randomized, placebo-controlled, phase 3 clinical trial in over 112,604 Chinese healthy participants (aged 16 to 65 years) and demonstrated a very high efficacy of approximately 94–100% with a good safety profile. HEV 239 is composed of a truncated HEV capsid protein, p239, derived from a HEV genotype 1 isolate. It was licensed under Hecolin, Xiamen Innovax Biotech, Xiamen in China, and is currently the only available vaccine. It is approved for high-risk groups and will soon be available to other countries which are highly endemic for HEV. While most cases of hepatitis E in this study were caused by HEV genotype 4 alone, given the single serotype of HEV, it is widely understood that protection extends to all four human genotypes [112, 113]. In light of the mortality associated with HEV genotype 1 infection among pregnant mothers and children with underlying liver disease, vaccine efforts have thus far focused on HEV prevention among such high-risk groups in endemic areas.

Although immunization with HEV vaccine (Hecolin, Xiamen Innovax Biotech, Xiamen, China) demonstrated long-term efficacy at 4.5 years against HEV, the lifelong durability of vaccine-induced immunity has not been demonstrated [113]. As such, while theoretically useful among pregnant women and travelers to endemic regions, the role for vaccine in preventing HEV infection in non-endemic areas (where other genotypes predominate) has not been investigated. Future research using preventive vaccine is required for other genotypes, particularly genotypes 3 and 4 in recipients prior to solid organ or bone marrow transplant recipients [86].

14.9 Summary

Hepatitis E virus is an increasingly recognized cause of viral hepatitis worldwide and an emerging global public health concern. The recognized global distribution of this disease, its high mortality among pregnant women, the severity of autochthonous HEV infection, and the ability of the virus to induce chronic infections among immunocompromised hosts make HEV increasingly relevant in the setting of increasing global flooding events and an ever-increasing number of immunocompromised hosts and solid organ transplant survivors worldwide. Keys to identifying cases of viral hepatitis include a high index of suspicion, knowledge of the geographic distribution where the patients or their families have lived or traveled, personal hygiene, immunocompromising conditions, and risk factors for zoonotic infection. Special precautionary measures are indicated for individuals at high risk for severe illness who may be traveling to known endemic regions and in the setting of HEV outbreaks. Immunocompromised hosts in western countries should be made aware of the zoonotic and food risks associated with autochthonous HEV. In addition, caution should be taken when interpreting HEV serology since different assays can differ in their sensitivity and specificity. Children who are immunosuppressed or receive blood products may have false-negative or false- positive anti-HEV antibodies, respectively; therefore both serological and nucleic acid-based HEV tests are needed for accurate interpretation. Specific antiviral treatment is available for children with persistent or chronic hepatitis E to prevent the development of liver cirrhosis, hepatic failure, and graft loss in solid organ transplantation or other extrahepatic complications.

References

1. Hyams KC (2002) New perspectives on hepatitis E. Curr Gastroenterol Rep 4(4):302–307
2. Mushahwar IK (2008) Hepatitis E virus: molecular virology, clinical features, diagnosis, transmission, epidemiology, and prevention. J Med Virol 80(4):646–658
3. Takahashi M, Okamoto H (2014) Features of hepatitis E virus infection in humans and animals in Japan. Hepatol Res 44(1):43–58
4. Dalton HR et al (2008) Hepatitis E: an emerging infection in developed countries. Lancet Infect Dis 8(11):698–709
5. Mirazo S et al (2014) Indigenous hepatitis E virus genotype 1 infection, Uruguay. Emerg Infect Dis 20(1):171–173
6. Buisson Y et al (2000) Identification of a novel hepatitis E virus in Nigeria. J Gen Virol 81.(Pt 4:903–909
7. van Cuyck-Gandre H et al (1997) Characterization of hepatitis E virus (HEV) from Algeria and Chad by partial genome sequence. J Med Virol 53(4):340–347
8. Tam AW et al (1991) Hepatitis E virus (HEV): molecular cloning and sequencing of the full-length viral genome. Virology 185(1):120–131
9. Dalton HR et al (2008) Autochthonous hepatitis E in Southwest England: natural history, complications and seasonal variation, and hepatitis E virus IgG seroprevalence in blood donors, the elderly and patients with chronic liver disease. Eur J Gastroenterol Hepatol 20(8):784–790
10. Banks M et al (2004) Evidence for the presence of hepatitis E virus in pigs in the United Kingdom. Vet Rec 154(8):223–227
11. World Health Organization (2014) Hepatitis E (Factsheet No. 280). World Health Organization
12. Mizuo H et al (2005) Possible risk factors for the transmission of hepatitis E virus and for the severe form of hepatitis E acquired locally in Hokkaido, Japan. J Med Virol 76(3):341–349
13. Okamoto H (2007) Genetic variability and evolution of hepatitis E virus. Virus Res 127(2):216–228
14. Williams TP et al (2001) Evidence of extrahepatic sites of replication of the hepatitis E virus in a swine model. J Clin Microbiol 39(9):3040–3046
15. Tsarev SA et al (1994) Successful passive and active immunization of cynomolgus monkeys against hepatitis E. Proc Natl Acad Sci U S A 91(21):10198–10202
16. Clayson ET et al (1995) Viremia, fecal shedding, and IgM and IgG responses in patients with hepatitis E. J Infect Dis 172(4):927–933
17. Kumar RM et al (2001) Sero-prevalence and mother-to-infant transmission of hepatitis E virus among pregnant women in the United Arab Emirates. Eur J Obstet Gynecol Reprod Biol 100(1):9–15
18. Navaneethan U, Al Mohajer M, Shata MT (2008) Hepatitis E and pregnancy: understanding the pathogenesis. Liver Int 28(9):1190–1199
19. Emerson SU, Purcell RH (2001) Recombinant vaccines for hepatitis E. Trends Mol Med 7(10):462–466
20. Tang X et al (2011) Structural basis for the neutralization and genotype specificity of hepatitis E virus. Proc Natl Acad Sci U S A 108(25):10266–10271
21. Jeblaoui A et al (2013) Genotype 4 hepatitis e virus in France: an autochthonous infection with a more severe presentation. Clin Infect Dis 57(4):e122–e126
22. Saravanabalaji S et al (2009) Viral load, antibody titers and recombinant open reading frame 2 protein-induced TH1/TH2 cytokines and cellular immune responses in self-limiting and fulminant hepatitis e. Intervirology 52(2):78–85
23. Srivastava R et al (2011) Adaptive immune responses during acute uncomplicated and fulminant hepatitis E. J Gastroenterol Hepatol 26(2):306–311
24. Nguyen HT et al (2012) A naturally occurring human/hepatitis E recombinant virus predominates in serum but not in faeces of a chronic hepatitis E patient and has a growth advantage in cell culture. J Gen Virol 93.(Pt 3:526–530
25. Mishra N, Walimbe AM, Arankalle VA (2013) Hepatitis E virus from India exhibits significant amino acid mutations in fulminant hepatic failure patients. Virus Genes 46(1):47–53
26. Krawczynski K (1993) Hepatitis E. Hepatology 17(5):932–941
27. Peron JM et al (2007) Fulminant liver failure from acute autochthonous hepatitis E in France: description of seven patients with acute hepatitis E and encephalopathy. J Viral Hepat 14(5):298–303
28. Nagasaki F et al (2005) A case of acute hepatitis with positive autoantibodies who actually had hepatitis E virus infection. Hepatol Res 32(2):134–137
29. Sylvan SP et al (1995) Hepatitis E in patients with chronic autoimmune liver disease. JAMA 273(5):377–378
30. Wendum D et al (2005) Acute hepatitis E: a cause of lymphocytic destructive cholangitis. Hum Pathol 36(4):436–438
31. Khuroo MS (1980) Study of an epidemic of non-a, non-B hepatitis. Possibility of another human hepatitis virus distinct from post-transfusion non-a, non-B type. Am J Med 68(6):818–824
32. World Health Organization (2012) Prevention and control of viral hepatitis: a framework for global action. World Health Organization. www.who.int/topics/hepatitis
33. Jacobsen KH, Wiersma ST (2010) Hepatitis a virus seroprevalence by age and world region, 1990 and 2005. Vaccine 28(41):6653–6657
34. World Health Organization (2010) The global prevalence of hepatitis E virus infection and susceptibility: a systematic review. www.who/int/vaccines-documents/
35. Franco E et al (2012) Hepatitis a: epidemiology and prevention in developing countries. World J Hepatol 4(3):68–73
36. Kumar A et al (2004) Hepatitis E in pregnancy. Int J Gynaecol Obstet 85(3):240–244

37. Favorov MO et al (1992) Serologic identification of hepatitis E virus infections in epidemic and endemic settings. J Med Virol 36(4):246–250
38. Khuroo MS, Khuroo MS, Khuroo NS (2016) Transmission of hepatitis E virus in developing countries. Viruses 8(9):E253
39. Kumar S et al (2013) Hepatitis E virus: the current scenario. Int J Infect Dis 17(4):e228–e233
40. Tsega E et al (1992) Acute sporadic viral hepatitis in Ethiopia: causes, risk factors, and effects on pregnancy. Clin Infect Dis 14(4):961–965
41. Kane MA et al (1984) Epidemic non-a, non-B hepatitis in Nepal. Recovery of a possible etiologic agent and transmission studies in marmosets. JAMA 252(22):3140–3145
42. Khuroo MS et al (1983) Acute sporadic non-a, non-B hepatitis in India. Am J Epidemiol 118(3):360–364
43. Patra S et al (2007) Maternal and fetal outcomes in pregnant women with acute hepatitis E virus infection. Ann Intern Med 147(1):28–33
44. Strand RT et al (2003) Infectious a etiology of jaundice among pregnant women in Angola. Scand J Infect Dis 35(6–7):401–403
45. Stoszek SK et al (2006) Hepatitis E antibody seroconversion without disease in highly endemic rural Egyptian communities. Trans R Soc Trop Med Hyg 100(2):89–94
46. Echevarria JM et al (2013) Hepatitis E virus infection in Latin America: a review. J Med Virol 85(6):1037–1045
47. Lopes Dos Santos DR et al (2010) First report of a human autochthonous hepatitis E virus infection in Brazil. J Clin Virol 47(3):276–279
48. Tsang TH et al (2000) Acute hepatitis E infection acquired in California. Clin Infect Dis 30(3):618–619
49. Mansuy JM et al (2004) Hepatitis E in the south west of France in individuals who have never visited an endemic area. J Med Virol 74(3):419–424
50. Dalton HR et al (2007) Locally acquired hepatitis E in chronic liver disease. Lancet 369(9569):1260
51. Hoofnagle JH, Nelson KE, Purcell RH (2012) Hepatitis E. N Engl J Med 367(13):1237–1244
52. Kamar N et al (2012) Hepatitis E. Lancet 379(9835):2477–2488
53. Tei S et al (2003) Zoonotic transmission of hepatitis E virus from deer to human beings. Lancet 362(9381):371–373
54. Meng XJ (2010) Hepatitis E virus: animal reservoirs and zoonotic risk. Vet Microbiol 140(3–4):256–265
55. Christou L, Kosmidou M (2013) Hepatitis E virus in the Western world–a pork-related zoonosis. Clin Microbiol Infect 19(7):600–604
56. Barnaud E et al (2012) Thermal inactivation of infectious hepatitis E virus in experimentally contaminated food. Appl Environ Microbiol 78(15):5153–5159
57. Cossaboom CM et al (2016) Risk factors and sources of foodborne hepatitis E virus infection in the United States. J Med Virol 88(9):1641–1645
58. Colson P et al (2010) Pig liver sausage as a source of hepatitis E virus transmission to humans. J Infect Dis 202(6):825–834
59. Verghese VP, Robinson JL (2014) A systematic review of hepatitis E virus infection in children. Clin Infect Dis 59(5):689–697
60. Kuniholm MH et al (2009) Epidemiology of hepatitis E virus in the United States: results from the third National Health and nutrition examination survey, 1988–1994. J Infect Dis 200(1):48–56
61. Teshale EH et al (2015) Decline in hepatitis E virus antibody prevalence in the United States from 1988–1994 to 2009–2010. J Infect Dis 211(3):366–373
62. Faber MS et al (2012) Hepatitis E virus seroprevalence among adults, Germany. Emerg Infect Dis 18(10):1654–1657
63. Fischler B et al (2016) Hepatitis E in children: a position paper by the ESPGHAN hepatology committee. J Pediatr Gastroenterol Nutr 63(2):288–294
64. Meng QF et al (2015) Seroprevalence and risk factors of hepatitis E virus infection among children in China. J Med Virol 87(9):1573–1577
65. Liu P et al (2012) Phylogenetic analysis of 626 hepatitis E virus (HEV) isolates from humans and animals in China (1986–2011) showing genotype diversity and zoonotic transmission. Infect Genet Evol 12(2):428–434
66. Bendall R et al (2010) A comparison of two commercially available anti-HEV IgG kits and a re-evaluation of anti-HEV IgG seroprevalence data in developed countries. J Med Virol 82(5):799–805
67. Krumbholz A et al (2014) Prevalence of hepatitis E virus antibodies in children in Germany. Pediatr Infect Dis J 33(3):258–262
68. Robson SC et al (1992) Hospital outbreak of hepatitis E. Lancet 339(8806):1424–1425
69. Psichogiou M et al (1996) Hepatitis E virus (HEV) infection in haemodialysis patients. The multicentre Haemodialysis cohort study on viral hepatitis. Nephrol Dial Transplant 11(6):1093–1095
70. Hewitt PE et al (2014) Hepatitis E virus in blood components: a prevalence and transmission study in Southeast England. Lancet 384(9956):1766–1773
71. Colson P et al (2007) Transfusion-associated hepatitis E, France. Emerg Infect Dis 13(4):648–649
72. Halac U et al (2012) Chronic hepatitis E infection in children with liver transplantation. Gut 61(4):597–603
73. Hoerning A et al (2012) Prevalence of hepatitis E virus infection in pediatric solid organ transplant recipients–a single-center experience. Pediatr Transplant 16(7):742–747
74. Kamar N et al (2014) Hepatitis E virus infection. Clin Microbiol Rev 27(1):116–138
75. Mast EE, Purdy MA, Krawczynski K (1996) Hepatitis E. Baillieres Clin Gastroenterol 10(2):227–242
76. Fiore S, Savasi V (2009) Treatment of viral hepatitis in pregnancy. Expert Opin Pharmacother 10(17):2801–2809

77. Khuroo MS, Kamili S (2003) Aetiology, clinical course and outcome of sporadic acute viral hepatitis in pregnancy. J Viral Hepat 10(1):61–69
78. Khuroo MS et al (1981) Incidence and severity of viral hepatitis in pregnancy. Am J Med 70(2):252–255
79. Arora NK et al (1996) Acute viral hepatitis types E, a, and B singly and in combination in acute liver failure in children in North India. J Med Virol 48(3):215–221
80. Jagadisan B et al (2012) Acute on chronic liver disease in children from the developing world: recognition and prognosis. J Pediatr Gastroenterol Nutr 54(1):77–82
81. Crossan CL et al (2014) Hepatitis E virus in patients with acute severe liver injury. World J Hepatol 6(6):426–434
82. Manka P et al (2015) Hepatitis E virus infection as a possible cause of acute liver failure in Europe. Clin Gastroenterol Hepatol 13(10):1836–1842 e2; quiz e157–8
83. Lau JY et al (1995) Detection of hepatitis E virus genome and gene products in two patients with fulminant hepatitis E. J Hepatol 22(6):605–610
84. Munne MS et al (2006) Molecular characterization of hepatitis E virus in three acute liver failure cases in children in Argentina. Acta Gastroenterol Latinoam 36(3):125–130
85. Goto K et al (2006) Prevalence of hepatitis E virus infection in Japanese children. J Pediatr Gastroenterol Nutr 42(1):89–92
86. Arends JE et al (2014) Hepatitis E: an emerging infection in high income countries. J Clin Virol 59(2):81–88
87. Haagsma EB et al (2008) Chronic hepatitis E virus infection in liver transplant recipients. Liver Transpl 14(4):547–553
88. Kamar N et al (2011) Factors associated with chronic hepatitis in patients with hepatitis E virus infection who have received solid organ transplants. Gastroenterology 140(5):1481–1489
89. Gerolami R et al (2011) Treatment of severe acute hepatitis E by ribavirin. J Clin Virol 52(1):60–62
90. Bouts AH, Schriemer PJ, Zaaijer HL (2015) Chronic hepatitis E resolved by reduced immunosuppression in pediatric kidney transplant patients. Pediatrics 135(4):e1075–e1078
91. Bazerbachi F et al (2016) Extra-hepatic manifestations associated with hepatitis E virus infection: a comprehensive review of the literature. Gastroenterol Rep (Oxf) 4(1):1–15
92. Kamar N et al (2011) Hepatitis E virus and neurologic disorders. Emerg Infect Dis 17(2):173–179
93. Kamar N et al (2012) Hepatitis E virus and the kidney in solid-organ transplant patients. Transplantation 93(6):617–623
94. Motte A et al (2012) Hepatitis E in three immunocompromized children in southeastern France. J Clin Virol 53(2):162–166
95. Aggarwal R (2013) Diagnosis of hepatitis E. Nat Rev Gastroenterol Hepatol 10(1):24–33
96. Gupta P et al (2012) Immunohistochemistry for the diagnosis of hepatitis E virus infection. J Viral Hepat 19(2):e177–e183
97. Mirazo S et al (2014) Transmission, diagnosis, and management of hepatitis E: an update. Hepat Med 6:45–59
98. Lhomme S et al (2016) Hepatitis E pathogenesis. Viruses 8(8):E212
99. Sue PK et al (2015) Variability of hepatitis E serologic assays in a pediatric liver transplant recipient: challenges to diagnosing hepatitis E virus infection in the United States. Transpl Infect Dis 17(2):284–288
100. Pas SD et al (2013) Diagnostic performance of selected commercial HEV IgM and IgG ELISAs for immunocompromised and immunocompetent patients. J Clin Virol 58(4):629–634
101. Aggarwal R et al (2000) Duration of viraemia and faecal viral excretion in acute hepatitis E. Lancet 356(9235):1081–1082
102. Khuroo MS, Dar MY (1992) Hepatitis E: evidence for person-to-person transmission and inability of low dose immune serum globulin from an Indian source to prevent it. Indian J Gastroenterol 11(3):113–116
103. Peron JM et al (2011) Acute autochthonous hepatitis E in western patients with underlying chronic liver disease: a role for ribavirin? J Hepatol 54(6):1323–1324 author reply 1324-5
104. Pischke S et al (2010) Hepatitis E virus infection as a cause of graft hepatitis in liver transplant recipients. Liver Transpl 16(1):74–82
105. Schildgen O, Muller A, Simon A (2008) Chronic hepatitis E and organ transplants. N Engl J Med 358(23):2521–2522. author reply 2522
106. Parvez MK (2013) Chronic hepatitis E infection: risks and controls. Intervirology 56(4):213–216
107. Saab S et al (2004) Outcomes of acute rejection after interferon therapy in liver transplant recipients. Liver Transpl 10(7):859–867
108. Kamar N et al (2014) Ribavirin for chronic hepatitis E virus infection in transplant recipients. N Engl J Med 370(12):1111–1120
109. Mjahed K et al (2006) Acute fatty liver of pregnancy. Arch Gynecol Obstet 274(6):349–353
110. Chibber RM, Usmani MA, Al-Sibai MH (2004) Should HEV infected mothers breast feed? Arch Gynecol Obstet 270(1):15–20
111. Shrestha MP et al (2007) Safety and efficacy of a recombinant hepatitis E vaccine. N Engl J Med 356(9):895–903
112. Zhu FC et al (2010) Efficacy and safety of a recombinant hepatitis E vaccine in healthy adults: a large-scale, randomised, double-blind placebo-controlled, phase 3 trial. Lancet 376(9744):895–902
113. Zhang J et al (2015) Long-term efficacy of a hepatitis E vaccine. N Engl J Med 372(10):914–922

Viral Causes of Acute Liver Failure in Children

15

Robert H. Squires

Abstract

Acute liver failure is a rare but devastating clinical condition. A viral cause of acute liver failure is the most common etiology worldwide, with hepatitis A being the most prevalent. In both developed and developing countries, the vaccines against viral hepatitis have reduced the frequency of disease as well as ALF. Testing for viral causes of ALF is often incomplete, and establishing a diagnosis for some viral etiologies can be challenging. With therapies available for viruses such as herpes simplex, adenovirus, and hepatitis B, it is imperative that a thorough diagnostic evaluation occur in children with ALF. Emergence of diseases, such as dengue, in developed countries requires a heightened vigilance to identify rare diseases not typically encountered.

Keywords

Acute liver failure · Virus · Hepatitis A · Hepatitis B · Hepatitis D · Hepatitis E · Herpes simplex virus · Enterovirus · Cytomegalovirus · Adenovirus · Epstein-Barr virus · Parvovirus B19 · Human herpes virus-6 · Influenza · Dengue · Liver transplant

R. H. Squires (✉)
University of Pittsburgh School of Medicine, Pittsburgh, PA, USA

Children's Hospital of Pittsburgh of UPMC, Pittsburgh, PA, USA
e-mail: squiresr@upmc.edu

15.1 Introduction

Acute liver failure (ALF) in children is a rare, often devastating, clinical condition in which a previously healthy child of any age experiences rapid deterioration of liver function with outcomes ranging from complete recovery, liver transplantation, or death. Treatment is largely supportive. There are a few conditions amenable to specific therapy that could alter the course of the disease. Examples include acute acetaminophen toxicity, Wilson disease, tyrosinemia, gestational alloimmune liver disease, and some viruses such as herpes simplex.

Many aspects of ALF in children remain complex and not fully understood, including definition, etiologies, natural history, prognostic indicators, and outcomes. The Pediatric Acute Liver Failure Study Group (PALFSG) was established by the National Institutes of Health/National Institute of Diabetes and Digestive and Kidney Diseases to study this life-threatening condition in children [1]. An unexpected early challenge for pediatricians was to establish entry criteria, because hepatic encephalopathy, which is a defining criteria for adults with acute liver failure, may not be clinically evident or may only

M.-H. Chang, K. B. Schwarz (eds.), *Viral Hepatitis in Children*,
https://doi.org/10.1007/978-981-13-0050-9_15

develop as a terminal event in children. These pediatric experts settled on the following entry criteria for the PALF study: [1] no evidence of chronic liver disease, [2] laboratory evidence of acute liver injury, and [3] coagulopathy not corrected by parenteral vitamin K, with or without encephalopathy. This last criterion was separated by severity of the coagulopathy. The criteria were met for any child with an international normalized ration (INR) or prothrombin time (PT) ≥2 or ≥20 s, respectively. For cases where the coagulopathy was less severe, where the INR or PT was ≥1.5 or ≥15 s, but <2 or <20 s, clinical evidence of hepatic encephalopathy was additionally required.

15.2 Etiology for ALF

One of the earliest reports of ALF in the pediatric age group described 31 children with only 4 diagnoses: paracetamol (acetaminophen) (n = 3), mushroom poisoning (n = 1), halothane (n = 1), and "acute viral hepatitis, hepatitis B surface antigen negative" (n = 26) [2]. Currently, the specific entities or conditions causing PALF are multiple and are grouped into broad categories that include viral, drug-related, metabolic/genetic, immune-mediated, shock, miscellaneous, and indeterminate.

Viral causes of PALF are well described but less commonly diagnosed than other etiologies among children in North America and Britain. The prodrome associated with ALF often includes nonspecific symptoms including fever, malaise, nausea, vomiting, or diarrhea. Such symptoms in children often suggest a viral process. But proving a viral cause can be problematic as many childhood viruses are ubiquitous. Thus laboratory findings may suggest the presence of common viruses, such as Epstein-Barr virus, parvovirus B19, and cytomegalovirus, but it is challenging to ascertain whether such a virus is the principal cause of liver injury or a nonculpable bystander. Additionally, the identification of previously unrecognized liver-injurious viruses has slowed. Several years ago, as more viral pathogens were recognized, many experts suggested a proposed diagnostic category called non-A-G hepatitis [3]. The obvious implication was that there were yet-to-be-identified viral pathogens. But efforts to identify novel viruses associated with ALF have not been successful [4, 5]. In general, more recent terminology has changed from the term non-A-G hepatitis to the broader term of indeterminate status.

The quest to increase the understanding of etiologies for ALF is obviously ongoing. Reasons for failure to make a specific diagnosis for ALF in children are multifactorial and include an incomplete diagnostic evaluation due to death, transplant, or clinical improvement, a diagnosis that was not considered, or the existence of novel etiologies not yet described [6, 7].

15.3 Viral Testing

Diagnostic tests to establish a viral etiology for ALF in children are listed in Table 15.1. For some conditions, such as hepatitis A, B, and E, the presence of serologies consistent with an acute infection in the context of ALF would establish a viral cause for the ALF. However, in circumstances in which the presumptive virus is ubiquitous within a population and rarely associated with ALF, such as Epstein-Barr virus, parvovirus, and cytomegalovirus, a more complete evaluation that would include evidence of active liver involvement would be needed to confidently establish the diagnosis. Unfortunately, testing for a viral etiology is often incomplete leaving the potential for treatable conditions, such as herpes simplex, hepatitis B, and adenovirus, to go undiagnosed [7].

15.4 Hepatitis A Virus

Human hepatitis A virus (HAV) is the most common cause of viral hepatitis worldwide [8]. Once thought to be an enterovirus within the family *Picornaviridae*, HAV was subsequently given its own genus (*Hepatovirus*) along with the only other member, Simian hepatitis A virus. There are currently three principal genotypes, each sub-

Table 15.1 Diagnostic tests to establish a viral etiology for acute liver failure

Viral agent	Diagnostic studies
Hepatitis A	Hepatitis A IgM
Hepatitis B	Hepatitis B surface antigen
	Hepatitis B viral DNA
	Hepatitis B core antigen IgM
Hepatitis D	Hepatitis D antibody IgM
	Hepatitis D viral RNA
	Liver
	Immunohistochemistry
Hepatitis E	Hepatitis E IgM
	Hepatitis E IgG + viral RNA
Herpes simplex virus	HSV PCR in blood
	HSV identified in blood culture
	HSV identified in liver culture
	HSV liver immunohistochemistry (+)
Enterovirus	Enterovirus PCR in blood
	Coxsackie PCR in blood
	Echovirus PCR in blood
	Liver tissue culture
Adenovirus	Adenovirus PCR in blood
	Liver tissue
	Culture (+)
	Viral inclusions identified
	Immunohistochemical stain (+)
Parvovirus B19	Parvovirus B19 blood PCR
	Parvovirus B19 IgM
Hepatitis C	Hepatitis C PCR
Cytomegalovirus	CMV IgM
	CMV blood PCR
	Liver
	Culture (+)
	Viral inclusions identified
	Immunohistochemical stain (+)
Epstein-Barr virus	EBV blood PCR (+)
	EBV viral capsule antigen IgM
	Liver
	Epstein-Barr-encoded RNA (EBER) in situ hybridization
Human herpes virus 6	HHV-6 viral PCR from blood
	HHV-6 antibody, IgM
	Liver
	Immunohistochemistry stain (+)
	HHV-6 PCR from tissue extract
Influenza	Respiratory viral panel
	Exclusion of other causes of ALF
	Acetaminophen toxicity
	Metabolic, immune mediated
Dengue	Dengue viral PCR
	Dengue antibody, IgM
	Dengue NS1 antigen

classified as A and B, with genotypes I and III being the most common [9]. Transmission of HAV is fecal-oral and facilitated by poor personal hygiene and sanitation. Outbreaks of HAV have been associated with contaminated seafood, farm products, and vegetables [10].

Infection with HAV in a susceptible host generally has a brief, asymptomatic course in children. In adults the course can be more clinically apparent with fever, jaundice, and malaise. HAV infection is typically self-limited with clinical symptoms lasting only a week or so, but relapsing or prolonged symptoms can occur. Lifelong immunity follows resolution of the acute HAV episode.

Acute liver failure develops in less than 1% of patients with acute HAV infection. Several factors have been identified that may place a patient at increased risk for developing HAV-associated ALF. Elderly individuals appear to be at a heightened risk relative to other age groups. Having an underlying chronic liver disease, such as hepatitis B, at the time of an acute HAV infection is also a known risk factor for more severe disease resulting in death or liver transplantation. Viral factors, such as genotype or mutations within the viral genome, do not appear to influence outcome [11]. Somewhat counterintuitively, a low or absent viral load at the time of presentation was associated with poor outcome [11, 12]. This would suggest that a rapid and overwhelming immune response against HAV could result in sufficient collateral damage to hepatocytes to cause massive hepatocellular necrosis and liver failure. Whole genome sequencing of nine adults with HAV-associated ALF identified a variety of coding and noncoding host genetic variants, some of which could be involved in immune, inflammatory, or apoptotic activity [13]. Therefore, the complex host immune response to HAV may be an important risk factor for disease severity.

Despite the rarity of ALF in HAV, the high prevalence of HAV worldwide makes it a major factor as a cause of ALF. Assessing international data, 7 developing regions reported 416 patients with PALF between 1982 and 2003; 227 (55%) had HAV as the identified etiology (Table 15.2) [14–20]. In contrast, PALFSG data from North America and Britain identified only 5/703 (0.7%) with the diagnosis of HAV-associated ALF [6].

There is no specific treatment for HAV, but there is a good prevention strategy. Introduction of the HAV vaccine in 1995 resulted in a dramatic reduction in acute HAV infection as well as acute liver failure in developed and developing countries [21]. Focusing on adults, Taylor et al. found that between 1988 and 2005, the frequency of patients receiving a liver transplant for HAV

Table 15.2 Etiology of acute liver failure in different countries

Diagnosis	South America, India, China [14–20] 1982–2003 (*N* = 416) (%)	North America/United Kingdom [6] 1999–2006 (*N* = 703) (%)
Indeterminate	97 (23)	329 (46.8)
Viral	300 (72)	45 (6.4)
Hepatitis A	227 (55)	5 (0.7)
Hepatitis B	20 (5)	2 (0.3)
Hepatitis C	0	0
Hepatitis E	30 (7)	0
Coinfection	21 (5)	0
Other	2 (0.5)	38 (4.9)
Drug related	7 (2)	111 (16)
Acetaminophen		88 (13)
Other		23 (3.3)
Autoimmune	8 (2)	48 (6.8)
Metabolic	2 (0.5)	68 (9.7)
Wilson	2	23 (3.3)
Other		45 (6.4)
Other	2 (0.5)	102 (14.5)

decreased from 0.7% to 0.1% ($p < .001$) and the proportion of adult patients enrolling in the ALFSG with the etiology of HAV decreased from 5% to 0.8% [22]. In children, one study from Argentina reported a similar decline in HAV-associated ALF and liver transplant following implementation of a universal hepatitis A vaccine program [23]. In this study, baseline annual cases of HAV-associated ALF ranged from 12 to 30 per year between 2000 and 2005. After universal immunization was implemented in 2005, there were no reported cases of HAV-associated ALF from November 2006 through December 2008.

Vaccination against HAV, administered as two injections 6 months apart, is now recommended for all children 12 months of age. Universal vaccination for adults has not yet been undertaken but is recommended for high-risk populations such as those with a chronic liver condition, intravenous drug exposure, contact at work or at home with international adoptees, or traveling to an area where HAV is endemic (see also Chap. 6).

15.5 Hepatitis B Virus

Hepatitis B virus (HBV) is an enigmatic, small DNA virus with eight genotypes (A-H) and myriad clinical features that vary by age of viral acquisition [24–26]. Transmission is generally associated with blood, semen, or other body fluid from an infected person entering the body of a susceptible host. Infants born to HBsAg- and HBeAg-positive mothers are at highest risk for vertical transmission (70–90%), while those born to HBsAg-positive and HBeAg-negative mothers are at lower risk (10–40%). If infants are infected with HBV, 90% will develop a chronic HBV infection [27]. In contrast, acute HBV infection acquired in older children and adults is often self-limited with complete clinical recovery accompanied by clearance of hepatitis B surface antigen (HBsAg) and appearance of antibodies (anti-HBs) [28]. Clinical features, HBV serologies, and HBV DNA are used to generally characterize four phases of chronic HBV infection: immune tolerant, immune active, inactive carrier, and reactivation (see also Chap. 7).

Acute liver failure develops in approximately 1% of patients infected with HBV alone [10]. PALFSG data showed ALF due to HBV was determined to be the final diagnosis in 2 of 703 (0.3%) tested for HBV [6]. Children with ALF due to HBV are more likely to die if the HBV DNA is absent in the serum and the serum bilirubin level is very high (mean 535 umol/L or 31.5 mg/dl) [29]. Other risk factors for developing ALF include rapid disappearance or absence of HBV DNA and HBsAg (similar to HAV), co-consumption of alcohol, acetaminophen or methamphetamines, and perhaps being infected with HBV genotype D. Individuals with chronic HBV infection who receive immunosuppressive therapy (e.g., systemic corticosteroids, chemotherapy) are at increased risk for activation of quiescent HBV and development of ALF, and, if it occurs, survival is poor beyond 21 days [30].

Prevention of perinatal HBV transmission is an integral part of the effort. This involves universal screening of pregnant women during each pregnancy and the provision of immunoprophylaxis for infants born to infected mothers, including hepatitis B vaccine and hepatitis B immune globulin. Routine vaccination of all infants with the first dose starting at birth will protect older children.

For a case of ALF due to HBV, uncertainty still surrounds treatment decisions [31]. Data on treatment are limited to small case studies. Initiation of antiviral therapy, and transfer to a liver transplant center, should be considered for those patients with acute severe HBV infection associated with significant liver injury and persistent INR over 1.5 despite parenteral vitamin K. For those with advanced ALF and progressive encephalopathy, it is unclear that antiviral therapy will alter the clinical course or ultimate need for liver transplantation. However, if antiviral agents can reduce the viral load prior to or after liver transplantation, recurrence of HBV following transplantation could be delayed. Guidelines from the American Association for the Study of Liver Diseases (AASLD) [32] and the European Association for the Study of the Liver (EASL)

[33] recommend treatment, currently entecavir or tenofovir, for immune active disease and evidence of severe liver injury.

15.6 Hepatitis C Virus

Hepatitis C virus (HCV) is a distinctly rare cause of ALF. Some experts have suggested HCV may not be a primary cause of ALF in the absence of coinfection or confounding nonviral factor [10]. A recent report by Reuben et al. found only 3 cases of HCV among 2070 North American subjects enrolled in the acute liver failure study with the site investigator assigning the final diagnosis [34]. Published reports of HCV-associated ALF are limited to case studies [35, 36]. In a provocative report from Kanzaki et al. [36], one subject received treatment with methylprednisolone for optic neuritis and presented 5 days later with fever and ALF. Following liver transplantation, he was found to have HCV, and retrospectively a PCR test for HCV on pretransplant serum suggested recent infection, suggesting the possibility of an acute HCV process.

15.7 Hepatitis D Virus

Hepatitis D virus (HDV) is a small, aberrant, RNA virus with a life cycle that requires HDV to be encased in a HBV surface antigen-positive coat. HDV infection can present either as a concomitant infection with HBV (coinfection) or as a secondary infection in a patient with chronic HBV (superinfection) [37]. Severe acute hepatitis or ALF occurs more commonly in HBV-HDV coinfected patients. HDV superinfection is more commonly associated with acceleration of hepatic fibrosis and cirrhosis, but ALF can also occur. HDV is endemic in many developing countries. HDV was found to be the underlying cause for a fulminant hepatitis previously known as Labrea hepatitis or black fever among indigenous people living in the Amazon basin [38]. In fulminant cases, serum levels of HDV antigen can be in the undetectable range with the only positive finding being positive nuclear staining of hepatocytes for HDV in infected individuals [37].

15.8 Hepatitis E Virus

Hepatitis E virus (HEV) is a single-stranded RNA virus with distinctive clinical phenotypes associated with the geographic distribution of HEV genotype [39]. A recent study has identified seven HEV genotypes, with only genotypes 1, 2, 3, 4, and 7 known to infect humans [40]. In the absence of a known animal reservoir, HEV genotypes 1 and 2 appear to infect only humans and are endemic within developing countries in tropical climates [39, 41]. HEV 1 is responsible for most cases in Asia, while HEV 2 is more prevalent in Africa and Central America. The virus is typically transmitted under conditions of poor sanitation via human fecal contamination of drinking water. HEV genotypes 3 and 4 infections are most common in developed countries and occur as a consequence of ingesting contaminated meat (e.g., pigs, rabbit, wild boar, deer), milk, or shell fish [39]. The clinical course is generally mild and often asymptomatic [39, 41] (see also Chap. 14).

Clinical features of HEV infections in endemic areas range from asymptomatic to acute liver failure. HEV-associated ALF was thought to be more severe among pregnant women [42]. However, a single-site study from India involving 1005 participants with ALF of reproductive age challenged that dogma [43]. Investigators found that, among women of child-bearing age, HEV occurred more frequently in pregnant women compared to nonpregnant women (59.4% vs 30.4%); however mortality was similar (53.8% v 57.2%). Why pregnant women appear to be more susceptible to HEV-associated ALF than nonpregnant women is unclear, but alterations in immune responses to HEV may contribute to these differences [44].

HEV rarely, if ever, causes acute liver failure in adults in the United States. A study by the ALFSG found that 294/681 (43.4%) participants tested positive for anti-HEV IgG, suggesting a previous exposure to the virus [45]. However, while just 3/681 (0.4%) tested positive for anti-HEV IgM, all were HEV-RNA negative and had other putative diagnoses. Like hepatitis A, acute HEV infection can cause acute decompensation of a chronic liver disease. Unlike hepatitis A, it may also be associated with chronic hepatitis in immunocompromised patients [39].

Treatment proposals have included ribavirin either alone [46] or in combination with pegylated interferon [47], but treatment failure has been reported, and specific guidelines or recommendations are not established [48].

15.9 Herpes Simplex Virus

Herpes simplex virus (HSV) is transmitted to the newborn at or around the time of delivery. In up to 80% of cases, the mother is unaware or has no evidence of an active perineal infection with a high proportion of mothers acquiring the infection in the last trimester [49]. The majority of infants who acquire HSV in the newborn period have localized disease involving the skin, eyes, or oral cavity [50]. Disseminated disease, that often involves the liver and central nervous system, can occur in up to 20% of cases. Beyond the neonatal period, HSV is most commonly transmitted by sexual intercourse or oral sex with an infected individual. Disseminated HSV can develop in immunocompromised hosts and rarely in immunocompetent individuals. Disseminated HSV-1 and HSV-2 can result in ALF.

The clinical presentation of disseminated disease in the newborn typically begins within 3 to 7 days after birth with nonspecific symptoms of poor feeding, lethargy, and fever leading to evidence of multisystem dysfunction. Cutaneous lesions are often not present, and the presenting phenotype is similar to an infant with bacterial sepsis or a metabolic crisis. Outcomes are poor in HSV-associated ALF with death occurring in 25% of cases [51].

In recent years, acyclovir is typically started at first presentation, along with broad spectrum antibiotics and other supportive care, and continued until HSV-PCR results of blood and/or spinal fluid are known. This approach avoids unnecessary delay in initiating potentially life-saving treatment [52]. A delayed or missed diagnosis is, unfortunately, more common among patients outside the newborn period [53]. Given its excellent safety profile, acyclovir is also recommended in all patients presenting with ALF, particularly those with serum aminotransferase levels over 750–1000 IU/L.

The PALFSG reported on 148 participants who were less than 90 days of age at enrollment. Data shows that HSV accounted for 12.8% of all cases of ALF in this age group making it the second most common identified cause of ALF, behind gestational alloimmune liver disease (a.k.a. neonatal iron storage disease) [54]. While more common in newborns, ALF due to HSV occurs in children of all age groups [55, 56]. Because there is a specific treatment, HSV should be considered strongly as part of the diagnostic evaluation for PALF. This is especially true in adolescents with ALF, who may or may not be known to be sexually active, even those without a known or suspected altered immune system.

Liver transplant has been successfully performed in HSV associated ALF, even those with active viremia [51, 53, 57]. However, long-term sequelae such as seizures, developmental delay, and posttransplant death can also occur. It has been recommended that acyclovir be continued indefinitely following transplant given the risk of recurrence.

15.10 *Enterovirus*

The genus *Enterovirus* includes over 120 genetically distinct viruses [58]. All are transmitted enterally, as suggested by the name. They are associated with clinical manifestations that range from mild gastroenteritis to encephalitis, flaccid paralysis, cardiomyopathy, and liver failure. Species associated with human disease are grouped into four categories (A–D) based on genetic and clinical manifestations and include coxsackievirus, enterovirus, and echovirus. As newer viruses are identified and given the genetic overlap for many, a recent approach to simplify the taxonomy is to use “EV” followed by consecutive numbers. For example, EV-D68 was associated with a respiratory outbreak, and EV-A71 was found to cause outbreaks for hand, foot, and mouth disease.

Enteroviruses were found to account for 34/139 (24%) sepsis-like events among neonates in Kuwait with the only death reported due to ALF [59]. Sundaram et al. found enteroviruses to be the second most common viral cause of ALF in newborns [54]. In a case series of 16 neonates with EV-associated ALF, myocarditis ($n = 5$) and encephalitis ($n = 4$) were complicating features [60]. While the case fatality rate reached 31% in this series, survivors appear to have had complete normalization of liver function and an absence of long-term sequelae.

Currently, there is no approved antiviral therapy for enterovirus infections [61]. Results of a randomized, double-masked, placebo-controlled trial of pleconaril in neonates with EV sepsis recently reported a shorter time to a negative EV culture and PCR as well as a greater survival among pleconaril recipients [62]. While the percentage of deaths among EV-confirmed subjects receiving pleconaril (7/31; 23%) was lower than placebo (5/12, 42%), this did not reach statistical significance ($p = .26$). Newer antiviral therapies are being investigated [61]. Liver transplantation for EV-associated ALF has been reported in at least two patients; with posttransplant follow-up, only one had documented neurodevelopmental deficiencies [63, 64].

15.11 Adenovirus

Adenovirus (AV) is a common infection among healthy children manifested by self-limited upper and lower respiratory tract infections and pneumonia [65]. It is rarely associated with ALF in immunocompetent individuals. In a case series of 143 children with a positive culture or direct fluorescent assay, one immunocompetent child developed acute liver injury and was considered for liver transplantation. However, the child recovered following treatment with cidofovir, and a liver transplant was avoided [65]. In another case report, a healthy 23-month-old, recently treated with trimethoprim/sulfamethoxazole (TMS) for a urinary tract infection, developed ALF and pancytopenia following an upper respiratory infection due to AV cultured from a nasal swab [66]. While she recovered spontaneously, it is possible the child's symptoms could have been related to drug toxicity from TMS.

More commonly, AV-associated ALF occurs in immunocompromised patients; particularly those who have received a solid organ or bone marrow transplant [67]. Children receiving chemotherapy for leukemia or lymphoma are also at risk. Mortality rates are high among immunocompromised patients with AV-associated ALF, reaching 63% in some cases [67]. Having a high index of suspicion for early detection and treatment with cidofovir offers the best chance for surviving this malicious virus [65, 68].

15.12 Cytomegalovirus

Cytomegalovirus (CMV) is associated with severe hepatitis and liver failure in patients with immunodeficiency or receiving immunosuppressive medications. Less commonly, CMV can cause acute hepatitis, and rarer still acute liver failure, in immunocompetent individuals. Infants less than 12 months of age appear particularly vulnerable to invasive CMV disease [69].

Cholestasis and hepatosplenomegaly are common features [70]. CMV PCR testing can detect latent viral infection which makes PCR testing highly sensitive in detecting virus but much less specific in relating viral presence with the patient's symptoms. Therefore, other measures are needed for reassurance that CMV is causing liver disease in a patient, such as serologic evidence of a recent infection (e.g., positive CMV-IgM) or liver tissue with detectable CMV inclusions.

There are no specific guidelines for initiation of antiviral therapy for CMV liver disease. Patients can resolve their liver disease spontaneously without antiviral therapy, but ganciclovir or valganciclovir has been used at times with variable success [70].

15.13 Epstein-Barr Virus

Primary Epstein-Barr (EBV) infection is associated with a broad range of liver involvement. Virtually all individuals with EBV infection have at least mild elevation of serum aminotransferase levels [71]. Cholestatic hepatitis is less common and ALF is rare. EBV-related ALF was identified in 4/1882 (0.21%) adult subjects [72], while 8/986 (0.8%) pediatric ALF subjects had a final diagnosis of EBV (unpublished). As with CMV, EBV-associated liver disease is more common in children receiving immunosuppression for solid organ or bone marrow transplant or with a primary immunodeficiency. Immunocompromised children naive to EBV are at risk at the time of primary infection, and those previously exposed to EBV are at risk for viral reactivation. However, immunocompetent children can also develop acute liver injury or liver failure.

Similar to patients with CMV, establishing EBV as the principal cause for liver injury requires not only detection of virus by EBV PCR techniques but also serological evidence of current or recent viral infection and histological evidence of EBV hepatitis using Epstein-Barr-encoded RNA (EBER) in situ hybridization staining of liver tissue [69, 72]. EBV-associated ALF occurs primarily in older patients but has been identified in all age groups over 1 year of age. Liver transplantation has been performed successfully in EBV-associated ALF [72].

EBV-associated hemophagocytic lymphohistiocytosis is a multisystem inflammatory condition associated with multisystem organ failure, including ALF, and carries a high mortality rate of over 70% [73]. In addition to intensive care management to support failing organ systems, chemotherapy using corticosteroids, etoposide, and cyclosporine either alone or in combination has been used [74]. Combining the chemotherapeutic regime with rituximab may have added benefit [75]. Bone marrow transplantation may also need to be considered in some circumstances [76].

15.14 Human Herpesvirus-6

Human herpesvirus 6 (HHV-6) infects individuals of all ages, manifesting as exanthema subitum in infants and a mononucleosis-like syndrome in older children and adults [77]. The clinical illness is typically self-limited, and serological evidence of a previous infection is seen in the majority of adults. Reactivation of HHV-6 can occur following immunosuppression with the implication that low levels of virus may be present for an extended period of time following primary infection [77].

Similar to other common ubiquitous latent viruses such as EBV and CMV, association of causality for an episode of ALF is challenging [69, 77]. Chevret et al. found evidence of HHV-6 in liver biopsy specimens in pediatric subjects with ALF of indeterminate (5/6; 83%) and known cause that was not HHV-6 related (2/4; 50%) as well children with chronic liver disease that was either acutely decompensated (3/3; 100%) or stable (2/10; 20%) [78]. This suggests HHV-6 may be associated with acute decompensation of chronic liver disease and ALF of indeterminate cause. Alternatively, it may be present as a bystander from a previous infection. Given the small numbers and incomplete viral load data for most patients, further study is needed to assess causality in an individual patient. For individuals with evidence of HHV-6 pre-liver transplant, up to 50% have recurrence of infection but appears to have no significant impact on long-term graft or patient survival [79].

15.15 Influenza A

Influenza A is a seasonal acute respiratory virus associated with prolonged fever, cough, anorexia, and myalgia. It is not typically associated with acute liver injury or liver failure. Whitworth et al. reported four pediatric cases of severe liver injury and liver failure associated with influenza [80]. All survived with their native livers. While none had toxic acetaminophen levels measured, all patients had chronic exposure to acetaminophen, which is a known hepatotoxin [81]. A liver biopsy in one patient had histologic evidence of central lobular necrosis, a finding associated with acetaminophen toxicity, as well as microvesicular steatosis which is suggestive of a possible mitochondrial disorder. In a murine influenza model, investigators found clinical evidence of hepatitis with elevated serum aminotransferase levels and liver histology that revealed foci of inflammation that included antigen-specific CD8+ T cells accompanied by hepatocyte apoptosis, but no evidence of virus was detected in liver tissue [82]. The mechanism of influenza A-associated liver injury is likely multifactorial and includes acetaminophen exposure as well as an immune-mediated liver injury.

15.16 Dengue Virus

Dengue virus, an arbovirus transmitted by the *Aedes* mosquito, is endemic in tropical nations around the world. Also known as breakbone fever, symptoms can range from a mild self-limited illness to a severe form that includes hemorrhagic fever and shock [83]. The liver is particularly affected with some evidence of liver injury in the majority of patients. Serum aminotransferase levels rise during the course of the illness and peak after 6–7 days of illness [84]. Therefore, early assessment of liver tests may not capture the eventual degree of liver injury or function. Progression to ALF is often, but not always, associated with shock, and patients with this degree of liver injury have a high mortality rate. Dengue-associated ALF occurs in all age groups, but children appear to be particularly susceptible as it is a major cause of ALF in children in Thailand and other Southeast Asian countries [83, 85]. The majority of cases of dengue reported from the United States are individuals with a recent travel history to an endemic area. However, and importantly, at least three cases of dengue have been locally acquired in 50 states of the United States, with one death due to dengue-associated hemophagocytic lymphohistiocytosis [86].

15.17 Parvovirus

Over 50% of adolescents and virtually all elderly individuals have evidence of a previous parvovirus B19 (PV) infection. The virus requires aspects of the host's cell replicating machinery and prefers actively dividing cells, such as erythrocyte progenitor cells, for propagation. Most infections are subclinical, but diseases caused by PV include Fifth's disease, arthropathy, transient aplastic crises, chronic anemia, hydrops fetalis, and congenital anemia [87]. Mild elevations of serum aminotransferase levels can be seen in children with Fifth's disease, but whether PV causes ALF remains uncertain [87].

Case reports and small case series have associated PV with ALF. In a report of 48 children in India with ALF, 19 tested positive of PV mRNA in liver tissue. Survival was common among subjects with only PV (6/19), while few subjects survived who were coinfected with hepatitis A, B, C, and/or E (3/13) [88]. However, the high prevalence of PV infection among children accompanied by the observation that PV DNA can be found in the liver and other tissues months following an infection raises uncertainty as to the role of PV in causing ALF [87]. While there are reports of PV causing ALF-associated aplastic anemia [89, 90], other investigators have found that the prevalence of PV DNA in liver tissue was similar among patients with diverse diagnoses such as ALF, ALF-associated aplastic anemia, hepatitis B, and hepatitis C [91]. This suggests that finding PV DNA in liver tissue is not sufficient to assign causality. A study in adults with ALF found no evidence of PV as a cause of ALF in North America [4].

15.18 Summary

Geography, patient age, and immunocompetency are the principal factors that influence prioritization for viral testing in children with acute liver failure. Therefore a reasoned approach to diagnostic viral testing should be undertaken to avoid unneeded tests and, at times, confusing results that can add more confusion than certainty relative to the actual diagnosis of ALF.

Together, hepatitis A, B, D, and E are the most common causes of ALF in poor or developing countries. Worldwide access to affordable vaccination programs and potable water will significantly decrease these deadly infections among vulnerable populations. Serologic evidence of HEV is increasing in developed countries, but confirmatory RNA testing is difficult to obtain and rarely present. Children in developed countries are at increased risk for HAV and HBV if they live in areas with low vaccination rates or live within an area where an outbreak has occurred. Dengue is endemic in tropical nations, but as tropical conditions encroach upon other areas of the world, such as the Gulf Coast of the United States, clinicians in these areas should maintain a heightened awareness of this potential pathogen. Interestingly, HCV is rarely, if ever, a cause of ALF in children, and other causes of ALF should continue to be pursued.

Herpes simplex virus and enterovirus tests should be performed on all children <3 months of age presenting with ALF and marked elevation of serum aminotransferase levels. High-risk populations for ALF due to HSV include neonates and infants <1 month of age, adolescents with a history of consensual oral or genital sex, and children of any age who have been raped or sexually abused. In all these cases, acyclovir should be started at presentation and continued until testing for HSV is negative.

Children with an inherited or acquired immunodeficiency who also experience acute hepatic decompensation should be tested for EBV, CMV, and adenovirus. Immunocompetent children typically develop mild clinical symptoms or a subclinical infection with these agents, although case reports and case series identified individuals who developed ALF. The relatively high frequency of these viruses, as well as HHV6, PV, and influenza within a community accompanied by its rare association with ALF in immunocompetent children, should prompt a continued search for other causes of ALF until a definitive viral cause is established, such as tissue confirmation (e.g., liver biopsy).

References

1. Squires RH Jr, Shneider BL, Bucuvalas J, Alonso E, Sokol RJ, Narkewicz MR, Dhawan A et al (2006) Acute liver failure in children: the first 348 patients in the pediatric acute liver failure study group. J Pediatr 148:652–658
2. Psacharopoulos HT, Mowat AP, Davies M, Portmann B, Silk DB, Williams R (1980) Fulminant hepatic failure in childhood: an analysis of 31 cases. Arch Dis Child 55:252–258
3. Whitington PF, Alonso EM (2001) Fulminant hepatitis in children: evidence for an unidentified hepatitis virus. J Pediatr Gastroenterol Nutr 33:529–536
4. Lee WM, Brown KE, Young NS, Dawson GJ, Schlauder GG, Gutierrez RA, Fontana R et al (2006) Brief report: no evidence for parvovirus B19 or hepatitis E virus as a cause of acute liver failure. Dig Dis Sci 51:1712–1715
5. Umemura T, Tanaka E, Ostapowicz G, Brown KE, Heringlake S, Tassopoulos NC, Wang RY et al (2003) Investigation of SEN virus infection in patients with cryptogenic acute liver failure, hepatitis-associated aplastic anemia, or acute and chronic non-A-E hepatitis. J Infect Dis 188:1545–1552
6. Narkewicz MR, Dell Olio D, Karpen SJ, Murray KF, Schwarz K, Yazigi N, Zhang S et al (2009) Pattern of diagnostic evaluation for the causes of pediatric acute liver failure: an opportunity for quality improvement. J Pediatr 155:801–806 e801
7. Schwarz KB, Dell Olio D, Lobritto SJ, Lopez MJ, Rodriguez-Baez N, Yazigi NA, Belle SH et al (2014) Analysis of viral testing in nonacetaminophen pediatric acute liver failure. J Pediatr Gastroenterol Nutr 59:616–623
8. Koff RS, Hepatitis A (1998) Lancet 351:1643–1649
9. Aggarwal R, Goel A (2015) Hepatitis A: epidemiology in resource-poor countries. Curr Opin Infect Dis 28:488–496
10. Manka P, Verheyen J, Gerken G, Canbay A (2016) Liver failure due to acute viral hepatitis (A-E). Visc Med 32:80–85
11. Ajmera V, Xia G, Vaughan G, Forbi JC, Ganova-Raeva LM, Khudyakov Y, Opio CK et al (2011) What factors determine the severity of hepatitis A-related acute liver failure? J Viral Hepat 18:e167–e174
12. Lee HW, Chang DY, Moon HJ, Chang HY, Shin EC, Lee JS, Kim KA et al (2015) Clinical factors and viral load influencing severity of acute hepatitis A. PLoS One 10:e0130728
13. Long D, Fix OK, Deng X, Seielstad M, Lauring AS, Acute Liver Failure Study G (2014) Whole genome sequencing to identify host genetic risk factors for severe outcomes of hepatitis a virus infection. J Med Virol 86:1661–1668
14. Moreira-Silva SF, Frauches DO, Almeida AL, Mendonca HF, Pereira FE (2002) Acute liver failure in children: observations in Vitoria, Espirito Santo State, Brazil. Rev Soc Bras Med Trop 35:483–486

15. Fonseca JC, Souza RA, Brasil LM, Araujo JR, Ferreira LC (2004) Fulminant hepatic failure in children and adolescents in Northern Brazil. Rev Soc Bras Med Trop 37:67–69
16. Ciocca M, Ramonet M, Cuarterolo M, Lopez S, Cernadas C, Alvarez F (2008) Prognostic factors in paediatric acute liver failure. Arch Dis Child 93:48–51
17. Samanta T, Ganguly S (2007) Aetiology, clinical profile and prognostic indicators for children with acute liver failure admitted in a teaching hospital in Kolkata. Trop Gastroenterol 28:135–139
18. Poddar U, Thapa BR, Prasad A, Sharma AK, Singh K (2002) Natural history and risk factors in fulminant hepatic failure. Arch Dis Child 87:54–56
19. Liu CL, Fan ST, Lo CM, Tam PK, Saing H, Wei WI, Yong BH et al (2003) Live donor liver transplantation for fulminant hepatic failure in children. Liver Transpl 9:1185–1190
20. Uribe M, Buckel E, Ferrario M, Godoy J, Blanco A, Hunter B, Ceresa S et al (2003) Epidemiology and results of liver transplantation for acute liver failure in Chile. Transplant Proc 35:2511–2512
21. Koff RS (2006) Fulminant hepatitis A: disappearing, but not soon enough. Hepatology 44:1397–1399
22. Taylor RM, Davern T, Munoz S, Han SH, McGuire B, Larson AM, Hynan L et al (2006) Fulminant hepatitis A virus infection in the United States: incidence, prognosis, and outcomes. Hepatology 44:1589–1597
23. Cervio G, Trentadue J, D'Agostino D, Luque C, Giorgi M, Armoni J, Debbag R (2011) Decline in HAV-associated fulminant hepatic failure and liver transplant in children in Argentina after the introduction of a universal hepatitis A vaccination program. Hepat Med 3:99–106
24. Liang TJ (2009) Hepatitis B: the virus and disease. Hepatology 49:S13–S21
25. Haber BA, Block JM, Jonas MM, Karpen SJ, London WT, McMahon BJ, Murray KF et al (2009) Recommendations for screening, monitoring, and referral of pediatric chronic hepatitis B. Pediatrics 124:e1007–e1013
26. Pan CQ, Duan ZP, Bhamidimarri KR, Zou HB, Liang XF, Li J, Tong MJ (2012) An algorithm for risk assessment and intervention of mother to child transmission of hepatitis B virus. Clin Gastroenterol Hepatol 10:452–459
27. Gentile I, Borgia G (2014) Vertical transmission of hepatitis B virus: challenges and solutions. Int J Womens Health 6:605–611
28. Sorrell MF, Belongia EA, Costa J, Gareen IF, Grem JL, Inadomi JM, Kern ER et al (2009) National Institutes of Health consensus development conference statement: management of hepatitis B. Hepatology 49:S4–S12
29. Chan PC, Chen HL, Kong MS, Huang FC, Lee HC, Lin CC, Liu CC et al (2005) Factors affecting the mortality of pediatric fulminant hepatic failure in relation to hepatitis B virus infection. J Gastroenterol Hepatol 20:1223–1227
30. Karvellas CJ, Cardoso FS, Gottfried M, Reddy KR, Hanje AJ, Ganger D, Lee WM et al (2017) HBV-associated acute liver failure after immunosuppression and risk of death. Clin Gastroenterol Hepatol 15:113–122
31. Tillmann HL, Hadem J, Leifeld L, Zachou K, Canbay A, Eisenbach C, Graziadei I et al (2006) Safety and efficacy of lamivudine in patients with severe acute or fulminant hepatitis B, a multicenter experience. J Viral Hepat 13:256–263
32. Terrault NA, Bzowej NH, Chang KM, Hwang JP, Jonas MM, Murad MH, American Association for the Study of Liver D (2016) AASLD guidelines for treatment of chronic hepatitis B. Hepatology 63:261–283
33. European Association For The Study Of The L (2012) EASL clinical practice guidelines: management of chronic hepatitis B virus infection. J Hepatol 57:167–185
34. Reuben A, Tillman H, Fontana RJ, Davern T, McGuire B, Stravitz RT, Durkalski V et al (2016) Outcomes in adults with acute liver failure between 1998 and 2013: an observational cohort study. Ann Intern Med 164:724–732
35. Farci P, Alter HJ, Shimoda A, Govindarajan S, Cheung LC, Melpolder JC, Sacher RA et al (1996) Hepatitis C virus-associated fulminant hepatic failure. N Engl J Med 335:631–634
36. Kanzaki H, Takaki A, Yagi T, Ikeda F, Yasunaka T, Koike K, Miyake Y et al (2014) A case of fulminant liver failure associated with hepatitis C virus. Clin J Gastroenterol 7:170–174
37. Xue MM, Glenn JS, Leung DH (2015) Hepatitis D in children. J Pediatr Gastroenterol Nutr 61:271–281
38. Bensabath G, Hadler SC, Soares MC, Fields H, Dias LB, Popper H, Maynard JE (1987) Hepatitis delta virus infection and Labrea hepatitis. Prevalence and role in fulminant hepatitis in the Amazon Basin. JAMA 258:479–483
39. Hartl J, Wehmeyer MH, Pischke S (2016) Acute hepatitis E: two sides of the same coin. Viruses 8:299
40. Smith DB, Simmonds P, Izopet J, Oliveira-Filho EF, Ulrich RG, Johne R, Koenig M et al (2016) Proposed reference sequences for hepatitis E virus subtypes. J Gen Virol 97:537–542
41. Price J (2014) An update on hepatitis B, D, and E viruses. Top Antivir Med 21:157–163
42. Cevrioglu AS, Altindis M, Tanir HM, Aksoy F (2004) Investigation of the incidence of hepatitis E virus among pregnant women in Turkey. J Obstet Gynaecol Res 30:48–52
43. Bhatia V, Singhal A, Panda SK, Acharya SK (2008) A 20-year single-center experience with acute liver failure during pregnancy: is the prognosis really worse? Hepatology 48:1577–1585
44. Pal R, Aggarwal R, Naik SR, Das V, Das S, Naik S (2005) Immunological alterations in pregnant women with acute hepatitis E. J Gastroenterol Hepatol 20:1094–1101
45. Fontana RJ, Engle RE, Scaglione S, Araya V, Shaikh O, Tillman H, Attar N et al (2016) The role of hepa-

titis E virus infection in adult Americans with acute liver failure. Hepatology 64:1870–1880
46. Hajji H, Gerolami R, Solas C, Moreau J, Colson P (2013) Chronic hepatitis E resolution in a human immunodeficiency virus (HIV)-infected patient treated with ribavirin. Int J Antimicrob Agents 41:595–597
47. Dalton HR, Keane FE, Bendall R, Mathew J, Ijaz S (2011) Treatment of chronic hepatitis E in a patient with HIV infection. Ann Intern Med 155:479–480
48. Donnelly MC, Scobie L, Crossan CL, Dalton H, Hayes PC, Simpson KJ (2017) Review article: hepatitis E-a concise review of virology, epidemiology, clinical presentation and therapy. Aliment Pharmacol Ther 46:126
49. Corey L, Wald A (2009) Maternal and neonatal herpes simplex virus infections. N Engl J Med 361:1376–1385
50. Kropp RY, Wong T, Cormier L, Ringrose A, Burton S, Embree JE, Steben M (2006) Neonatal herpes simplex virus infections in Canada: results of a 3-year national prospective study. Pediatrics 117:1955–1962
51. McGoogan KE, Haafiz AB, Gonzalez Peralta RP (2011) Herpes simplex virus hepatitis in infants: clinical outcomes and correlates of disease severity. J Pediatr 159:608–611
52. Verma A, Dhawan A, Zuckerman M, Hadzic N, Baker AJ, Mieli-Vergani G (2006) Neonatal herpes simplex virus infection presenting as acute liver failure: prevalent role of herpes simplex virus type I. J Pediatr Gastroenterol Nutr 42:282–286
53. Norvell JP, Blei AT, Jovanovic BD, Levitsky J (2007) Herpes simplex virus hepatitis: an analysis of the published literature and institutional cases. Liver Transpl 13:1428–1434
54. Sundaram SS, Alonso EM, Narkewicz MR, Zhang S, Squires RH (2011) Characterization and outcomes of young infants with acute liver failure. J Pediatr 159:813–818 e811
55. Ichai P, Roque Afonso AM, Sebagh M, Gonzalez ME, Codes L, Azoulay D, Saliba F et al (2005) Herpes simplex virus-associated acute liver failure: a difficult diagnosis with a poor prognosis. Liver Transpl 11:1550–1555
56. Levitsky J, Duddempudi AT, Lakeman FD, Whitley RJ, Luby JP, Lee WM, Fontana RJ et al (2008) Detection and diagnosis of herpes simplex virus infection in adults with acute liver failure. Liver Transpl 14:1498–1504
57. Twagira M, Hadzic N, Smith M, Ramaswamy M, Verma A, Dhawan A, Knisely AS et al (2004) Disseminated neonatal herpes simplex virus (HSV) type 2 infection diagnosed by HSV DNA detection in blood and successfully managed by liver transplantation. Eur J Pediatr 163:166–169
58. Lugo D, Krogstad P (2016) Enteroviruses in the early 21st century: new manifestations and challenges. Curr Opin Pediatr 28:107–113
59. Ahmad S, Dalwai A, Al-Nakib W (2013) Frequency of enterovirus detection in blood samples of neonates admitted to hospital with sepsis-like illness in Kuwait. J Med Virol 85:1280–1285
60. Abzug MJ (2001) Prognosis for neonates with enterovirus hepatitis and coagulopathy. Pediatr Infect Dis J 20:758–763
61. Bauer L, Lyoo H, van der Schaar HM, Strating JR, van Kuppeveld FJ (2017) Direct-acting antivirals and host-targeting strategies to combat enterovirus infections. Curr Opin Virol 24:1–8
62. Abzug MJ, Michaels MG, Wald E, Jacobs RF, Romero JR, Sanchez PJ, Wilson G et al (2016) A randomized, double-blind, placebo-controlled trial of Pleconaril for the treatment of neonates with enterovirus Sepsis. J Pediatr Infect Dis Soc 5:53–62
63. Grabhorn E, Richter A, Fischer L, Ganschow R (2008) Emergency liver transplantation in neonates with acute liver failure: long-term follow-up. Transplantation 86:932–936
64. Miyata I, Hanaoka N, Okabe N, Fujimoto T, Sakamoto S, Kasahara M, Saitoh A (2014) Echovirus 3 as another enterovirus causing life-threatening neonatal fulminant hepatitis. J Clin Virol 59:132–134
65. Rocholl C, Gerber K, Daly J, Pavia AT, Byington CL (2004) Adenoviral infections in children: the impact of rapid diagnosis. Pediatrics 113:e51–e56
66. Matoq A, Salahuddin A (2016) Acute hepatitis and pancytopenia in healthy infant with adenovirus. Case Rep Pediatr 2016:8648190
67. Schaberg KB, Kambham N, Sibley RK, Higgins JP (2017) Adenovirus hepatitis: Clinicopathologic analysis of 12 consecutive cases from a single institution. Am J Surg Pathol 41:810
68. Cimsit B, Tichy EM, Patel SB, Rosencrantz R, Emre S (2012) Treatment of adenovirus hepatitis with cidofovir in a pediatric liver transplant recipient. Pediatr Transplant 16:E90–E93
69. Tsunoda T, Inui A, Iwasawa K, Oikawa M, Sogo T, Komatsu H, Ito Y et al (2017) Acute liver dysfunction not resulting from hepatitis virus in immunocompetent children. Pediatr Int 59:551
70. Hasosah MY, Kutbi SY, Al-Amri AW, Alsahafi AF, Sukkar GA, Alghamdi KJ, Jacobson K (2012) Perinatal cytomegalovirus hepatitis in Saudi infants: a case series. Saudi J Gastroenterol 18:208–213
71. Shkalim-Zemer V, Shahar-Nissan K, Ashkenazi-Hoffnung L, Amir J, Bilavsky E (2015) Cholestatic hepatitis induced by Epstein-Barr virus in a pediatric population. Clin Pediatr (Phila) 54:1153–1157
72. Mellinger JL, Rossaro L, Naugler WE, Nadig SN, Appelman H, Lee WM, Fontana RJ (2014) Epstein-Barr virus (EBV) related acute liver failure: a case series from the US acute liver failure study group. Dig Dis Sci 59:1630–1637
73. Maakaroun NR, Moanna A, Jacob JT, Albrecht H (2010) Viral infections associated with haemophagocytic syndrome. Rev Med Virol 20:93–105

74. Kogawa K, Sato H, Asano T, Ohga S, Kudo K, Morimoto A, Ohta S et al (2014) Prognostic factors of Epstein-Barr virus-associated hemophagocytic lymphohistiocytosis in children: report of the Japan Histiocytosis Study Group. Pediatr Blood Cancer 61:1257–1262
75. Stefanou C, Tzortzi C, Georgiou F, Timiliotou C (2016) Combining an antiviral with rituximab in EBV-related haemophagocytic lymphohistiocytosis led to rapid viral clearance; and a comprehensive review. BMJ Case Rep 2016
76. Kunitomi A, Kimura H, Ito Y, Naitoh K, Noda N, Iida H, Sao H (2011) Unrelated bone marrow transplantation induced long-term remission in a patient with life-threatening Epstein-Barr virus-associated hemophagocytic lymphohistiocytosis. J Clin Exp Hematop 51:57–61
77. Harma M, Hockerstedt K, Lautenschlager I (2003) Human herpesvirus-6 and acute liver failure. Transplantation 76:536–539
78. Chevret L, Boutolleau D, Halimi-Idri N, Branchereau S, Baujard C, Fabre M, Gautheret-Dejean A et al (2008) Human herpesvirus-6 infection: a prospective study evaluating HHV-6 DNA levels in liver from children with acute liver failure. J Med Virol 80:1051–1057
79. Harma M, Hockerstedt K, Lautenschlager I (2013) The long-term outcomes of patients transplanted due to acute liver failure with hepatic human herpesvirus-6 infection. Transplant Proc 45:1910–1912
80. Whitworth JR, Mack CL, O'Connor JA, Narkewicz MR, Mengshol S, Sokol RJ (2006) Acute hepatitis and liver failure associated with influenza A infection in children. J Pediatr Gastroenterol Nutr 43:536–538
81. Leonis MA, Alonso EM, Im K, Belle SH, Squires RH, Pediatric Acute Liver Failure Study G (2013) Chronic acetaminophen exposure in pediatric acute liver failure. Pediatrics 131:e740–e746
82. Polakos NK, Cornejo JC, Murray DA, Wright KO, Treanor JJ, Crispe IN, Topham DJ et al (2006) Kupffer cell-dependent hepatitis occurs during influenza infection. Am J Pathol 168:1169–1178 quiz 1404–1165
83. Samanta J, Sharma V (2015) Dengue and its effects on liver. World J Clin Case 3:125–131
84. Fernando S, Wijewickrama A, Gomes L, Punchihewa CT, Madusanka SD, Dissanayake H, Jeewandara C et al (2016) Patterns and causes of liver involvement in acute dengue infection. BMC Infect Dis 16:319
85. Poovorawan Y, Hutagalung Y, Chongsrisawat V, Boudville I, Bock HL (2006) Dengue virus infection: a major cause of acute hepatic failure in Thai children. Ann Trop Paediatr 26:17–23
86. Sharp TM, Gaul L, Muehlenbachs A, Hunsperger E, Bhatnagar J, Lueptow R, Santiago GA et al (2014) Fatal hemophagocytic lymphohistiocytosis associated with locally acquired dengue virus infection – New Mexico and Texas, 2012. MMWR Morb Mortal Wkly Rep 63:49–54
87. Young NS, Brown KE (2004) Parvovirus B19. N Engl J Med 350:586–597
88. Dwivedi M, Manocha H, Tiwari S, Tripathi G, Dhole TN (2009) Coinfection of parvovirus b19 with other hepatitis viruses leading to fulminant hepatitis of unfavorable outcome in children. Pediatr Infect Dis J 28:649–650
89. Langnas AN, Markin RS, Cattral MS, Naides SJ (1995) Parvovirus B19 as a possible causative agent of fulminant liver failure and associated aplastic anemia. Hepatology 22:1661–1665
90. Bathla L, Grant WJ, Mercer DF, Vargas LM, Gebhart CL, Langnas AN (2014) Parvovirus associated fulminant hepatic failure and aplastic anemia treated successfully with liver and bone marrow transplantation. A report of two cases. Am J Transplant 14:2645–2650
91. Wong S, Young NS, Brown KE (2003) Prevalence of parvovirus B19 in liver tissue: no association with fulminant hepatitis or hepatitis-associated aplastic anemia. J Infect Dis 187:1581–1586

16 Emerging New Therapies for Viral Hepatitis

Pei-Yi Su and Chiaho Shih

Abstract

Viral hepatitis can be caused by infection with different viruses, including hepatitis A virus (HAV), hepatitis B virus (HBV), hepatitis C virus (HCV), hepatitis D virus (HDV), and hepatitis E virus (HEV). In this chapter, we summarized current treatments and new emerging therapies for viral hepatitis in general, with a particular focus on chronic hepatitis B. Acute hepatitis is most commonly managed with supportive care symptomatically. Recently, chronic infection with HCV can be cured at a high efficacy with combinations of antivirals via oral intake. Unlike HCV, eradication of HBV in chronic hepatitis B patients remains a challenge. We reviewed here recent advances of new strategies for HBV therapy, including the inhibition of viral entry, the destruction or silencing of HBV covalently closed circular DNA (cccDNA), and the approach of breaking immune tolerance. Combinations of different therapeutic strategies could improve the cure rate of chronic hepatitis B.

Keywords

Chronic infection · Combination therapy · Covalently closed circular DNA (cccDNA) · Hepatitis B virus · Immune tolerance · Viral entry

P.-Y. Su · C. Shih (✉)
Institute of Biomedical Sciences, Academia Sinica, Taipei, Taiwan
e-mail: cshih@ibms.sinica.edu.tw

16.1 HAV

So far, there are no specific antivirals for HAV infection. Treatment for acute hepatitis A is mainly by supportive therapies symptomatically [1]. In most cases, infected patients can clear HAV spontaneously without persistent infection and recurrent liver damage. Formaldehyde- inactivated HAV vaccine (Table 16.1) is effective against clinically apparent hepatitis A in recent decades [2–4]. In China and India, live attenuated HAV vaccines have been shown to be safe and highly protective against clinical infection in recent years [4–6]. Of note, potential inhibitors against HAV replication, such as JAK2 and sirtuin inhibitors, are also under active investigation [7, 8] (Table 16.2).

16.2 HCV

Infection with HCV often results in chronic infection. Interferon-based treatment at an early stage of HCV infection could help viral clearance [12]. As shown in Table 16.1, IFN alpha combined with ribavirin treatment has been a major therapy for a long while [13]. However,

M.-H. Chang, K. B. Schwarz (eds.), *Viral Hepatitis in Children*,
https://doi.org/10.1007/978-981-13-0050-9_16

the effects on viral clearance and the sustained virological response (SVR) rate are variable between genotypes (gt) and populations. In 2011, the first-generation direct-acting antivirals (DAAs), such as telaprevir and boceprevir, were introduced for HCV therapy. So far, DAAs for HCV can be divided into three classes based on their different targets of viral proteins: (a) NS3/4A protease inhibitors, such as telaprevir, boceprevir, simeprevir, asunaprevir, grazoprevir, and paritaprevir (of note telaprevir and boceprevir were not FDA-approved given the side effects); (b) NS5B polymerase inhibitors, such as sofosbuvir and dasabuvir, and (c) NS5A inhibitors, such as ledipasvir, daclatasvir, velpatasvir, ombitasvir, and elbasvir [14]. For example, the combination treatment of velpatasvir and sofosbuvir for 12 weeks can cure up to 97–100% for all HCV genotypes, including gt 1a, 1b, 2, 3, 4, 5, and 6 [15, 16]. Similarly, the cure rate of the combination treatment of grazoprevir and elbasvir is around 92–99% for gt 1a and 1b and near 100% for gt 4 [17]. For further information about HCV therapeutics, please refer to many excellent reviews in literature as well as Chap. 11 by Green and Murray.

Table 16.1 Conventional medicine for viral hepatitis

	Treatments	Vaccine
HAV	Supportive care	Available
HBV	Interferon alpha/pegylated interferon	Available
	Nucleos(t)ide analogs	
HCV	PEG-IFN and ribavirin	Available
	Direct-acting antivirals (DAAs)	
	NS3/4A protease inhibitors	
	NS5B polymerase inhibitors	
	NS5A inhibitors	
HDV	Interferon alpha	HBV vaccine
	Supportive care	
HEV	Supportive care	Phase IV clinical trials

16.3 HDV

There are no specific drugs for hepatitis D. PEG-IFN alpha treatment can facilitate viral clearance in chronic hepatitis D in 25–30% of patients (Table 16.1); however, PEG-IFN alpha treatment combined with adefovir has shown no improved efficacy [18–20]. Here, we summarized the new HDV prodrugs at the late preclinical or clinical

Table 16.2 New emerging prodrugs for hepatitis A, D, and E

	Drug name	Mechanism/target	Status	References
HAV	AZD1480	Host factor: JAK2	Cell models	Jiang et al. [7]
	Sirtinol	Host factor: sirtuin	Cell models	Kanda et al. [8]
HDV	Myrcludex B (pre-S1 peptide)	Entry inhibitor	Phases I–II	NCT02888106[a]
				NCT02637999
	Rep 2139	HBsAg	Phase II	NCT02233075
				NCT02726789
	Lonafarnib	Viral prenylation	Phase II	NCT02430194
				NCT02430181
	ALN-HDV	RNAi	Preclinical	Koh et al. [9]
	Pegylated interferon lambda	Immunomodulator	Phase II	NCT02765802
HEV	Ribavirin	Guanosine (ribonucleic) analog	Phase IV	NCT02558114
	Sofosbuvir + ribavirin	Nucleotide analog	Cell models	Dao et al. [10]
	MPA (mycophenolic acid)	Inosine monophosphate dehydrogenase inhibitor	Cell models	Wang et al. [11]
	Cyclophilins A and B	The targets of cyclosporine A	Cell models	Wang et al. [11]

[a]Identifier for ClinicalTrials.gov

stage in Table 16.2. The potent new therapies include the entry inhibitor of HBV/HDV, HBsAg inhibitor, the prenylation inhibitor [9], and RNAi gene silencer specific for HDV and immunomodulator (PEG-IFN lambda) [19]. So far, there is no vaccine available for HDV, but the HBV vaccination can be used for effective protection against HDV, a parasite virus of HBV.

16.4 HEV

Similar to other viral hepatitis, patients with acute HEV infection can clear the virus spontaneously after a certain period. In some rare cases, acute HEV infection could lead to severe liver failure and damage. Short-term treatment with ribavirin is safe and effective for acute HEV infection [21]. However, ribavirin treatment in pregnant women may increase the risk of stillbirths, abortions, premature distribution, and maternal or fetal death [22]. Ribavirin treatment for severe acute HEV infection is being tested in Phase IV clinical trials (Table 16.2; https://clinicaltrials.gov/ct2/show/NCT02558114).

Organ transplant patients with chronic hepatitis E can be treated in two steps. The first step is to reduce immunosuppression in these patients, which can help to clear virus up to 30% of patients [23]. Treatment with MPA (mycophenolic acid; inosine monophosphate dehydrogenase inhibitor) and cyclosporine A (target at cyclophilins A and B) has also been shown to inhibit HEV replication [11] (Table 16.2). The second step is to use ribavirin for further treatment [23–25]. Continuous treatment of ribavirin for 3 months can achieve an SVR rate up to 78%, and extended treatment for 6 months can achieve an SVR up to 85% [26]. The in vitro combination treatment of ribavirin and sofosbuvir can significantly increase the efficacy of HEV inhibition [10]. Combination treatment in vivo for HEV is still under investigation. Because HEV appeared to have an anti-interferon mechanism, treatment with type I, II, and III IFN should be carefully assessed [24]. A promising vaccine candidate for HEV is in Phase IV clinical trials in China and Bangladesh (https://clinicaltrials.gov/ct2/show/NCT02584543; https://clinicaltrials.gov/ct2/show/NCT02759991).

16.5 HBV

Similar to other viral hepatitis, acute HBV patients are treated with supporting care symptomatically [27]. Most patients with acute HBV can recover spontaneously. At present, HBV vaccination is a well-established, safe, and effective practice worldwide. However, 5–15% of vaccine recipients are estimated to be nonresponders. For HBV chronic infection, there are two most common types of treatment (Table 16.1): interferon alpha (IFN-α) and nucleos(t)ide analogs (NAs; lamivudine, entecavir, emtricitabine, telbivudine, adefovir, and tenofovir) [28]. Long-term treatment with NAs can frequently select for drug-resistant variants, and IFN treatment is notorious for its side effects [29]. In brief, current HBV therapy using either interferon or polymerase inhibitors (NAs) cannot cure HBV at a high efficacy. Lifelong therapy with NAs is often needed to suppress HBV in patients who maintain a very low level of HBV DNA in the liver. It is therefore very important and urgent to develop new antiviral therapies for chronic hepatitis B.

16.6 HBV Life Cycle

HBV is the smallest DNA animal virus, which replicates through a RNA intermediate. In HBV life cycle (Fig. 16.1), HBV attaches to the host cell surface and binds with its entry receptor NTCP (sodium taurocholate cotransporting polypeptide). After viral entry, HBV undergoes an uncoating step to remove its envelope proteins. Capsid particles containing the relaxed circular (RC) DNA genome can traffic to the nucleus and release the RC DNA. In the nucleus, RC DNA can be converted into cccDNA (covalently closed circular DNA). This cccDNA form can serve as a template for viral mRNA transcription. It is very difficult to clear cccDNA from the nucleus of

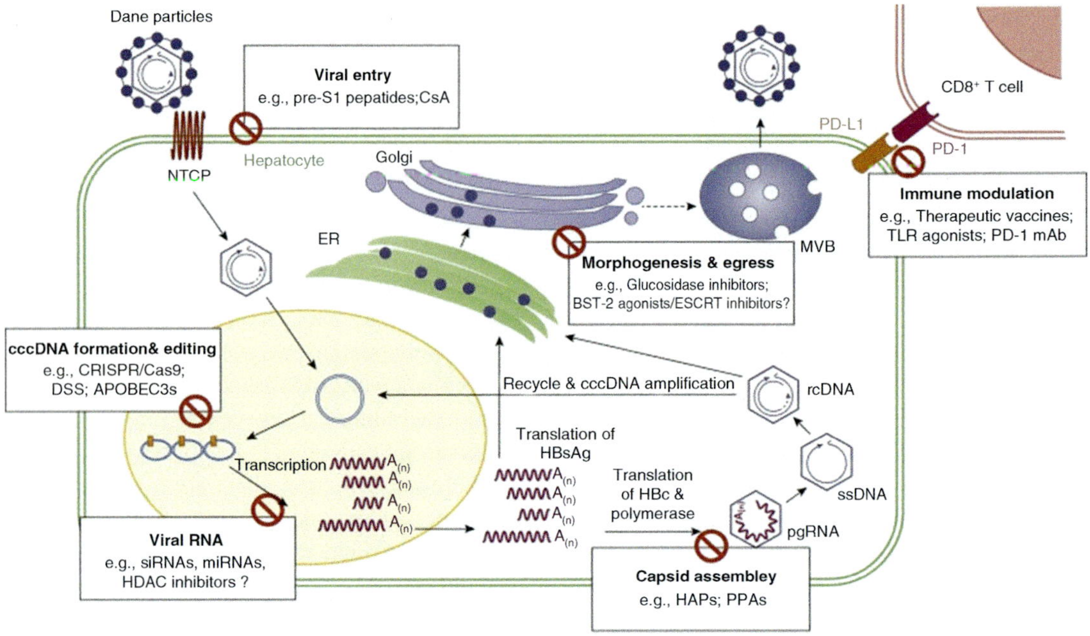

Fig. 16.1 A cartoon illustration of six major potential targets in HBV life cycle for therapeutic research: (1) viral entry, by targeting at the cellular NTCP receptor or the viral preS1 ligand; (2) covalently closed circular (ccc) DNA, by genome editing or prevention from cccDNA biogenesis; (3) viral RNA, by RNA interference or chromatin modification; (4) core particle (capsid) assembly, by modification of capsid assembly and pgRNA encapsidation; (5) envelopment and virion secretion, by inhibiting morphogenesis and egress of virions; and (6) host immunity, by breaking the liver immune tolerance or by reactivation of innate or humoral immunity. The conventional interferon-α treatment and polymerase inhibitors are not included here [30, 31]. Abbreviations: *CsA* cyclosporine A, *DSS* disubstituted sulfonamide, *HAPs* heteroaryldihydropyrimidines, *PPAs* phenylpropenamides. (Reproduced with permission from Ref. [32])

infected hepatocytes. It is this cccDNA reservoir that is responsible for chronic hepatitis B [33]. In the cytoplasm, HBV core protein, polymerase, and the pregenomic RNA (pgRNA) can assemble into an icosahedral particle, where pgRNA can be reverse transcribed into an RC DNA genome. Mature capsids containing RC DNA can either traffic back into nucleus for more cccDNA amplification or assemble with envelope proteins for virion secretion (Fig. 16.1).

Persistent infection with HBV can cause liver inflammation, injury, fibrosis, cirrhosis, liver failure, and hepatocellular carcinoma (HCC). Although the current antiviral therapy of chronic hepatitis B can reduce the risk of cirrhosis and HCC [30, 34], as mentioned earlier, it remains a challenge to eradicate HBV from patients. We summarized here new emerging therapies against HBV in Table 16.3. As illustrated in Fig. 16.1, potential antiviral targets include the inhibition of viral entry, formation of cccDNA, RNA interference, capsid assembly, virion secretion, and breaking immune tolerance in chronic carriers.

16.7 Viral Entry Inhibitors

HBV uses the viral pre-S1 domain of the large envelope proteins (LHBs) to bind with its entry receptor, cellular NTCP [56]. Pre-S1 peptide is an entry inhibitor shown to inhibit HBV and HDV infection in vitro [57, 58]. In a humanized mouse model, this pre-S1 peptide can inhibit

Table 16.3 New emerging therapies for hepatitis B

Drug name	Mechanism/target	Sponsor	Status	References
Myrcludex B (pre-S1 peptide)	Entry inhibitor	Hepatera Ltd.	Phases I–II	NCT02888106[a]
				NCT02881008
Cyclosporine A	Entry inhibitor		Cell models	Watashi et al. [35], Nkongolo et al. [36] and Shimura et al. [37]
CRISPR/Cas9	cccDNA		Cell models and animal models	Kennedy et al. [38], Lin et al. [39], Lin et al. [40], Liu et al. [41] and Moyo et al. [42]
ARB-1467	SiRNA (target viral RNAs)	Arbutus Biopharma	Phase II	http://investor.arbutusbio.com/releasedetail.cfm?ReleaseID=1003823
ARC-520	SiRNA (target viral RNAs)	Arrowhead Pharmaceuticals	Phase IIa	NCT02452528
				NCT02065336
				NCT02577029
ALN-HBV	SiRNA (target viral RNAs)	Alnylam Pharmaceuticals	Phases I–II	NCT02826018
miR-130a	miRNA (target host factor)		Animal models	Huang et al. [43]
miR-125a-5p, miR-199a	miRNA (target host factor)		Cell models	Lamontagne et al. [44]
GLS4 (morphothiadin; HAPs derivatives)	Viral assembly inhibitor	HEC Pharma	Phase II	Wu et al. [45]
				Schinazi and Asselah [46]
AT-130 (PPAs derivatives)	Viral assembly inhibitor		Preclinical	Katen et al. [47]
				Schinazi and Asselah [46]
NVR 3–778 (NVR1221)	Viral assembly inhibitor	Janssen	Phase Ib	NCT02112799
				NCT02401737
α-glucosidase inhibitor (iminosugar derivatives)	Virion secretion inhibitor		Preclinical	Lazar et al. [48], Chang et al. [49] and Simsek et al. [50]
ESCRT components	Virion secretion inhibitor		Cell models and animal models	Kian Chua et al. [51], Lambert et al. [52] and Chou et al. [53]
GS 4774	Therapeutic vaccine	Gilead Sciences	Phase II	NCT02174276
				NCT01943799
INO-1800	Therapeutic vaccine	Inovio Pharmaceuticals	Phase I	NCT02431312

(continued)

Table 16.3 (continued)

Drug name	Mechanism/target	Sponsor	Status	References
ABX203	Therapeutic vaccine	Abivax S.A.	Phase II–III	NCT02249988
TG1050	Therapeutic vaccine	Transgene	Phase I	NCT02428400
Anti-PD-L1	Immunotherapy		Animal models	Tzeng et al. [54]
				Liu et al. [55]
GS-9620 (vesatolimod)	TLR-7 agonist	Gilead Sciences	Phase II	NCT02579382
				NCT02166047
RO6864018 (RG7795, ANA773)	TLR-7 agonist	Roche	Phase II	NCT02391805
SB 9200	RIG-1 and NOD2 agonist	Spring Bank Pharmaceuticals	Phase II	NCT02751996
CYT107	Recombinant human IL-7	National Cancer Institute (NCI)	Phases I–II	NCT01027065
				NCT01339000

[a]Identifier for ClinicalTrials.gov

both HBV infection and intrahepatic virus spreading [59]. The studies of myristoylated pre-S1 peptide (Myrcludex B) for HBV patients are currently in Phase I–II clinical trials (Table 16.3; https://clini-caltrials.gov/ct2/show/NCT02888106; https://clinicaltrials.gov/ct2/show/NCT02881008). Cyclosporine A (CsA) is an FDA-approved immunomodulator. This compound can serve as another entry inhibitor by blocking the interaction between HBV pre-S1 peptide and NTCP [35, 36]. Recently, one study identified a new CsA derivative, which can selectively inhibit HBV entry without the side effect of interfering with the NTCP transporter activity [37]. Furthermore, proanthocyanidin and its analogs can directly act on LHBs and thus represent a new class of hepatitis B and D virus entry inhibitors [60]. In addition to pre-S1 peptide and CsA, there are several other NTCP entry inhibitors, including FDA-approved drugs (ezetimibe and irbesartan), bile acids (e.g., tauroursodeoxycholic acid), and tricyclic polyketide [61–63]. In addition to directly targeting at the NTCP molecule or the pre-S1 peptide, some drug candidates can reduce NTCP expression [63], such as retinoic acid receptor (RAR) antagonist (Ro41-5253).

Potential limitations of entry inhibitors need to be discussed. First, while entry inhibitors can strongly inhibit HBV reinfection [59], they cannot eradicate viral cccDNA and persistent infection. Second, NTCP may not be the only receptor for HBV entry. For example, HepG2 cells expressing NTCP variant p. Ser267Phe (S267F) are resistant to in vitro HBV infection [61]. However, HBsAg+ patients carrying the infection-resistant S267F allele of NTCP can be found in Asia [64, 65]. Therefore, a therapeutic strategy by targeting NTCP may not completely prevent HBV infection. Overall, while entry inhibitors alone may not be sufficient to eradicate cccDNA and abolish chronic infection, combination with other therapeutics merits further investigation.

16.8 Elimination of HBV cccDNA by Exogenous Nuclease Digestion

It is generally believed that cccDNA is the major reason for HBV persistent infection and drug resistance. To target cccDNA is one of the best strategies for HBV eradication. The approaches for cccDNA destruction could be by zinc finger nucleases (ZFNs), transcription activator-like effector nucleases (TALENs), and the clustered regularly interspaced short palindromic repeats (CRISPR)/Cas9 system [66]. For example, in a Phase I clinical trial of HIV infection, a ZFN was used to target HIV entry co-receptor CCR5 [67]. Both ZFNs and TALENs have been used to cleave the hepadnaviral cccDNA [68, 69]. Similarly, the CRISPR/Cas9 system has also been widely tested for HBV treatment [38–42]. In this genome editing approach, it is a good practice to design multiple target sites at evolutionarily conserved regions among different HBV genotypes [41].

Despite the fact that genome editing is a fashionable tool for research, it is not without limitations. First, the direct or indirect effect of CRISPR/Cas9 treatment needs to be more carefully distinguished. In particular, the specificity of CRISPR/Cas9 is not perfect, and it is known for its low stringency in base pairing and frequent off-target effects [70, 71]. Can CRISPR/Cas9 distinguish between integrated linear HBV DNA from episomal cccDNA? If not, host chromosomes could be cleaved and damaged at integrated HBV DNA sites by CRISPR/Cas9 in HBV-infected hepatocytes. Clinical trials using ZFN to target CCR5 (the HIV co-receptor) are ongoing [67]. It is hopeful that ZFN- or Cas9-damaged chromosomes can be repaired timely and efficiently by host cells. Second, CRISPR-/Cas9-resistant HBV variants could emerge from the selection by CRISPR/Cas9 treatment. Therefore, multiple sgRNAs targeting at multiple sites should be considered [72]. Of note,

CRISPR-/Cas9-resistant HIV mutants have been reported recently [73]. Third, the amount of cccDNA molecules should always be measured before and after CRISPR/Cas9 treatment. In addition to quantitative PCR assay, it is most convincing if cccDNA can be characterized by Southern blot analysis. Fourth, in the in vivo delivery of CRISPR/Cas9 and sgRNA to hepatocytes in the liver, the therapeutic efficacy also depends on the efficiency of the delivery vehicles. Unless a very high percentage of infected hepatocytes can be transduced with CRISPR/Cas9 in the liver, the therapeutic efficacy in vivo could be an issue. Fifth, it is unclear whether the naked form and minichromosomes of cccDNA can be equally targeted and cleaved by CRISPR/Cas9. Different versions of Cas9 with improved features in genome editing are already around the corner [38]. It would be interesting to see whether new versions of CRISPR/Cas9 can circumvent all these issues in the future.

16.9 Epigenetic Silencing of HBV cccDNA Expression

The episomal cccDNA of hepadnaviruses was shown to exist as a minichromosome [74, 75]. Transcription of HBV cccDNA can be epigenetically regulated by cytokines and histone deacetylase (HDAC) inhibitors [76]. However, controversy over the effect of HDAC inhibitors on HBV replication needs to be resolved [77, 78]. Another controversy is about the correlation between cccDNA methylation and viral replication in chronic HBV patients [79, 80]. At present, it is unclear how the HDAC inhibitors could selectively affect the expression of cccDNA minichromosomes, but not the excessive background of host chromosomes. In fact, HDAC inhibitors are known to reduce platelet counts and for the side effect of reactivation of latent HSV or EBV [81, 82]. Unless these serious side effects can be properly managed, it may not be possible to repurpose HDAC inhibitors against cccDNA transcription in patients.

16.10 RNA Interference

Both siRNAs and miRNAs are new tools for gene silencing. In nature, miRNAs play important roles in development and diseases [83, 84]. At present, a number of siRNA and miRNA candidates are being tested in clinical trials for human diseases [85, 86] (Table 16.3). For example, miRNA-122 is highly abundant in the liver and is required for HCV replication. Miravirsen is a drug that can deplete miR-122. In a clinical trial, miravirsen therapy effectively reduced HCV RNA levels in patients with no side effects and drug resistance [86]. Furthermore, patients with Crohn's disease were treated with oral intake of a SMAD7 antisense oligonucleotide. These patients showed higher rates of remission and clinical response than the control [87]. In another human cancer clinical trial, miR-34 mimics are being tested as tumor suppressors [88].

ARC-520 is a cholesterol-conjugated siRNA drug against HBV [75]. It can significantly suppress viral expression and replication in cell culture and animal models [89]. A Phase IIa clinical trial reported that this drug was nontoxic, and treated patients displayed a reduced level of HBV surface antigen for nearly 2 months [90].

The replication of HBV can be inhibited by several cellular miRNAs, such as miR-130a [43], miR-125a-5p, and miR-199a [44]. MiR-130a was shown to target at PPARγ and PGC1α, which are important coactivators for HBV transcription [43]. It will be important to further demonstrate in animal models whether these miRNAs can inhibit HBV propagation.

16.11 Allosteric Modulators of Capsid Assembly

Two prototype capsid inhibitors include heteroaryldihydropyrimidines (HAPs) [91, 92] and phenylpropenamides (PPAs) [47]. Derivatives of these compounds are currently being tested in preclinical or clinical trials [46, 93]. GLS4 (morphothiadin) is another derivative related to the

HAP compound BAY41-4109 but with greatly increased potency (IC50 or EC50) and significantly reduced toxicity [45]. NVR-010-001-E2 is a stereoisomer of GLS4. These drugs cannot only interfere with pgRNA encapsidation leading to the formation of empty capsids but also affect capsid stability and morphology. It is relevant to know whether these capsid inhibitors can work across all HBV genotypes and whether drug-resistant variants will emerge after drug selection. In natural infection, HBc can assemble into icosahedral particles of either smaller (180-mer) or larger (240-mer) sizes [94]. It remains critical to know whether these drugs can target at both larger- and smaller-sized particles.

16.12 Inhibition of Virion Secretion

Another therapeutic strategy is to target virion secretion. Three examples can be cited here. First, HBV virions need HBsAg envelope for secretion. HBsAg is a glycoprotein. Endoplasmic reticulum (ER) is the factory for protein glycosylation. Available compounds which can perturb glycosylation include α-glucosidase inhibitors [48], iminosugar derivatives, and related glycolipids [49]. Indeed, inhibition of HBsAg glycosylation can reduce egress of infectious virions [50]. Potential side effects of this type of compound include gastrointestinal illness [49].

The endosomal sorting complex required for transport (ESCRT) is an important cellular machinery for the sorting and trafficking of ubiquitinated cargos. In the second example, we focus on the ESCRT machinery [95]. Dominant-negative ESCRT mutants, such as VPS4, can hamper the secretion of HBV virions [51, 52]. Furthermore, treatment with siRNAs specific for a number of ESCRT factors can strongly down-regulate HBV transcription and replication [51, 53]. Recently, the ESCRT-0 factor HGS was shown to have a dual role in silencing HBV RNA transcription and promoting the release of naked capsids [53]. By HGS co-transfection, HBV exhibited a significantly reduced level of nucleocapsids and secreted virions [53]. In addition, α-taxilin was shown to be important for HBV virion secretion [96]. In brief, these host factors and the ESCRT machinery are promising targets for developing virion morphogenesis inhibitors.

The third example is BST-2/tetherin. This is an IFN-inducible host factor. BST-2/tetherin can restrict viral morphogenesis and secretion, such as HIV [97]. Three recent reports demonstrated that tetherin can also restrict HBV virion secretion, albeit their reported efficiencies are different [98–100]. At present, part of the tetherin protein structure is known [101], and this could provide an opportunity for a bioinformatics-based drug research. In theory, tetherin agonists could reduce the amount of virions in the blood circulation. Overall, virion release is a druggable target, which can be further developed by interference with envelope protein glycosylation, ESCRT machinery, or enhancement of tetherin/BST-2 restriction.

16.13 Immunotherapy by Therapeutic Vaccination

T cell exhaustion has been considered as a primary cause for the lack of viral clearance in the liver chronically infected with HBV [102]. The main goal of immunotherapy is to refresh the tolerant host immunity and restore an effective level of the HBV-specific T cell population. To this end, one approach is to treat chronic carriers with therapeutic vaccines [103]. In Phase I clinical studies, therapeutic vaccination yields no satisfactory outcome in terms of HBeAg seroconversion rate or the reduction of viral DNA titers [104, 105]. While the heterologous prime-boost vaccination can induce a potent T cell response [106], it is equally important to have a sustained level of cytotoxic T lymphocytes (CTL) in the liver. In this regard, it is noteworthy that aggregates of CD11b + myeloid cells could contribute to the maintenance of HBc-specific CTLs in the liver [107].

In a cohort of lamivudine-treated Caucasian patients, good therapeutic efficacy was obtained by using combined DNA vaccine containing a mixture of various HBV ORFs and immunomodulator IL-12 [108]. The rationale for the inclusion of IL12 is because it is an important cytokine for survival and differentiation of HBV-specific CTLs [109]. In a Phase I trial of adefovir-treated Korean patients, however, a further modified DNA vaccine exhibited a weak response [110]. Another Phase III clinical trial was conducted by using the alum adjuvant and an HBsAg-HBIG complex. Again, the efficacy needs further improvement [111]. Additional clinical trials of therapeutic vaccines can be cited such as the Phase II–III trials with ABX203 and nucleos(t) ide analogs in HBeAg-negative chronic carriers (http://clinicaltrials.gov/ct2/show/NCT02249988), the Phase I trial with INO-1800 regimens in entecavir and/or tenofovir-treated carriers (http://clinicaltrials.gov/ct2/show/NCT02431312), and the Phase I trial with TG1050 in tenofovir or entecavir-treated carriers (http://clinicaltrials.gov/ct2/show/NCT02428400). Given such active clinical research on therapeutic vaccination, it is hopeful that one can soon achieve the goal of breaking the immune tolerance in HBV chronic carriers.

16.14 Immunotherapy Against Immune Checkpoints

Treatment of cancer patients with an antibody specific for PD-1 (programmed cell death-1) has been shown to break immune tolerance [112]. This PD-1 blockade approach can restore virus-specific CD8 T cells in inactive HBV carrier patients [113]. Similarly, a sophisticated combination therapy was conducted using a woodchuck model chronically infected with woodchuck hepatitis B virus (WHV) [55]. The WHV titer in these woodchucks was first reduced by treatment with entecavir for 7 months. Therapeutic vaccinations were conducted repeatedly by injecting plasmid DNA-expressing WHV core and surface antigens at around 3 months after entecavir was initiated. Finally, an anti-PD-L1 antibody was administered three times on week 24. This triple combination approach produced encouraging results in some of the treated woodchucks, including WHsAg seroconversion, disappearance of serum WHV DNA, and an increased level of WHV core antigen-specific CD8 T cells. It remains to be investigated whether other immune checkpoint molecules, such as Tim-3 [114], CD244/CD48 [115], CTLA-4 [116], and the Axl pathway [117], can also serve as druggable targets for immunotherapy.

Despite the encouraging result from this woodchuck therapy, several issues need to be addressed. First, is WHV cccDNA still detectable in the hepatocytes of seroconverted woodchucks? Second, how can the therapeutic efficacy be improved? Finally, what could be the mechanism behind this PD-1/PD-L1 blockade leading to the evolution from immune tolerance to immune clearance? What could be the mechanism for the reactivation or repopulation of HBV-specific CD8 T cells? Does the rejuvenated immune clearance involve any other arms of the innate or adaptive immune systems [118]? In addition to the reported adversary effects, such as pneumonitis, liver injury, and endocrine dysfunction [119], can the treatment with anti-PD-1/PD-L1 antibody induce fulminant hepatitis after breaking the tolerance? One caveat here is to first reduce viral titers to low levels, prior to combination treatment with the antibody specific for immune checkpoints. The concept here is that immune-mediated liver injury needs to be "optimized" for safety and viral clearance.

16.15 Other Immune Modulators

With one exception of TLR2, most ligands for TLRs could inhibit HBV replication in the HBV transgenic model [120]. Therefore, endogenous IFN can be induced for viral clearance by injecting TLR ligands [121, 122]. The notorious side effect of IFN therapy is likely due to the nonselective systemic exposure to exogenous IFN. TLR agonists can be given by the oral route and thus can be more restricted to the liver and gut, instead of the whole body. For example, oral intake of GS-9620, a TLR7 agonist, can decrease HBV DNA and protein markers in both serum and liver in a chimpanzee model [123]. In another example, GS-9620 increased the numbers of immune cells and enhanced IFN response and seroconversion rate to anti-WHsAg status in the woodchuck model [124]. There is so far no reported toxicity of GS-9620. Agonists for other TLRs can also increase innate immunity and decrease viral titer [125]. GS-9620 is now in Phase II clinical trials (https://clinicaltrials.gov/ct2/show/NCT02579382; https://clinicaltrials.gov/ct2/show/NCT02166047).

In addition to activating innate immunity via exogenous ligands, therapeutic cytokines, including IL-7, IL-12, and IL-21, can be another option for immunotherapy. IL-7 is important for the development of B cells, T cells, and dendritic cell subsets. Treatment of chronic hepatitis B patients using human IL-7 (CYT107) is ongoing in a Phase I–II clinical trials (http://www.clinicaltrials.gov/ct2/show/NCT01027065). IL21 has pleiotropic functional roles in B cell differentiation, virus-specific antibody production, and maintenance of CD8+ T cell homeostasis [126]. Phase I and II clinical trials of IL-21 are still ongoing in cancer patients [127], and if successful, IL-21 therapy may be extended to clinical trials of hepatitis B patients [128]. There is no doubt that more therapeutic cytokines will be available in the near future.

16.16 Other Therapeutic Strategies in Development

A number of potential drug targets are still at their infancy for drug development. For example, β-thujaplicinol and hydroxylated tropolones are inhibitors for ribonuclease H of HBV genotypes B, C, and D [129]. Additive and synergistic effects were observed, when these RNase H antagonists were used in combination with other inhibitors. Similarly, the potential to block cccDNA formation has been evaluated. Two sulfonamide compounds were reported to be inhibitors for cccDNA production [130]. Another example, the conversion from rcDNA to cccDNA, was inhibited by depletion of the endogenous TDP2 (tyrosyl-DNA-phosphodiesterase) [131, 132]. By inducing cytidine-to-uracil hypermutation, APOBEC (apolipoprotein B mRNA editing catalytic polypeptide) can suppress HBV replication [133]. It is therefore natural to ask whether APOBEC3 agonists, such as IFN-α and lymphotoxin-β receptor agonists, could selectively inactivate cccDNA by inducing extensive editing [134–136]. Two caveats here are as follows: (1) APOBEC-induced mutations could promote the occurrence of immune escape or drug-resistant HBV variants; and (2) the host genome could be injured by potential off-target effect of APOBEC. Lastly, the intracellular loop of cccDNA amplification and capsid recycling can be drug targets for further research [137, 138]. Overall, these emerging new strategies are based on new targets against HBV persistence.

16.17 Summary

Current HBV treatment cannot cure or eradicate virus from patients. Alternative approaches need to be invented [103, 139, 140]. We summarized the current status of emerging new strategies in HBV therapy (Fig. 16.1). For entry inhibitors, significant progress has been made in developing a new derivative of cyclosporine, which can uncouple the desired antiviral effect from the deleterious effect on NTCP-mediated bile salt transport [37]. It is also encouraging that a new antiviral proanthocyanidin and its analogs can directly act on the preS1 domain of LHBs, instead of the cellular NTCP [60]. To target the preexisting cccDNA in patients, the current approach includes the digestion or modification of cccDNA (CRISPR-/Cas9- or APOBEC-edited) and the prevention of de novo cccDNA formation. As for breaking immune tolerance, promising strategies include TLR agonists, therapeutic cytokines, and therapeutic vaccination. Most likely, combination therapy for HBV should deliver a higher cure rate than monotherapy [141, 142]. Given the highly active research in the control and eradication of HBV in academia and industry, there is good reason to be hopeful that a cure or a functional cure will be possible in the near future.

References

1. Martin A, Lemon SM (2006) Hepatitis A virus: from discovery to vaccines. Hepatology 43:S164–S172. https://doi.org/10.1002/hep.21052
2. Werzberger A et al (1992) A controlled trial of a formalin-inactivated hepatitis A vaccine in healthy children. N Engl J Med 327:453–457. https://doi.org/10.1056/NEJM199208133270702
3. Innis BL et al (1994) Protection against hepatitis A by an inactivated vaccine. JAMA 271:1328–1334
4. WHO (2017) Hepatitis A-vaccine. http://www.who.int/ith/vaccines/hepatitisA/en/
5. Zhang X et al (2016) Comparison of immune persistence among inactivated and live attenuated hepatitis a vaccines 2 years after a single dose. Hum Vaccin Immunother 12:2322–2326. https://doi.org/10.1080/21645515.2015.1134069
6. Rao S, Mao JS, Motlekar S, Fangcheng Z, Kadhe G (2016) A review of immunogenicity and tolerability of live attenuated Hepatitis A vaccine in children. Hum Vaccin Immunother 12:3160–3165. https://doi.org/10.1080/21645515.2016.1216286
7. Jiang X et al (2015) The JAK2 inhibitor AZD1480 inhibits hepatitis A virus replication in Huh7 cells. Biochem Biophys Res Commun 458:908–912. https://doi.org/10.1016/j.bbrc.2015.02.058
8. Kanda T et al (2015) The sirtuin inhibitor sirtinol inhibits hepatitis A virus (HAV) replication by inhibiting HAV internal ribosomal entry site activity. Biochem Biophys Res Commun 466:567–571. https://doi.org/10.1016/j.bbrc.2015.09.083
9. Koh C et al (2015) Oral prenylation inhibition with lonafarnib in chronic hepatitis D infection: a proof-of-concept randomised, double-blind, placebo-controlled phase 2A trial. Lancet Infect Dis 15:1167–1174. https://doi.org/10.1016/S1473-3099(15)00074-2
10. Dao Thi VL et al (2016) Sofosbuvir inhibits hepatitis E virus replication in vitro and results in an additive effect when combined with ribavirin. Gastroenterology 150:82–85 e84. https://doi.org/10.1053/j.gastro.2015.09.011
11. Wang Y et al (2014) Calcineurin inhibitors stimulate and mycophenolic acid inhibits replication of hepatitis E virus. Gastroenterology 146:1775–1783. https://doi.org/10.1053/j.gastro.2014.02.036
12. Gerlach JT et al (2003) Acute hepatitis C: high rate of both spontaneous and treatment-induced viral clearance. Gastroenterology 125:80–88
13. European Association for the Study of the, L (2011) EASL clinical practice guidelines: management of hepatitis C virus infection. J Hepatol 55:245–264. https://doi.org/10.1016/j.jhep.2011.02.023
14. Chan J, Chung RT (2017) Perspectives on HCV: current therapeutic regimens and drug-drug interactions. Clin Pharmacol Drug Dev 6:147–163. https://doi.org/10.1002/cpdd.338
15. Feld JJ et al (2015) Sofosbuvir and velpatasvir for HCV Genotype 1, 2, 4, 5, and 6 Infection. N Engl J Med 373:2599–2607. https://doi.org/10.1056/NEJMoa1512610
16. Foster GR et al (2015) Sofosbuvir and velpatasvir for HCV Genotype 2 and 3 Infection. N Engl J Med 373:2608–2617. https://doi.org/10.1056/NEJMoa1512612
17. Zeuzem S et al (2015) Grazoprevir-elbasvir combination therapy for treatment-naive cirrhotic and noncirrhotic patients with chronic hepatitis C virus genotype 1, 4, or 6 infection: a randomized trial. Ann Intern Med 163:1–13. https://doi.org/10.7326/M15-0785
18. Heidrich B, Manns MP, Wedemeyer H (2013) Treatment options for hepatitis delta virus infection. Curr Infect Dis Rep 15:31–38. https://doi.org/10.1007/s11908-012-0307-z
19. Bahcecioglu IH, Sahin A (2017) Treatment of delta hepatitis: today and in the future – a review. Infect Dis (Lond) 49:241–250. https://doi.org/10.1080/23744235.2016.1271998
20. Petersen J, Thompson AJ, Levrero M (2016) Aiming for cure in HBV and HDV infection. J Hepatol 65:835–848. https://doi.org/10.1016/j.jhep.2016.05.043
21. Gerolami R et al (2011) Treatment of severe acute hepatitis E by ribavirin. J Clin Virol 52:60–62. https://doi.org/10.1016/j.jcv.2011.06.004
22. El Sayed Zaki M, El Razek MM, El Razek HM (2014) Maternal-fetal hepatitis E transmission: is it underestimated? J Clin Transl Hepatol 2:117–123. https://doi.org/10.14218/JCTH.2014.00006
23. Kamar N et al (2010) Influence of immunosuppressive therapy on the natural history of genotype 3 hepatitis-E virus infection after organ transplantation. Transplantation 89:353–360. https://doi.org/10.1097/TP.0b013e3181c4096c
24. Wedemeyer H, Pischke S, Manns MP (2012) Pathogenesis and treatment of hepatitis E virus infection. Gastroenterology 142:1388–1397 e1381. https://doi.org/10.1053/j.gastro.2012.02.014
25. Mallet V et al (2010) Brief communication: case reports of ribavirin treatment for chronic hepatitis E. Ann Intern Med 153:85–89. https://doi.org/10.7326/0003-4819-153-2-201007200-00257
26. Abravanel F, Lhomme S, Rostaing L, Kamar N, Izopet J (2015) Protracted fecal shedding of HEV during ribavirin therapy predicts treatment relapse. Clin Infect Dis 60:96–99. https://doi.org/10.1093/cid/ciu742
27. Liang T, Hepatitis J (2009) B: the virus and disease. Hepatology 49:S13–S21. https://doi.org/10.1002/hep.22881
28. Terrault NA et al (2016) AASLD guidelines for treatment of chronic hepatitis B. Hepatology 63:261–283. https://doi.org/10.1002/hep.28156
29. European Association for the Study of the, L (2012) EASL clinical practice guidelines: Management of

chronic hepatitis B virus infection. J Hepatol 57:167–185. https://doi.org/10.1016/j.jhep.2012.02.010
30. Chen YC, Liaw YF (2016) Pharmacotherapeutic options for hepatitis B. Expert Opin Pharmacother 17:355–367. https://doi.org/10.1517/14656566.2016.1118056
31. Devi U, Locarnini S (2013) Hepatitis B antivirals and resistance. Curr Opin Virol 3:495–500. https://doi.org/10.1016/j.coviro.2013.08.006
32. Shih C, Chou S-F, Yang C-C, Huang J-Y, Choijilsuren G, Jhou R-S (2016) Control and eradication strategies of hepatitis B virus. Trends Microbiol 24(9):739–749
33. Nassal M (2015) HBV cccDNA: viral persistence reservoir and key obstacle for a cure of chronic hepatitis B. Gut 64:1972–1984. https://doi.org/10.1136/gutjnl-2015-309809
34. Chiang CJ et al (2015) Significant reduction in end-stage liver diseases burden through the national viral hepatitis therapy program in Taiwan. Hepatology 61:1154–1162. https://doi.org/10.1002/hep.27630
35. Watashi K et al (2014) Cyclosporin A and its analogs inhibit hepatitis B virus entry into cultured hepatocytes through targeting a membrane transporter, sodium taurocholate cotransporting polypeptide (NTCP). Hepatology 59:1726–1737. https://doi.org/10.1002/hep.26982
36. Nkongolo S et al (2014) Cyclosporin A inhibits hepatitis B and hepatitis D virus entry by cyclophilin-independent interference with the NTCP receptor. J Hepatol 60:723–731. https://doi.org/10.1016/j.jhep.2013.11.022
37. Shimura S et al (2016) Cyclosporin derivatives inhibit hepatitis B virus entry without interfering with NTCP transporter activity. J Hepatol. https://doi.org/10.1016/j.jhep.2016.11.009
38. Kennedy EM, Kornepati AV, Cullen BR (2015) Targeting hepatitis B virus cccDNA using CRISPR/Cas9. Antivir Res 123:188–192. https://doi.org/10.1016/j.antiviral.2015.10.004
39. Lin G, Zhang K, Li J (2015) Application of CRISPR/Cas9 technology to HBV. Int J Mol Sci 16(26):077–26086. https://doi.org/10.3390/ijms161125950
40. Lin SR et al (2014) The CRISPR/Cas9 system facilitates clearance of the intrahepatic HBV templates in vivo. Mol Ther Nucleic Acids 3:e186. https://doi.org/10.1038/mtna.2014.38
41. Liu X, Hao R, Chen S, Guo D, Chen Y (2015) Inhibition of hepatitis B virus by the CRISPR/Cas9 system via targeting the conserved regions of the viral genome. J Gen Virol 96:2252–2261. https://doi.org/10.1099/vir.0.000159
42. Moyo B, Bloom K, Scott T, Ely A, Arbuthnot P (2017) Advances with using CRISPR/Cas-mediated gene editing to treat infections with hepatitis B virus and hepatitis C virus. Virus Res. https://doi.org/10.1016/j.virusres.2017.01.003
43. Huang JY et al (2015) MicroRNA-130a can inhibit hepatitis B virus replication via targeting PGC1alpha and PPARgamma. RNA 21:385–400. https://doi.org/10.1261/rna.048744.114
44. Lamontagne J, Steel LF, Bouchard MJ (2015) Hepatitis B virus and microRNAs: Complex interactions affecting hepatitis B virus replication and hepatitis B virus-associated diseases. World J Gastroenterol 21:7375–7399. https://doi.org/10.3748/wjg.v21.i24.7375
45. Wu G et al (2013) Preclinical characterization of GLS4, an inhibitor of hepatitis B virus core particle assembly. Antimicrob Agents Chemother 57:5344–5354. https://doi.org/10.1128/AAC.01091-13
46. Schinazi RF, Asselah T (2017) From HCV to HBV cure. Liver Int 37(Suppl 1):73–80. https://doi.org/10.1111/liv.13324
47. Katen SP, Tan Z, Chirapu SR, Finn MG, Zlotnick A (2013) Assembly-directed antivirals differentially bind quasiequivalent pockets to modify hepatitis B virus capsid tertiary and quaternary structure. Structure 21:1406–1416. https://doi.org/10.1016/j.str.2013.06.013
48. Lazar C et al (2007) Treatment of hepatitis B virus-infected cells with alpha-glucosidase inhibitors results in production of virions with altered molecular composition and infectivity. Antivir Res 76:30–37. https://doi.org/10.1016/j.antiviral.2007.04.004
49. Chang J, Block TM, Guo JT (2013) Antiviral therapies targeting host ER alpha-glucosidases: current status and future directions. Antivir Res 99:251–260. https://doi.org/10.1016/j.antiviral.2013.06.011
50. Simsek E, Lu X, Ouzounov S, Block TM, Mehta AS (2006) alpha-Glucosidase inhibitors have a prolonged antiviral effect against hepatitis B virus through the sustained inhibition of the large and middle envelope glycoproteins. Antivir Chem Chemother 17:259–267
51. Kian Chua P, Lin MH, Shih C (2006) Potent inhibition of human Hepatitis B virus replication by a host factor Vps4. Virology 354:1–6. https://doi.org/10.1016/j.virol.2006.07.018
52. Lambert C, Doring T, Prange R (2007) Hepatitis B virus maturation is sensitive to functional inhibition of ESCRT-III, Vps4, and gamma 2-adaptin. J Virol 81:9050–9060. https://doi.org/10.1128/JVI.00479-07
53. Chou SF, Tsai ML, Huang JY, Chang YS, Shih C (2015) The Dual Role of an ESCRT-0 Component HGS in HBV Transcription and Naked Capsid Secretion. PLoS Pathog 11:e1005123. https://doi.org/10.1371/journal.ppat.1005123
54. Tzeng HT et al (2012) PD-1 blockage reverses immune dysfunction and hepatitis B viral persistence in a mouse animal model. PLoS One 7:e39179. https://doi.org/10.1371/journal.pone.0039179
55. Liu J et al (2014) Enhancing virus-specific immunity in vivo by combining therapeutic vaccination and PD-L1 blockade in chronic hepadnaviral infection. PLoS Pathog 10:e1003856. https://doi.org/10.1371/journal.ppat.1003856

56. Yan H et al (2012) Sodium taurocholate cotransporting polypeptide is a functional receptor for human hepatitis B and D virus. Elife 1:e00049. https://doi.org/10.7554/eLife.00049
57. Gripon P, Cannie I, Urban S (2005) Efficient inhibition of hepatitis B virus infection by acylated peptides derived from the large viral surface protein. J Virol 79:1613–1622. https://doi.org/10.1128/JVI.79.3.1613-1622.2005
58. Barrera A, Guerra B, Notvall L, Lanford RE (2005) Mapping of the hepatitis B virus pre-S1 domain involved in receptor recognition. J Virol 79:9786–9798. https://doi.org/10.1128/JVI.79.15.9786-9798.2005
59. Volz T et al (2013) The entry inhibitor Myrcludex-B efficiently blocks intrahepatic virus spreading in humanized mice previously infected with hepatitis B virus. J Hepatol 58:861–867. https://doi.org/10.1016/j.jhep.2012.12.008
60. Tsukuda S et al (2017) A new class of hepatitis B and D virus entry inhibitors, proanthocyanidin and its analogs, that directly act on the viral large surface proteins. Hepatology 65:1104–1116. https://doi.org/10.1002/hep.28952
61. Yan H et al (2014) Viral entry of hepatitis B and D viruses and bile salts transportation share common molecular determinants on sodium taurocholate cotransporting polypeptide. J Virol 88:3273–3284. https://doi.org/10.1128/JVI.03478-13
62. Kaneko M et al (2015) A novel tricyclic polyketide, vanitaracin A, specifically inhibits the entry of hepatitis B and D viruses by targeting sodium taurocholate cotransporting polypeptide. J Virol 89(11):945–11953. https://doi.org/10.1128/JVI.01855-15
63. Yan H, Liu Y, Sui J, Li W (2015) NTCP opens the door for hepatitis B virus infection. Antivir Res 121:24–30. https://doi.org/10.1016/j.antiviral.2015.06.002
64. Hu HH et al (2016) The rs2296651 (S267F) variant on NTCP (SLC10A1) is inversely associated with chronic hepatitis B and progression to cirrhosis and hepatocellular carcinoma in patients with chronic hepatitis B. Gut 65:1514–1521. https://doi.org/10.1136/gutjnl-2015-310686
65. Peng L et al (2015) The p.Ser267Phe variant in SLC10A1 is associated with resistance to chronic hepatitis B. Hepatology 61:1251–1260. https://doi.org/10.1002/hep.27608
66. White MK, Hu W, Khalili K (2015) The CRISPR/Cas9 genome editing methodology as a weapon against human viruses. Discov Med 19:255–262
67. Gu WG (2015) Genome editing-based HIV therapies. Trends Biotechnol 33:172–179. https://doi.org/10.1016/j.tibtech.2014.12.006
68. Zimmerman KA, Fischer KP, Joyce MA, Tyrrell DL (2008) Zinc finger proteins designed to specifically target duck hepatitis B virus covalently closed circular DNA inhibit viral transcription in tissue culture. J Virol 82:8013–8021. https://doi.org/10.1128/JVI.00366-08
69. Bloom K, Ely A, Mussolino C, Cathomen T, Arbuthnot P (2013) Inactivation of hepatitis B virus replication in cultured cells and in vivo with engineered transcription activator-like effector nucleases. Mol Ther 21:1889–1897. https://doi.org/10.1038/mt.2013.170
70. Fu Y et al (2013) High frequency off-target mutagenesis induced by CRISPR-Cas nucleases in human cells. Nat Biotechnol 31:822–826. https://doi.org/10.1038/nbt.2623
71. Kuscu C, Arslan S, Singh R, Thorpe J, Adli M (2014) Genome-wide analysis reveals characteristics of off-target sites bound by the Cas9 endonuclease. Nat Biotechnol 32:677–683. https://doi.org/10.1038/nbt.2916
72. Wang J et al (2015) Dual gRNAs guided CRISPR/Cas9 system inhibits hepatitis B virus replication. World J Gastroenterol 21:9554–9565. https://doi.org/10.3748/wjg.v21.i32.9554
73. Wang Z et al (2016) CRISPR/Cas9-derived mutations both inhibit HIV-1 replication and accelerate viral escape. Cell Rep 15:481–489. https://doi.org/10.1016/j.celrep.2016.03.042
74. Bock CT, Schranz P, Schroder CH, Zentgraf H (1994) Hepatitis B virus genome is organized into nucleosomes in the nucleus of the infected cell. Virus Genes 8:215–229
75. Newbold JE et al (1995) The covalently closed duplex form of the hepadnavirus genome exists in situ as a heterogeneous population of viral minichromosomes. J Virol 69:3350–3357
76. Koumbi L, Karayiannis P (2015) The epigenetic control of hepatitis B virus modulates the outcome of infection. Front Microbiol 6:1491. https://doi.org/10.3389/fmicb.2015.01491
77. Pollicino T et al (2006) Hepatitis B virus replication is regulated by the acetylation status of hepatitis B virus cccDNA-bound H3 and H4 histones. Gastroenterology 130:823–837. https://doi.org/10.1053/j.gastro.2006.01.001
78. Liu F et al (2013) Alpha-interferon suppresses hepadnavirus transcription by altering epigenetic modification of cccDNA minichromosomes. PLoS Pathog 9:e1003613. https://doi.org/10.1371/journal.ppat.1003613
79. Guo Y, Li Y, Mu S, Zhang J, Yan Z (2009) Evidence that methylation of hepatitis B virus covalently closed circular DNA in liver tissues of patients with chronic hepatitis B modulates HBV replication. J Med Virol 81:1177–1183. https://doi.org/10.1002/jmv.21525
80. Kaur P et al (2010) DNA methylation of hepatitis B virus (HBV) genome associated with the development of hepatocellular carcinoma and occult HBV infection. J Infect Dis 202:700–704. https://doi.org/10.1086/655398
81. Falkenberg KJ, Johnstone RW (2014) Histone deacetylases and their inhibitors in cancer, neurological diseases and immune disorders. Nat Rev

Drug Discov 13:673–691. https://doi.org/10.1038/nrd4360
82. Duvic M, Dimopoulos M (2016) The safety profile of vorinostat (suberoylanilide hydroxamic acid) in hematologic malignancies: A review of clinical studies. Cancer Treat Rev 43:58–66. https://doi.org/10.1016/j.ctrv.2015.04.003
83. Mizuguchi Y, Takizawa T, Uchida E (2015) Host cellular microRNA involvement in the control of hepatitis B virus gene expression and replication. World J Hepatol 7:696–702. https://doi.org/10.4254/wjh.v7.i4.696
84. Lin S, Gregory RI (2015) MicroRNA biogenesis pathways in cancer. Nat Rev Cancer 15:321–333. https://doi.org/10.1038/nrc3932
85. Lam JK, Chow MY, Zhang Y, Leung SW (2015) siRNA Versus miRNA as Therapeutics for Gene Silencing. Mol Ther Nucleic Acids 4:e252. https://doi.org/10.1038/mtna.2015.23
86. Janssen HL et al (2013) Treatment of HCV infection by targeting microRNA. N Engl J Med 368:1685–1694. https://doi.org/10.1056/NEJMoa1209026
87. Kennedy BW (2015) Mongersen, an oral SMAD7 antisense oligonucleotide, and Crohn's disease. N Engl J Med 372:2461. https://doi.org/10.1056/NEJMc1504845#SA1
88. Bader AG (2012) miR-34 – a microRNA replacement therapy is headed to the clinic. Front Genet 3(120). https://doi.org/10.3389/fgene.2012.00120
89. Wooddell CI et al (2013) Hepatocyte-targeted RNAi therapeutics for the treatment of chronic hepatitis B virus infection. Mol Ther 21:973–985. https://doi.org/10.1038/mt.2013.31
90. Gish RG et al (2015) Synthetic RNAi triggers and their use in chronic hepatitis B therapies with curative intent. Antiviral Res 121:97–108. https://doi.org/10.1016/j.antiviral.2015.06.019
91. Stray SJ et al (2005) A heteroaryldihydropyrimidine activates and can misdirect hepatitis B virus capsid assembly. Proc Natl Acad Sci U S A 102:8138–8143. https://doi.org/10.1073/pnas.0409732102
92. Bourne C et al (2008) Small-molecule effectors of hepatitis B virus capsid assembly give insight into virus life cycle. J Virol 82(10):262–10,270. https://doi.org/10.1128/JVI.01360-08
93. Zeisel MB et al (2015) Towards an HBV cure: state-of-the-art and unresolved questions–report of the ANRS workshop on HBV cure. Gut 64:1314–1326. https://doi.org/10.1136/gutjnl-2014-308943
94. Steven AC et al (2005) Structure, assembly, and antigenicity of hepatitis B virus capsid proteins. Adv Virus Res 64:125–164. https://doi.org/10.1016/S0065-3527(05)64005-5
95. Hurley JH (2015) ESCRTs are everywhere. EMBO J 34:2398–2407. https://doi.org/10.15252/embj.201592484
96. Hoffmann J et al (2013) Identification of alpha-taxilin as an essential factor for the life cycle of hepatitis B virus. J Hepatol 59:934–941. https://doi.org/10.1016/j.jhep.2013.06.020
97. Evans DT, Serra-Moreno R, Singh RK, Guatelli JC (2010) BST-2/tetherin: a new component of the innate immune response to enveloped viruses. Trends Microbiol 18:388–396. https://doi.org/10.1016/j.tim.2010.06.010
98. Lv M et al (2015) Identification of BST-2/tetherin-induced hepatitis B virus restriction and hepatocyte-specific BST-2 inactivation. Sci Rep 5(11):736. https://doi.org/10.1038/srep11736
99. Yan R et al (2015) The interferon-inducible protein tetherin inhibits hepatitis B virus virion secretion. J Virol 89:9200–9212. https://doi.org/10.1128/JVI.00933-15
100. Miyakawa K et al (2015) Molecular dissection of HBV evasion from restriction factor tetherin: a new perspective for antiviral cell therapy. Oncotarget 6:21840–21852. https://doi.org/10.18632/oncotarget.4808
101. Schubert HL et al (2010) Structural and functional studies on the extracellular domain of BST2/tetherin in reduced and oxidized conformations. Proc Natl Acad Sci U S A 107(17):951–17956. https://doi.org/10.1073/pnas.1008206107
102. Guidotti LG, Isogawa M, Chisari FV (2015) Host-virus interactions in hepatitis B virus infection. Curr Opin Immunol 36:61–66. https://doi.org/10.1016/j.coi.2015.06.016
103. Kapoor R, Kottilil S (2014) Strategies to eliminate HBV infection. Future Virol 9:565–585. https://doi.org/10.2217/fvl.14.36
104. Vandepapeliere P et al (2007) Therapeutic vaccination of chronic hepatitis B patients with virus suppression by antiviral therapy: a randomized, controlled study of co-administration of HBsAg/AS02 candidate vaccine and lamivudine. Vaccine 25:8585–8597. https://doi.org/10.1016/j.vaccine.2007.09.072
105. Fontaine H et al (2015) Anti-HBV DNA vaccination does not prevent relapse after discontinuation of analogues in the treatment of chronic hepatitis B: a randomised trial–ANRS HB02 VAC-ADN. Gut 64:139–147. https://doi.org/10.1136/gutjnl-2013-305707
106. Kardani K, Bolhassani A, Shahbazi S (2016) Prime-boost vaccine strategy against viral infections: mechanisms and benefits. Vaccine 34:413–423. https://doi.org/10.1016/j.vaccine.2015.11.062
107. Huang LR et al (2013) Intrahepatic myeloid-cell aggregates enable local proliferation of CD8(+) T cells and successful immunotherapy against chronic viral liver infection. Nat Immunol 14:574–583. https://doi.org/10.1038/ni.2573
108. Yang SH et al (2006) Correlation of antiviral T-cell responses with suppression of viral rebound in chronic hepatitis B carriers: a proof-of-concept study. Gene Ther 13:1110–1117. https://doi.org/10.1038/sj.gt.3302751
109. Schurich A et al (2013) The third signal cytokine IL-12 rescues the anti-viral function of exhausted HBV-specific CD8 T cells. PLoS Pathog 9:e1003208. https://doi.org/10.1371/journal.ppat.1003208

110. Yoon SK et al (2015) Safety and immunogenicity of therapeutic DNA vaccine with antiviral drug in chronic HBV patients and its immunogenicity in mice. Liver Int 35:805–815. https://doi.org/10.1111/liv.12530
111. Xu DZ et al (2013) Results of a phase III clinical trial with an HBsAg-HBIG immunogenic complex therapeutic vaccine for chronic hepatitis B patients: experiences and findings. J Hepatol 59:450–456. https://doi.org/10.1016/j.jhep.2013.05.003
112. Fuller MJ et al (2013) Immunotherapy of chronic hepatitis C virus infection with antibodies against programmed cell death-1 (PD-1). Proc Natl Acad Sci U S A 110(15):001–15006. https://doi.org/10.1073/pnas.1312772110
113. Bengsch B, Martin B, Thimme R (2014) Restoration of HBV-specific CD8+ T cell function by PD-1 blockade in inactive carrier patients is linked to T cell differentiation. J Hepatol 61:1212–1219. https://doi.org/10.1016/j.jhep.2014.07.005
114. Wu W et al (2012) Blockade of Tim-3 signaling restores the virus-specific CD8(+) T-cell response in patients with chronic hepatitis B. Eur J Immunol 42:1180–1191. https://doi.org/10.1002/eji.201141852
115. Raziorrouh B et al (2010) The immunoregulatory role of CD244 in chronic hepatitis B infection and its inhibitory potential on virus-specific CD8+ T-cell function. Hepatology 52:1934–1947. https://doi.org/10.1002/hep.23936
116. Kumar S, Naqvi RA, Khanna N, Pathak P, Rao DN (2011) Th3 immune responses in the progression of leprosy via molecular cross-talks of TGF-beta, CTLA-4 and Cbl-b. Clin Immunol 141:133–142. https://doi.org/10.1016/j.clim.2011.06.007
117. Huang MT et al (2015) Feedback regulation of IFN-alpha/beta signaling by Axl receptor tyrosine kinase modulates HBV immunity. Eur J Immunol 45:1696–1705. https://doi.org/10.1002/eji.201445239
118. Li M et al (2015) Kupffer cells support Hepatitis B virus-mediated CD8+ T cell exhaustion via Hepatitis B core antigen-TLR2 interactions in mice. J Immunol 195:3100–3109. https://doi.org/10.4049/jimmunol.1500839
119. Topalian SL et al (2012) Safety, activity, and immune correlates of anti-PD-1 antibody in cancer. N Engl J Med 366:2443–2454. https://doi.org/10.1056/NEJMoa1200690
120. Isogawa M, Robek MD, Furuichi Y, Chisari FV (2005) Toll-like receptor signaling inhibits hepatitis B virus replication in vivo. J Virol 79:7269–7272. https://doi.org/10.1128/JVI.79.11.7269-7272.2005
121. Schwabe RF, Seki E, Brenner DA (2006) Toll-like receptor signaling in the liver. Gastroenterology 130:1886–1900. https://doi.org/10.1053/j.gastro.2006.01.038
122. Zhang X et al (2012) Preclinical development of TLR ligands as drugs for the treatment of chronic viral infections. Expert Opin Drug Discov 7:597–611. https://doi.org/10.1517/17460441.2012.689281
123. Lanford RE et al (2013) GS-9620, an oral agonist of Toll-like receptor-7, induces prolonged suppression of hepatitis B virus in chronically infected chimpanzees. Gastroenterology 144:1508–1517, 1517.e1501–1510. https://doi.org/10.1053/j.gastro.2013.02.003
124. Menne S et al (2015) Sustained efficacy and seroconversion with the Toll-like receptor 7 agonist GS-9620 in the Woodchuck model of chronic hepatitis B. J Hepatol 62:1237–1245. https://doi.org/10.1016/j.jhep.2014.12.026
125. Zhang E, Kosinska A, Lu M, Yan H, Roggendorf M (2015) Current status of immunomodulatory therapy in chronic hepatitis B, fifty years after discovery of the virus: search for the "magic bullet" to kill cccDNA. Antiviral Res 123:193–203. https://doi.org/10.1016/j.antiviral.2015.10.009
126. Yi JS, Du M, Zajac AJ (2009) A vital role for interleukin-21 in the control of a chronic viral infection. Science 324:1572–1576. https://doi.org/10.1126/science.1175194
127. Hashmi MH, Van Veldhuizen PJ (2010) Interleukin-21: updated review of Phase I and II clinical trials in metastatic renal cell carcinoma, metastatic melanoma and relapsed/refractory indolent non-Hodgkin's lymphoma. Expert Opin Biol Ther 10:807–817. https://doi.org/10.1517/14712598.2010.480971
128. Li Y, Tang L, Hou J (2015) Role of interleukin-21 in HBV infection: friend or foe? Cell Mol Immunol 12:303–308. https://doi.org/10.1038/cmi.2014.109
129. Tavis JE, Lomonosova E (2015) The hepatitis B virus ribonuclease H as a drug target. Antiviral Res 118:132–138. https://doi.org/10.1016/j.antiviral.2015.04.002
130. Cai D et al (2012) Identification of disubstituted sulfonamide compounds as specific inhibitors of hepatitis B virus covalently closed circular DNA formation. Antimicrob Agents Chemother 56:4277–4288. https://doi.org/10.1128/AAC.00473-12
131. Koniger C et al (2014) Involvement of the host DNA-repair enzyme TDP2 in formation of the covalently closed circular DNA persistence reservoir of hepatitis B viruses. Proc Natl Acad Sci U S A 111:E4244–E4253. https://doi.org/10.1073/pnas.1409986111
132. Cui X et al (2015) Does Tyrosyl DNA Phosphodiesterase-2 Play a Role in Hepatitis B Virus Genome Repair? PLoS One 10:e0128401. https://doi.org/10.1371/journal.pone.0128401
133. Janahi EM, McGarvey MJ (2013) The inhibition of hepatitis B virus by APOBEC cytidine deaminases. J Viral Hepat 20:821–828. https://doi.org/10.1111/jvh.12192
134. Lucifora J et al (2014) Specific and nonhepatotoxic degradation of nuclear hepatitis B virus cccDNA. Science 343:1221–1228. https://doi.org/10.1126/science.1243462
135. Chisari FV, Mason WS, Seeger C (2014) Virology. Comment on "Specific and nonhepatotoxic degrada-

tion of nuclear hepatitis B virus cccDNA". Science 344:1237. https://doi.org/10.1126/science.1254082
136. Xia Y, Lucifora J, Reisinger F, Heikenwalder M, Protzer U (2014) Virology. Response to comment on "Specific and nonhepatotoxic degradation of nuclear hepatitis B virus cccDNA". Science 344:1237. https://doi.org/10.1126/science.1254083
137. Li HC et al (2010) Nuclear export and import of human hepatitis B virus capsid protein and particles. PLoS Pathog 6:e1001162. https://doi.org/10.1371/journal.ppat.1001162
138. Yang CC, Huang EY, Li HC, Su PY, Shih C (2014) Nuclear export of human hepatitis B virus core protein and pregenomic RNA depends on the cellular NXF1-p15 machinery. PLoS One 9:e106683. https://doi.org/10.1371/journal.pone.0106683
139. Block TM, Rawat S, Brosgart CL (2015) Chronic hepatitis B: a wave of new therapies on the horizon. Antivir Res 121:69–81. https://doi.org/10.1016/j.antiviral.2015.06.014
140. Liang TJ et al (2015) Present and future therapies of hepatitis B: from discovery to cure. Hepatology 62:1893–1908. https://doi.org/10.1002/hep.28025
141. Wong PK et al (2008) Closed-loop control of cellular functions using combinatory drugs guided by a stochastic search algorithm. Proc Natl Acad Sci U S A 105:5105–5110. https://doi.org/10.1073/pnas.0800823105
142. Weiss A et al (2015) A streamlined search technology for identification of synergistic drug combinations. Sci Rep 5:14508. https://doi.org/10.1038/srep14508